Clinical Challenges in Orthopaedics:

The Knee

Edited by

Robin L. Allum, Colin M. Fergusson
and Neil P. Thomas

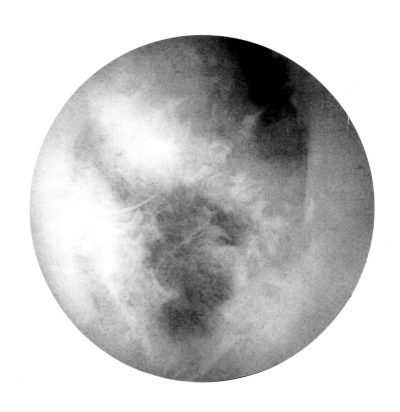

I S I S
MEDICAL
MEDIA

© 2000 by Isis Medical Media Ltd.
59 St Aldates
Oxford OX1 1ST, UK

First published 2000

British Library Cataloguing in Publication Data.
A catalogue record for this title is available from
the British Library.

ISBN 1 899066 63 2

Allum, R. L. (Robin)
Clinical Challenges in Orthopaedics: The Knee
Robin L. Allum, Colin M. Fergusson and Neil P. Thomas

Always refer to the manufacturer's Prescribing
Information before prescribing drugs cited in this book.

Commissioning Editor: Jonathan Gregory
Senior Editorial Controller: Sarah Carlson
Production Controller: Geoff Holdsworth

Medical illustration by
Oxford Illustrators

Indexed by
Laurence Errington

Typeset by
Creative Associates Ltd., UK

Colour reproduction by
Track Direct, London, UK

Produced by Phoenix Offset, HK
Printed in Hong Kong

Distributed in the USA by
Books International, Inc., PO Box 605,
Herndon, VA 20172, USA

Distributed in the rest of the world by
Plymbridge Distributors Ltd., Estover Road,
Plymouth PL6 7PY, UK

Contents

Contributors

Paul Aichroth MS FRCS
Consultant Orthopaedic Surgeon, Director, The Wellington Knee Surgery Unit, The Wellington Hospital, Wellington Place, London, UK

Robin L. Allum FRCS
Consultant Orthopaedic Surgeon, Wexham Park Hospital, Slough, UK

Vladimir Bobic MD
Consultant Orthopaedic Knee Surgeon, The Royal Liverpool University Hospitals, Broadgreen Hospital Knee Service, Thomas Drive, Liverpool, UK

David J. Dandy MD MChir FRCS
Consultant Orthopaedic Surgeon, Addenbrooke's Hospital, Cambridge, UK

George S. E. Dowd MD MCh(Orth) FRCS
Consultant Orthopaedic Surgeon, The Royal Free Hospital, The Wellington Knee Surgery Unit, The Wellington Hospital, Wellington Place, London, UK

Richard H. Fell MB BS FFARCS
Consultant Anaesthetist, Wexham Park Hospital, Slough, UK

Colin M. Fergusson MA FRCS
Consultant Orthopaedic Surgeon, Royal Berkshire Hospital, Reading, UK

Niall Flynn MB CHB FRCS(Orth)
Specialist Orthopaedic Registrar, North Hampshire Hospital, Basingstoke, UK

Richard W. Nutton MD FRCS
Consultant Orthopaedic Surgeon, Princess Margaret Rose Orthopaedic Hospital, Edinburgh, UK

Neil P. Thomas BSc FRCS
Consultant Orthopaedic Surgeon, North Hampshire Hospital and Hampshire Clinic, Basingstoke; Wessex Knee Unit, Wessex Nuffield Hospital, Chandlers Ford, Hampshire, UK

Andrew Unwin BSc FRCS(Orth)
Consultant Orthopaedic Surgeon, Heatherwood Hospital, Ascot, UK

Foreword

The subject of this book is well chosen, since the practising knee surgeon will confront at least one of the problems discussed here at least once a week. These 'clinical challenges' arise most often in relatively young and active patients who, from injury or premature degeneration, have lost the full use of a knee. Such problems cannot be solved by total replacement, which is so effective in older patients but which seldom provides normal function and may not withstand heavy use for long enough.

The surgeon should feel 'challenged' because the results of most of the procedures he can offer are not as predictable as those of joint replacement. Indeed, for many of the most widely used operations there is no firm evidence of their efficacy. Such evidence may come, eventually, from randomized controlled trials but few of these have yet been done and the multiplicity of variables is dishearteningly great.

In these circumstances, the clinician must depend upon his own judgement and on reports of the experiences of others. Their advice is not necessarily imprecise and it is notable that the experienced practitioners of knee surgery who have contributed chapters to this book have seldom felt able to offer exact prescriptions or simple algorhythms. The thoughful reader will also detect the implicit caveat that a knee that is still functioning, even if less than ideally, may be as easily made worse as better.

These difficulties are often compounded by the too optimistic expectations of popular belief, for instance, about the results of 'key-hole' surgery or of surgical repair of damaged articular cartilage. An exaggerated idea of the usefulness of their technology is, also, a feature of inexperienced surgeons. This collection of essays, by authors who can draw on a wide practical knowledge of their subject, should help the student of surgery towards a balanced approach in decision making and a properly modest estimate of his chances of success.

John Goodfellow MS FRCS
Consultant Orthopaedic Surgeon
Nuffield Orthopaedic Centre
Oxford

Introduction

The idea of this book was to ask experienced knee surgeons to focus their attention on a series of contentious issues which are faced regularly in clinical practice, but for which there are no easy solutions. The list of topics is not meant to be comprehensive but certainly covers most of the areas of current concern to us.

It is hoped that it will introduce experienced trainees and specialists in knee surgery to the decision-making processes of those of us facing difficult challenges in the subject. We have sought to discourage too proscriptive an approach, and the reliance on over-simple algorithms, and instead offer a balanced view supported by experience and appropriate up-to-date references.

We have also provided a distillation of their chapters in a few key points.

Our contributors have responded magnificently to the task, and amply rewarded our hopes for the book.

As editors, we have found the work to be interesting and highly educative, and we can only hope that the reader will be similarly rewarded.

R. L. Allum
C. M. Fergusson
N. P. Thomas

CHAPTER 1

Management of the young patient with an osteoarthritic knee

C. M. Fergusson

Introduction

At the end of the twentieth century, osteoarthritis remains an incurable disorder. Despite the advances in molecular biology, the increasing understanding of the genetic influences in osteoarthritis and developments in cytokine chemistry, we are still a long way from understanding all the mechanisms in the pathogenesis of osteoarthritis [1], and certainly from influencing them medically.

Dramatic advances in the arthroscopic management of soft tissue problems of the knee in the sportsperson, and increasing success in joint arthroplasty for the elderly arthritic patient, have raised popular expectations of what can be achieved in knee surgery. Young osteoarthritic patients (Fig. 1.1) are making greater demands on their knees in terms of sport and leisure activities, and when pain and disability afflict them they make increasing demands on the surgeon.

There are no simple solutions to osteoarthritis in the young, active person, but this chapter aims to provide a structured approach to the problem. However, there can be no simple algorithms of care, and each patient's condition must be taken strictly on its own merit.

This chapter deals specifically with the process of osteoarthritis, rather than specific osteochondral defects, in which there has been increasing interest.

Allografting [2], the use of woven carbon fibre pads [3], cultured autologous chondrocytes [4,5], and more recently the increasingly attractive osteochondral autograft transplantation [6], have all raised awareness of the potential possibilities of restoring articular surface at an earlier stage. Some of these techniques have received more media attention than their scientific and outcome studies would warrant. Although they remain an exciting

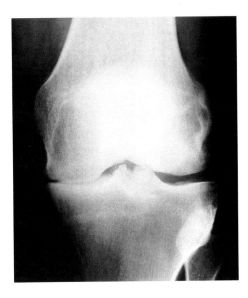

Figure 1.1 – *Medial osteoarthritis in a 36-year-old man.*

development in the field of knee surgery, at the present time they have no established role in the surgical management of the more generally arthritic knee joint.

Osteoarthritis

Osteoarthritis is a progressive age-related disorder. It is not simple 'wear and tear' in the joint, although this term is commonly used to try to explain the phenomenon to the patient. The osteoarthritic joint is metabolically, biochemically and structurally entirely different from the ageing joint, and anyone who has done hip surgery for both arthritic hips and neck-of-femur fractures can readily distinguish between the two.

Normal articular cartilage is made up of an elegant array of strong collagen fibres (type II) which contain hydrophilic proteoglycans which imbibe fluid and swell against the restricting net of the collagen. This provides a tense but flexible endurable material which not only has highly slippery properties in association with synovial fluid, but also remarkable ability to spread load, so that with increasing pressure high points of stress are diffused.

The articular surface contains living chondrocyte cells which maintain the chemical structure throughout adult life; these cells remain active even in osteoarthritis.

In osteoarthritis, disruption of the collagen and release of proteoglycan, swelling of the articular surface, subsequent fragmentation and debris formation, occur with ensuing inflammatory reaction from the synovium. Crystals may form and exacerbate the inflammatory condition, and in advanced cases subchondral bone sclerosis occurs, together with eburnation and cyst formation, fulfilling the typical radiographic criteria for osteoarthritis.

Although the latter cascade of events is readily identifiable, it is hard to define clearly whether the biochemical changes were the cause or effect. In trying to understand the aetiology of osteoarthritis, there are proponents for a primarily biochemical cause, failure in one of the glucosaminoglycans, failure of type II collagen, or purely mechanical factors. There is likely to be a combination of all these events, with the genetically predisposed individual having a more sensitive articular surface, whereby anatomical malalignments, anterior cruciate ligament (ACL) and meniscal injury [7] or direct trauma can then lead to a subsequent cascade of the osteoarthritic process [8]. In knee surgery, which attempts to preserve the meniscus and stabilise the young ligament-deficient's knee, it is easy to forget the important observation of Doherty *et al.* [9], who showed that those patients developing osteoarthritis after meniscectomy had developed osteoarthritis at other sites; the pure mechanical factor alone was therefore not the whole story.

One continuing clinical conundrum is the relationship of symptoms to the severity of disease, and it is impossible to predict how severe a patient's pain and disability will be purely on the radiological, or indeed, arthroscopic findings. This important fact needs to be borne in mind continually when advising patients on management of knee arthritis. Nevertheless, the overall prognosis, certainly for medial osteoarthritis of the knee, is a steady deterioration [10].

Clinical factors

Assessment of the patient

As with all knee problems, the assessment starts with clinical history, careful examination and X-ray. Most patients can be thoroughly assessed with these clinic-based approaches from the outset, although the value of further specialist investigations will be covered later. Overall, the purpose of this first clinic visit is to answer three broad questions: 1) is the knee the true source of the symptoms? 2) is the disease in the knee truly osteoarthritic? and 3) how disabled is the patient from the symptoms? Failure to address these points can tempt the surgeon to treat on the basis of the X-ray, with attendant disappointments.

History

The patient's age, occupation, sporting aspirations and expectations of treatment must be clearly established at the outset.

Any traumatic event which initiated the problem will indicate associated meniscal or ligamentous problems which may need addressing. The possible medico–legal implications should be established early if there was an industrial or accidental component to the onset.

Although different practitioners use the terms seizing, locking, jamming and giving way in slightly different ways, it is a useful discipline to try to establish whether the symptoms are broadly synovitic (i.e. pain predominating and pain after exercise and swelling) or mechanical, as these can help in determining subsequent management.

Level of pain

Patients' description of pain and, indeed, memory of it is variable and poorly quantifiable. An attempt should be made to establish the effect of pain on the patients' day-to-day life, rather than assess their description of the pain itself. Some individuals will describe being in 'absolute agony' and yet maintain a highly active working life without the need of analgesics; the converse is also true, with stoical types making light of their symptoms and yet rendered almost bed-bound with pain.

Functional assessment

It is easier to assess the patient based on actual functionality rather then relying on descriptions of pain alone. Activities of daily living should be specifically asked about (e.g. can the individual get around a supermarket and do their own shopping, manage a flight of stairs, walk half a mile, kneel for domestic tasks).

Although this degree of enquiry seems too detailed for what might appear initially to be a simple knee problem in a busy clinic, profound mistakes can be made in advising the wrong management for the wrong patient. A useful enquiry at this stage is to assess the patient's expectations of what the knee should feel like at their age and stage. This will give advanced warning of whether to anticipate realistic outcomes from surgical or conservative treatment.

Other related problems

After a detailed history regarding the knee and its effect on the patient's lifestyle, information should be sought on related inflammatory joint problems such as gout, psoriasis, colitis and any other specific inflammatory joint conditions. Direct enquiry about the status of the ipsilateral hip, groin and low back is essential. Patients with sciatica can often present at the knee clinic with a deep popliteal fossa ache and some calf pain, and the well-recognised problem of hip pain being felt in the knee is seen on a weekly basis in the clinic.

Examination

This should include assessments of:
- General condition
- Specific hip examination
- Gait
- Knee examination.

General condition

The patient's general health must be assessed with particular note to weight, presence of related phenomena such as psoriasis which in the patient's mind will have no connection with their knee problem, and evidence of other joint disease.

Hips

Proper examination of both hips should be conducted prior to laying the hands on the affected knee, and X-rays must be taken if there is any doubt about the knee symptoms arising from the hip joint.

Gait

While it is easy to concentrate on the patient on the clinical couch, the value of simply watching the patient walk must not be under-estimated. Hip problems, leg length discrepancy, varus and valgus angulation of the knee, slight muscle wasting or weakness, foot over-pronation or external rotation can all be very quickly and readily picked up in the clinic setting. The value of formal gait assessment in a proper laboratory will be discussed in relation to high tibial osteotomy later (see pp. 8–9).

Examination of the knee

This must include, with reference to the normal side, range of movement, stability, presence or absence of an effusion, points of tenderness along the joint lines and elsewhere and muscle wasting, which can be measured readily 12 cm above the patella with the leg straight. Asking the patient to locate the source of the symptoms with a finger is a valuable adjunct to the physical examination. A finger pointing accurately to the medial joint line may suggest degenerate meniscal pathology, whereas a hand clasped over the medial femoral condyle or patella and rubbed suggests a more diffuse problem.

X-rays

In advanced osteoarthritis, plain anteroposterior (AP) and lateral views may be enough to show the disease, but weight-bearing views in extension in the AP are essential to obtain an adequate impression of true joint space loss. They can often reveal dramatic disease, which an AP taken supine will not reveal. By the same token, although rarer, skyline views of the patella and intercondylar views can reveal joint space loss and, in the former case, patellofemoral arthritis is readily overlooked on simple AP and lateral views (Figs 1.2–1.7).

Further investigation of the young osteoarthritic knee

In most cases, the above clinical assessments and X-rays will be adequate for a full understanding of the patient's problem and will answer the three questions outlined at the beginning of the chapter. However, where there is doubt about the possible cause of symptoms, or the site of pain, it may be necessary to consider specialised tests.

Magnetic resonance imaging

Magnetic resonance imaging (MRI) is a very valuable tool in soft tissue problems of the knee, but has a limited place in the assessment of the osteoarthritic patient. It will, of course, pick up features of articular surface erosion, loose bodies, cysts and bone change, but it adds little to management in most cases. However, MRI may be considered if a degenerate meniscal tear is suspected on the clinical assessment, and the X-ray features are not too advanced. It must be borne in mind that over 40 years of age, degenerate menisci are seen in 20% and frank tears in 5% of the asymptomatic population. Finding a tear does not indicate arthroscopy, and its value can only be

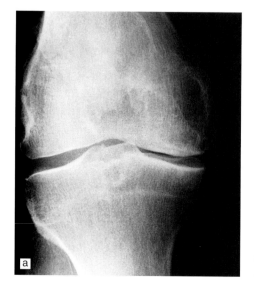
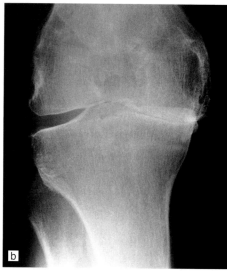

Figure 1.2 – *The importance of weight-bearing films is well illustrated in this individual in whom the medial compartment is seen to close down completely. (a) Normal supine AP film; (b) weight-bearing film.*

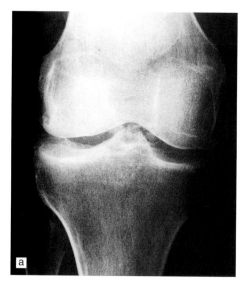
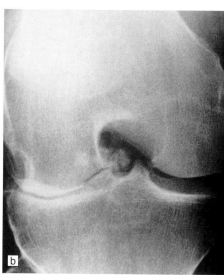

Figure 1.3 – *X-rays of an osteoarthritic lateral compartment in extension. The disease is less appreciable (a) than in the tunnel view (b), where in flexion the bones are seen in close apposition.*

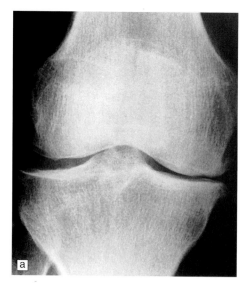
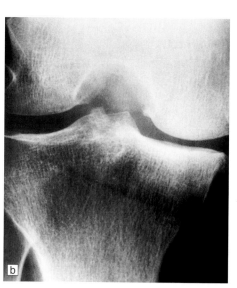

Figure 1.4 – *Medial compartment osteoarthritis appearing more noticeable in the extended position (a) than in the tunnel view (b), in contrast to that seen in the lateral disease of of Figure 1.3.*

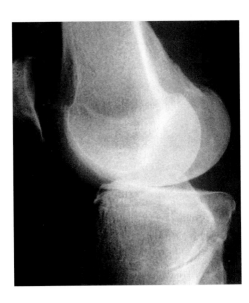

Figure 1.5 – *Lateral weight-bearing view of an osteoarthritic knee. This is not a usual view but shows clearly the anterior tibial contact of the bone in this case.*

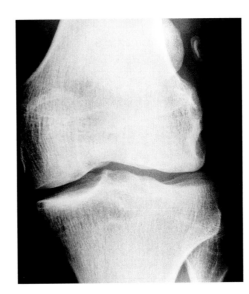

Figure 1.6 – *X-ray of an osteoarthritic knee showing a clear loose body in the superolateral part of the joint. This is one that could be responsible for mechanical symptoms and worthy of arthroscopic removal if indicated.*

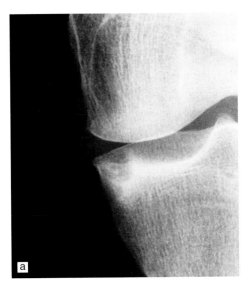
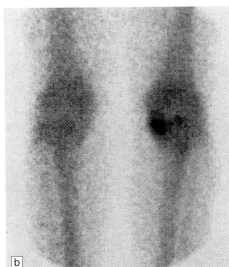
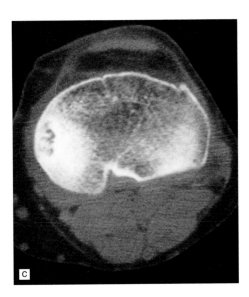

Figure 1.7 – *(a) Medial compartment of an osteoarthritic knee with a large medial plateau cyst. (b) Isotope scan of the same knee, showing a high 'hot-spot' at the cyst site. (c) Transverse CT cut showing the sclerotic bone around the cyst in the upper plateau.*

considered in conjunction with the full clinical picture.

Isotope scanning

This is a highly sensitive but rather non-specific investigation, but can be particularly useful in excluding rarities such as osteoid osteoma, metastatic bone disease and stress fractures. It can also be very helpful in the assessment of elderly poly-symptomatic individuals, rather than the younger group in question. If there are symptoms and signs suggestive of reflex sympathetic dystrophy, the isotope scan is particularly valuable (Fig. 1.7b).

Blood investigations

Blood tests are needed in exclusion of suspected arthropathy, and should include urate levels, erythrocyte sedimentation rate, C reactive protein, bone indices, rheumatoid factor and thyroid function tests if clinically indicated.

Treatment of the young osteoarthritic knee

Once the diagnosis is clear and the degree of disability and pain established, initial conservative treatment is almost always indicated. One notable exception is the presence of an obvious jamming, loose body within the joint, but this must be large, clearly visible on plain films, and obviously the cause of true mechanical jamming. X-ray reports available to most general practitioners often include the mention of small loose bodies. These are invariably detached but not loose and very rarely the cause of the patient's symptoms; immediate arthroscopy on these individuals will be disappointing.

Conservative treatment of osteoarthritis
The four cornerstones of conservative treatment are:
- Anti-inflammatory medication
- Physiotherapy
- Weight loss if necessary
- Exercise programme.

The efficacy of the first three measures is clearly established in the literature, and borne out by clinical experience. The value of the fourth is less easy to determine, but enhances the advice regarding the weight loss and physiotherapy regimes, and is very valuable in encouraging patients from the outset to come to terms with their problem and to maintain an active lifestyle. It answers many of their questions about what they should and should not do, and in particular how their condition relates to sporting activities.

Medication
Anti-inflammatory medication is the most effective way of controlling symptoms within the arthritic knee. Through its action on the inflammatory cascade, joint pain and swelling can be reduced and there is some early evidence that the newer generation of non-steroidal anti-inflammatory drugs (NSAIDs) may indeed have a protective effect on the articular cartilage, although it is too early to say whether this will have true long-term clinical benefits. The risk of side effects from the medication, in particular gastrointestinal upsets, is not to be overlooked, but patients regularly need reminding that the risks of being on anti-inflammatory drugs, even for many years, are tiny compared with undergoing major knee surgery such as osteotomy or arthroplasty. The biggest hurdle, however, is the need to counsel patients regarding the long-term use of drugs when they naturally want an instant solution, and feel they have come to see you to 'fix it with the telescope', rather than be advised on further drug usage.

Physiotherapy
There are huge benefits to be gained from proper techniques of modern exercise treatment and other modalities, such as interferential ultrasound, in the treatment of osteoarthritis. Once again the patient may dismiss this, having possibly been advised previously by a physiotherapist to do a few exercises, with little result. However, a course of clinic-based physiotherapy is an essential preliminary before considering more invasive techniques. Despite our broad recognition of this fact and regular use of physiotherapy, there are still too few published data from controlled trials of these modalities.

Weight loss
Although the literature does little to support the view that obesity increases the risk of osteoarthritis, there is a large body of evidence to suggest that being overweight increases the symptoms from an arthritic joint. Weight control is the most difficult conservative advice to give, and often so unsuccessful that practitioners may not even consider recommending it. Nevertheless, if one can achieve it, the benefits to an arthritic knee can be significant and long-lasting, as well as reducing the risks if subsequent surgery is needed. There is, however, little value in using it as an essential preliminary to further surgical treatment, as it is so often unsuccessful, and the benefits of surgery are usually as good, even if coming with greater risk.

Fitness
It is well recognised that regular exercise improves mood and pain control. It also enhances weight loss and will be valuable in supporting a physiotherapy regime involving muscle strengthening. Although it is impossible to prove its benefit, it answers patients' major concerns, which is what they can and cannot do with their joint. There is no evidence that the author can find in the literature that regular use of a limb speeds its degenerative features; if anything, the clinical impression is that the opposite is true. Recurrent trauma in high-speed twisting sports is a different matter, but regular walking, cycling or swimming should not wear out the joint any faster than a sedentary lifestyle. In trying to encourage a patient to come to terms with a painful, disabling and chronic condition, this can be an extremely important piece of advice, and often at odds with other practitioners' opinions. One is all too familiar with the scenario of the patient who complains that his doctor has advised him to give up his football, to which

his riposte is, 'But I am only 38 and other people I work with are still playing squash – it doesn't seem right or fair – I can't be written off as an old man at my age.' To advise an active but less violent lifestyle can aid the patient's acceptance of conservative treatment.

Failure to respond to conservative treatment

The above regime is used on all young arthritic patients over a 3- or 4-month period to rehabilitate the knee as much as possible with non-operative measures. The occasional orthosis is helpful in some unstable joints for certain activities. The author's practice does not include regular intra-articular steroid injection. This can cause significant damage and may accelerate articular surface loss. One possible exception is the peri-articular injection along the joint line to a single trigger point which has been unresponsive to local ultrasound and physiotherapy measures.

Further management

After a full course of proper conservative treatment, the patient is re-assessed, the level of symptoms established and his or her approach to coping strategies and lifestyle changes noted. In most cases there will have been a significant improvement in symptoms, and in the majority this will be considerable. For these individuals, reinforcement of the lifestyle changes and physiotherapy exercises is all that is required and, although there is a steady deterioration in the condition in most cases, no further action may need to be taken for several years. If there has been no response, or minimal help, the primary diagnosis of osteoarthritis needs reviewing, re-submitting the patient to the diagnostic mill and further special tests as indicated. The patient's symptoms and disability from them, expectations and co-operation with conservative treatment all need to be balanced before making further recommendations and, in particular, for surgical treatment. This is not a suitable task for a trainee.

None of the surgical treatments available at this stage, other than total joint replacement, carries any greater reported success rate than initial conservative treatment, and yet they are considerably more hazardous.

Indications for arthroscopy

There seems little doubt in the literature that arthroscopic wash-out and debridement can help in early arthritis of the joint, and 60% of patients gaining a short- to mid-term improvement in symptoms seems a reasonable summary of the literature search [11–16]. This alone is not sufficiently high to warrant arthroscopy as an initial treatment, but it can be a useful adjunct to the conservative package, especially as it gives increasing information about the severity of the disease and its site, which may help with further treatment planning [17], and may also allow a more accurate description of the disease process to help the patient cope with his or her symptoms. The debate really exists as to what a wash-out, debridement or chondroplasty can achieve. Some reports suggest that a simple wash-out alone is as valuable as any more invasive technique [18]. The word 'debridement' comes from the French, meaning to unbridle, i.e. set free, but it is increasingly used loosely to suggest the removal of arthritic debris. The former, however, is perhaps more accurate, in the words of our forefathers 'letting out the evil humors'. Probably by changing the biochemical 'soup' within the joint, and the inflammatory environment, we can break the cycle of the secondary reaction in osteoarthritis and improve the symptoms. In the face of conflicting literature on the subject it seems reasonable, however, to attend to any unstable meniscal fragment [19], remove any loose chondral flakes and loose bodies, and wash out the joint thoroughly. The efficacy of more extensive power synovectomy, chondroplasty or subchondral drilling has yet to be proved conclusively, and these procedures significantly increase the possible operative complications, with potential haemarthroses and longer operating times. Repeat arthroscopic procedures have a lower success rate than the first [13].

Synovial biopsy, however, may be a valuable procedure if there is any doubt about an inflammatory component to the problem which might be amenable to subsequent medical manipulation. Careful identification of the site and severity of the arthritic disease, the integrity of the ACL and posterior cruciate ligament (PCL), and the benefit of a good examination under anaesthesia (EUA) can all add to the knowledge base of the surgeon in possibly advising for subsequent treatment, e.g. the suitability for a unicompartmental arthroplasty. In isolated patellofemoral disease maltracking or marked lateral pressure, as against more widespread patellofemoral disease, may help in making further decisions regarding patellofemoral surgery if arthroscopic wash-out alone is unsuccessful.

The value of arthroscopy in the young osteoarthritic knee

At this juncture, therefore, arthroscopy is indicated if 1) there has been absolutely no improvement with properly controlled and conservative measures, and the patient's symptoms remain sufficiently disabling; 2) if there is a clear or suspected mechanical component to the problem, for example a symptomatic loose body or true medial or lateral joint line catching and jamming, even if some of the general symptoms have been improved with the conservative approach; 3) if there is some doubt about the severity or nature of the disease.

The presence of a meniscal tear on MRI scan is not, in its own right, an indication for arthroscopy. This diagnostic indication has to be considered in light of the other available investigations, but there is a group of individuals, typically heavy young men, in whom the symptoms are more severe than the X-rays give credit for, and in whom other tests have failed to identify another cause. Minor fibrillary change of the articular surface alone at arthroscopy would discourage one from taking the surgical treatment further, whereas occasionally localised chondral defects overlooked by the films may suggest more specific treatment, such as the newer techniques of autografting.

Open debridement of the arthritic knee

Techniques originally described by Pridie [20] and Magnuson [21] of debridement and drilling have been well established and give symptomatic benefit in the majority of individuals [22]. However, the reported success rate appears no higher than that of arthroscopic surgical treatment, and at some higher risk of complications and potential joint stiffness. There seems little reason to recommend their use now.

The value of osteotomy about the knee

Osteotomies around the knee for arthritis have a long history, but have fallen into some disrepute recently because of the significant success rate of arthroplasty, especially in the older age group, and the greater expectations of the patients accordingly. The results of osteotomies are rather unpredictable, and there are significant complications which include non-union, infection, complications with metalwork and common peroneal palsy. The necessity for plaster support postoperatively, and the subsequent rehabilitation extends the recovery time beyond that of a joint replacement. The benefits of osteotomy deteriorate with time, both symptomatically and in terms of the correction achieved. All of these issues have adversely affected the popularity of this procedure at the present time. The practical skill of the operating surgeon now spending more of his time doing arthroscopic and arthroplastic work may also be a factor, as well as our more rigorous outcome measures after surgical procedures. Nevertheless, there is a place for both lower femoral and high tibial osteotomy [23,24].

The approach in both is to over-correct limb alignment, reduce the increasing stresses in the arthritic compartment of the knee, and throw more weight across onto the less affected compartment. The patient gains an immediate cosmetic re-alignment of the limb, for which many seem surprisingly grateful, as well as a reduction in pain. By leaving the joint intact, future arthroplasty may be technically compromised but not impossible, and significant time may be bought before an inevitable joint replacement. Repeat osteotomy with good results has also been reported [25].

The success of these measures, however, is probably no more than 70% in most cases in terms of pain control, and this at the expense of a fairly significant undertaking with potential morbidity and complication rate.

Indications for high tibial osteotomy

High tibial osteotomy to correct a varus knee seems most valuable in the young, heavy male patient employed in a manual job, in whom conservative measures and arthroscopic debridement have been unsuccessful. Despite the relatively low success rate, the gains to be achieved in this approach are to maintain the man in his employment for as long as possible [26]. If he is unable to change to a sedentary lifestyle and occupation, the risks of failure and the surgery itself are worth taking. The more successful pain-relieving procedure of arthroplasty may not be a suitable alternative, as it may not allow the patient to return to heavy lifting, digging or kneeling tasks, or if it did, such activities could rapidly cause deterioration in the arthroplasty and requirement for early revision (Fig. 1.8).

To predict the possible success of the procedure more accurately in high tibial osteotomy, gait analysis has been shown to be valuable [27,28], and in an increasingly rare procedure with variable benefits, as much information as possible should be gleaned to

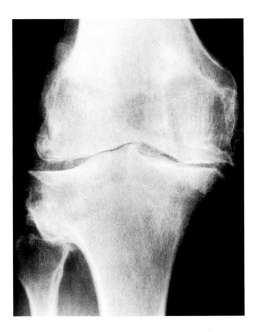

Figure 1.8 – *Weight-bearing view of an osteoarthritic knee taken before total knee arthroplasty. A previous dome osteotomy has been performed which allowed 7 years of relatively pain-free weight-bearing before the joint was replaced. The osteotomy has united soundly without too much upper tibial distortion and without metalwork in place to complicate the joint replacement.*

improve the success rate and understand the failures. It is the author's practice to obtain formal laboratory gait analysis before osteotomies, and regularly afterwards if there are any unexpected clinical outcomes. Occasionally, this approach has thrown up other important factors in the patient's gait which have been tackled non-operatively with success, for example, identifying problems in the foot and ankle during gait, which may contribute to the knee pain.

Lower femoral osteotomy

Low femoral osteotomy for a valgus knee with lateral compartment arthritis is less often indicated, as it is a less common condition, and normally follows arthritis secondary to lateral meniscectomy earlier in life. It can re-align the joint line so that it remains perpendicular to the alignment of the lower leg [24,29]. A small number of cases and studies have been reported in the literature, though the success rate in outcomes seems broadly similar [30].

Summary

The most suitable patients for osteotomy appear to be in earlier disease [31,32], younger patients who have a clear understanding of the likely outcomes and moderately

limited goals that can be achieved, and patients who earn a living from physical work and would thus be unsuitable for arthroplasty. Osteotomy seems less successful in the older patient with more advanced disease.

Techniques of osteotomy around the knee for osteoarthritis

Closing wedge high tibial osteotomy [33] has a well-established history and is quick and straightforward in experienced hands. However, it is usually combined with metalwork staple fixation which may cause subsequent problems, and distorts the upper tibial anatomy, which may influence future arthroplasty [34]. It is also performed through an oblique incision which may cause skin problems with subsequent midline incisions for joint replacement. The author's preferred technique is a dome osteotomy as originally described by Macquet [24] with fibular osteotomy. The dome has the advantages that it requires no metalwork, removes no bone and can, if necessary, be adjusted with manipulation under anaesthesia (MUA) or wedging if the position is unacceptable on X-ray. It is also conducted through a midline incision which can be re-used for arthroplasty at a later date, and distorts the anatomy of the upper metaphysis less. Over-correction to between 7° and 10° valgus is the aim.

In the rarer low femoral osteotomy, the standard technique is a closing wedge osteotomy, held with a Dynamic Condylar Screw (DCS) plate which allows immediate mobilisation and full weight-bearing.

In any osteotomy around the knee for osteoarthritis nowadays, consideration must be given to the fact that this will almost certainly be a prelude to a joint arthroplasty. This is in contradistinction to former days, when it was used as an alternative. In this regard, particular attention must be paid to skin flaps, preservation of well-positioned bone stock, and the avoidance of unnecessary metalwork. By the same token, sepsis must be rigorously treated to prevent it from becoming established and potentially threatening future arthroplasty.

Ligament deficiency and the young arthritic knee

This is a special situation which deserves mention in its own right. It is an increasingly common problem and a chronic ACL deficiency, especially associated with previous meniscal tearing and resection, can lead to development of arthritis in relatively young and active individuals. The initial management follows the same route of conservative therapy and many will come to arthroscopy for the above indications. The common pattern is a medial compartment arthritis in a slightly varus knee with an ACL-deficient knee.

The symptoms in these patients may be both synovitic, i.e. pain and swelling, as well as mechanical. The use of a specialist orthosis can be useful in specific patients with a single area of activity affected, but for day-to-day problems it is usually unhelpful. The debate is often between addressing the medial compartment osteoarthritis with high tibial osteotomy, or addressing the instability of the ACL reconstruction, or doing both together [35]. The latter is quite a significant surgical undertaking and, although it has been described, there seems little benefit over and above osteotomy alone. Although there is some dissenting opinion, the impression is that one should address the osteoarthritic component of the problem with an osteotomy, rather than try to tackle the instability first. It is the author's experience that in this latter case the recovery is slower, the effusion persists and the results certainly do not match those of ACL reconstruction in the uninvolved joint. There is insufficient support in the literature for clear guidance overall, and it seems reasonable to tackle the main form of symptoms with the appropriate procedure. If the arthritic component is significant, then addressing that with an osteotomy if indicated seems logical. If the patient is only getting episodes of pivoting and presents in an ACL-deficient pattern despite some X-ray change, then reconstruction of the ligament is advisable. Once again, careful and honest counselling in this group of patients is essential to avoid disappointment.

Expectations of joint replacement in younger patients

This is the real problem in management of osteoarthritic knees in younger people. There is an expectation that joint replacement will result in a normal knee. It is so obvious to them that patients do not even challenge the concept, and yet as surgeons, we know this is far from the truth. We can sometimes give them a better knee, but never a normal one. It is worth pointing out clearly that a normal knee to a 70-year-old is one which allows him or her to get around the golf course, to sit comfortably in front of a television, to walk to the shops and back, and to sleep well at night.

This is a very significant distance away from someone who sees their contemporaries run upstairs, play sport, and stand up 8 hours at a time in their professions. Joint replacement in these circumstances is almost always destined to disappoint. It is essential to spell out these issues and get a clear idea of the expectations of the patient before embarking on joint replacement, to make sure that the goals of the surgeon and the patient are realistically matched. Only then is it sensible to advise joint replacement in the young patient.

Despite all the above cautions, the results of modern joint arthroplasty in the young patient are reported as very good and equivalent to those in the older category [36–39], despite fairly high demands, though the survival of total knee replacements in the long term is reduced in those aged 65 and younger [40]. Despite some of the theoretical support for an uncemented device for the younger patient, there are few data in the literature to suggest that one should adopt a different approach in the younger patient than the older one in terms of surgical technique.

The use of unicondylar knee arthroplasty requires careful patient selection and choice of prosthesis for a successful result [41], but it offers only an alternative to a total knee replacement, not a halfway house in surgical management.

The risks of failure in the surgical approach of osteoarthritis of the knee in the young patient

Despite the recent excellent reports of joint replacement in the young patient, at every stage the surgeon's responsiblity is to re-assess the failures of any therapy, either conservative or surgical, rather than immediately stepping on to the next procedure. The worst scenario is the embittered, disappointed patient who has had multiple treatments for a relatively mildly arthritic joint caused by an industrial injury, for whom the level of indignation and anxiety are high. The author has seen one such 40-year-old end up with an above-knee amputation to try and manage the on-going problems, even in the face of a technically successful joint replacement.

Another example is a 50-year-old patient with medial compartment arthritis, a carpet fitter by trade, who begged for a joint replacement. He was not satisfied by explanations of the attendant risks and potential disappointments, and was supported by his wife who, at the same age, had already had a unicompartmental arthroplasty with great benefit. She failed to understand why joint replacement was not recommended for her husband. Only after it was pointed out that she lived an entirely sedentary life with minimal activity on the knee, no prolonged kneeling or vigorous heavy exercise, did she understand that her husband's situation was entirely different; there was little prospect that a joint replacement could return him to his previous level of activity, principally on all fours 8 hours a day (Figs 1.9, 1.10).

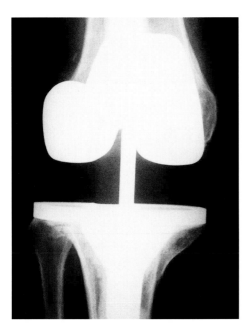

Figure 1.9 – *A revision total knee arthroplasty in a 40-year-old, in whom a previous cementless device had failed. Despite the functional success in this individual with a good recovery of pain-free move-ment, it is never-theless the drastic end result of what is fundamentally an articular cartilage disease.*

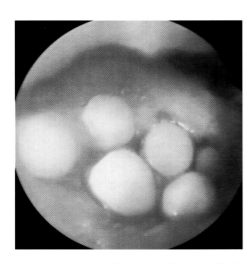

Figure 1.10 – *Arthroscopic photograph of a recent osteo-chondral graft (by kind permission of R. Dodds, OBE, FRCS). Whether in the long term osteochondral grafting in any of its forms, or chondrocyte culture will be the solution, their developments and the associated interest in the basic science of articular cartilage degeneration and repair is very welcome, as the biological approach to the young osteoarthritic knee must ultimately be better than the mechanical one (Fig. 1.9).*

Other agencies in the management of the young osteoarthritic knee

As the above section stresses, the temptation is to take a surgical line with all young arthritics, and yet this can lead to disappointment. The goal must be to try to keep the patient's own knee as long as possible and support him with all other measures. During the progression from conservative through to minor surgery, it is important to be constantly aware of any abnormal pain responses or the development of a true chronic pain syndrome if the symptoms and signs and X-ray features are not consistent. In this situation, the help of an established pain clinic can be extremely valuable. It can exclude specific conditions and treat them appropriately with guanethidine, for example in reflex sympathetic dystrophy, and can add significantly to the armamentarium of pain control with advice regarding analgesics as well as other agents such as antidepressants in small doses. Above all, it can help patients come to terms with a coping, rather than a curing, strategy. It is essential to keep close links with the pain specialists, if not a true combined clinic, to maintain at least inter-current appointments for a combined management approach, rather than use them as a final option when all else fails.

By the same token, the support of the rehabilitation specialist, industrial resettlement office and a knowledge of the disablement benefits will be an integral part of helping the young osteoarthritic patient in the absence of a cure for osteoarthritis, or a readily available surgical solution.

Key points

1. True primary osteoarthritis of the knee in a young person is relatively uncommon.
2. Symptomatic knees in young people with early degenerative joint disease are relatively frequent. Conservative and/or surgical treatment of an osteoarthritic knee will only be effective if arthritis is the genuine cause of symptoms.
3. Conservative treatment must be well structured and carefully followed through and medically supervised if it is to be successful.
4. Weight control, exercise programmes, physiotherapy and anti-inflammatory medication are the mainstays of conservative treatment.
5. Failure to respond at all to conservative therapy suggests an alternative diagnosis.

6. In the combination of an ACL-deficient knee with osteoarthritis, combined treatment appears no more effective than tackling the most symptomatic of the two with the appropriate operation.

7. Pain clinic help is valuable if there is any doubt about an abnormal pain response, as this will seriously compromise surgical treatment results.

8. Total knee arthroplasty is effective in the young patient, but good results rely heavily on very careful patient selection.

CHAPTER 2

The painful total knee replacement

A. Unwin

Introduction

The painful total knee replacement (TKR) is a challenging problem for the surgeon and the patient. This chapter addresses the causes and attempts to present a rationale for diagnosing the problem. It is emphasised that 'blind revision surgery' for painful knee replacements is rarely rewarding.

This chapter is concerned with the causes, diagnosis and treatment choices for the painful knee replacement after surgery, but does not refer to aseptic loosening of prosthetic components.

Causes of pain after TKR

- Infection
- Intra-articular problems
- Extra-articular problems
- Malalignment of the prosthesis
- Prosthetic instability
- Patellofemoral problems
- Neuropathic pain
- Miscellaneous causes
- No diagnosis.

Infection following total knee replacement

All painful knee replacements are infected until proven otherwise. Quoted incidences for infection after TKR vary from 1 to 12%. Rand and Bryan et al. [1,2] have quoted an incidence of 1.2% in 3000 primary knee replacements. The Swedish Knee Arthroplasty project quotes a deep infection rate after 12,118 primary knee replacements between 1975 and 1985 as 1.7% for osteoarthritis and 4.4% for rheumatoid arthritis [3]. The infection rate is increased in those with previous surgery, rheumatoid arthritis, obesity, male sex, oral steroid usage, diabetes, distal skin infections and ulceration [4], perioperative urinary tract instrumentation and/or infection, chronic renal failure, immunosuppression and neoplasia [5].

Although suspected by many, there is no direct correlation between early wound healing problems after knee replacement and subsequent prosthetic infection. Garner et al. [6] noted that 49 out of 220 knee replacements had an acute problem with wound healing. Thirty-five of the 41 cultures taken were negative. The commonest organism grown was *Staphylococcus epidermidis*. They found no correlation between wound healing and subsequent periprosthetic infection. Insall [7] also maintains that slight wound drainage occurs in up to 25% of replacements and does not predispose to deep infection.

The organisms associated with deep infection include:
- *Staphylococcus aureus* (58% of cases [8], 66% of cases [5])
- *Staphylococcus epidermidis* – perhaps under-recognised as a cause of infection
- *E.coli* – less common
- *Pseudomonas aeruginosa* – less common
- Mixed polymicrobial infection – especially in actively draining wounds
- Resistant bacterial strains in those patients administered chronic antibiotic treatment.

Early deep infection (within 3 months of implantation) is relatively uncommon. The diagnosis is usually obvious as long as antibiotics are not administered. Clinically, the patient exhibits severe and prolonged pain, fever, swelling and inflammation. The white cell count (WCC) and inflammatory indices (erythrocyte sedimentation rate (ESR) and C-reactive protein (CRP)) remain high after surgery.

Late deep infection is much more common. The patient may present with acute pain and swelling where there was previously a satisfactory arthroplasty, but in many cases the patient gives a history of a replacement that 'was never quite right'. Late infection may occasionally develop via haematogenous spread from a secondary focus.

The clinical features associated with periprosthetic infection are varied. Wilson *et al.* [5], in a study of 52 patients with infected TKRs, noted the following:

- 96% had considerable pain
- 77% had swelling of the knee
- 27% were pyrexial
- 27% had active drainage
- Average ESR was 63 mm/h
- Average WCC was 8.3
- 51 of 52 had a positive aspiration of knee fluid.

Radiological features in periprosthetic infection are unreliable. Infection is often present in the absence of radiological evidence of loosening. Large confluent lucencies are indicative of advanced infection.

The role of nuclear imaging in the diagnosis of infection after knee replacement is controversial. Technetium or gallium scans are not conclusive of infection. However, Henderson *et al.* [9] demonstrated that sequential technetium and citrate scans were useful in the diagnosis and differentiation of aseptic and septic loosening of TKRs. They also held that a painful TKR with a normal bone scan is probably not due to loosening or infection.

Aspiration is thought by many authorities to be an excellent method of diagnosis of infection after knee replacement surgery. Aspiration should be performed in an aseptic manner, either blindly or with X-ray guidance. Aspirates should be sent for smear, Gram staining and culture with sensitivities for aerobic and anaerobic bacilli, mycobacteria and fungi. Two or more organisms may be involved. If the neutrophil count is greater than 25,000 cells per mm^3 and the differential is more than 75%, infection should be suspected. In infection, the synovial glucose decreases and the synovial protein content increases. Aspiration is often negative due to antibiotic administration, which should be avoided in

the treatment of painful knee replacements without a definitive diagnosis. There is clear evidence to show that antibiotic suppression alone will not adequately manage an infected TKR [7]. Thus there is no rationale for the use of oral antibiotics in the management of established infection. Culture from drainage sites is not reliable, as there may be a secondary infection or skin flora contamination.

If an aspirate does not demonstrate infection, an open biopsy by arthroscopy or arthrotomy may be helpful. In addition to synovial and capsular tissue, the bone–cement interface also needs to be analysed at the time of biopsy. All biopsies should be sent for both histological and microbiological analysis. Intraoperative frozen sections can be useful, with neutrophilia indicative of bacterial infection.

Intra-articular problems causing pain after a TKR

Several intra-articular problems can cause pain after a TKR:

- *Overhanging components*, especially the tibial prosthesis, can cause localised pain. If disabling, revision of the relevant component may be necessary.
- *Recurrent haemarthroses* are not uncommon, and can closely resemble infection in their clinical presentation. The symptoms of pain, stiffness and swelling may arise several months after insertion of the prosthesis [10]. There are several postulated causes of these haemarthroses, but the two most likely are synovial impingement and knee laxity predisposing to the impingement. On aspiration, blood is evacuated. Management includes an arthroscopic synovectomy or, if this is unsuccessful, insertion of a thicker tibial component.
- *Patellar clunk syndrome* (see below), associated with posterior stabilised knees, and less prevalent with newer prosthetic designs. Responds well to arthroscopic debridement.
- *Popliteus impingement* – mechanical impingement of the prosthesis against the popliteus tendon, causing posterolateral pain and snapping. It is more common where there is lateral overhang of the tibial prosthesis, and especially in the valgus knee. This is a condition which should be excluded at the trial reduction. Where the components are inserted, resection of all or part of the popliteus tendon can alleviate the condition.

- *Impingement against osteophytes* – can produce pain or clunking, especially in very conforming types of knee prostheses. Resection of the osteophytes offers very good relief of symptoms [11].
- *Fabellar impingement* – similar to popliteus impingement. The fabella can impinge against either the femoral or tibial components. As with popliteus impingement, this condition can be diagnosed at trial reduction. If established, the fabella can be removed from within the lateral head of gastrocnemius, preferably by the posterolateral approach [12] or anteriorly.
- *Pseudomeniscus* – these soft tissue lesions can form between the femoral and tibial articulation, and are composed of fibrocartilage. They can be excised arthroscopically, and are one of the lesions that should be excluded if an arthroscopy is performed in the investigation of a painful TKR [13].
- *Persistent synovitis* – may occur in the inflammatory arthropathies where the synovium has been inadequately excised at the time of knee replacement surgery.
- *Loose bodies* – rare.
- *Gout and pseudogout* – rare.

Extra-articular problems causing pain after a TKR

- Intraoperative and postoperative fractures of the femur or tibia – these may occur on either the tibial plateaux or the femoral condyles. They are more common in osteoporotic bone.
- Femoral condyle fractures can occur where the prosthesis is driven hard onto soft bone, especially in rheumatoid arthritis. If the central portion of the femoral prosthesis is not cut accurately, a vertical split in the femur may occur. These fractures can usually be treated conservatively, although on occasions internal fixation or the addition of a femoral stem is required.
- Tibial fractures may occur with central stem designs, especially if the stem hole is undersized during preparation. The vast majority settle with conservative treatment.
- Periprosthetic fracture, usually in the distal femur, may result from a fall. There is controversy as to whether notching of the femur predisposes to supracondylar fracture. Ritter [14] is of the view that it does not. Fixation of these periprosthetic fractures can be demanding.

- *Stress fractures of the tibia* – these can occur after total knee replacement, especially in the rheumatoid patient with a valgus knee. They are difficult to diagnose on plain X-ray, but are shown well on bone scanning.
- *Patellar tendinitis.*
- *Pes anserinus bursitis* – usually with overhanging components.
- *Heterotopic ossification* – a not uncommon cause of a stiff, painful knee. The ossification usually occurs in the quadriceps, causing limited flexion. The condition is important to recognise, as it often resolves spontaneously, although it can cause persistent pain [15].

Malalignment as a cause of pain after total knee replacement

Malalignment can cause pain after knee replacement surgery, even in the absence of gross laxity or evidence of loosening. The more common malalignment patterns are:

- *Patellar subluxation* – the commonest cause of malalignment causing pain after a knee replacement (see page 17).
- *Strain of the medial collateral ligament* – this can occur if a knee replacement is positioned in a valgus position, especially if there is valgus laxity upon weight-bearing. For this reason alone, it is probably best to choose 5° rather than 7° of femoral component valgus in a valgus knee.
- *Tibial overload in a varus knee* – the medial tibial plateau can be overloaded where a knee replacement is positioned in excessive varus.
- *Rotational impingement.*

Instability as a cause of pain after total knee replacement

Although a knee replacement should not be too tight with full extension, or even hyperextension, possible at the end of the procedure, there is a danger of leaving knee replacements too lax – instability can be a potent cause of pain. Beware especially of merely addressing the extension gap and ignoring the flexion gap during trial reduction.

Unstable painful total knee replacements often require revision. There are four major types of instability after knee replacement surgery:

■ *Extensor instability* – the extension gap is larger than the prosthetic thickness. This is caused by component malposition or limb malalignment.
■ *Flexion instability* – the flexion gap is too large for the tibial component thickness.
■ *Medial/lateral instability.*
■ *Global instability.*

Extensor instability

Symmetrical extension instability

This occurs when the total component thickness is less than the extension gap between the bone ends, e.g. from excessive bone removal from the femur/tibia or after inadequate soft tissue tensioning of the collateral ligaments at the time of resection. It can occasionally be due to genu recurvatum or where extensive medial and lateral ligament releases have been performed.

Over-resection of tibial bone can be corrected by increasing the tibial polyethylene thickness, and this is a reasonably straightforward procedure.

Over-resection of the distal femur is more difficult to correct, requiring augmentation with blocks. This problem should not be managed by simply adding thickness to the tibial component, as this merely raises the joint line, alters ligament stability and creates a patella infera (Fig. 2.1).

Asymmetrical extension instability

This is a relatively common problem and is due to some degree of ligament asymmetry. The most common cause is a failure adequately to release a tight ligament, especially the medial collateral ligament in a varus knee.

Management involves an adequate soft tissue release and correction of any 'incorrect' component thickness.

Flexion instability

The flexion gap is too large for the thickness of the tibial component. This is associated with a posterior sag, anterior knee pain, increased polyethylene wear and 'start-up pain'. There are a number of causes:
■ The commonest cause is where the surgeon finds that there is a flexion contracture with the trial components and inappropriately uses a thinner tibial component or resects more tibia, rather than correctly resecting more femoral bone or performing a posterior capsulotomy.
■ The femoral component may be undersized antero–posteriorly. This can be managed using a larger femoral component with posterior augmentation if necessary.

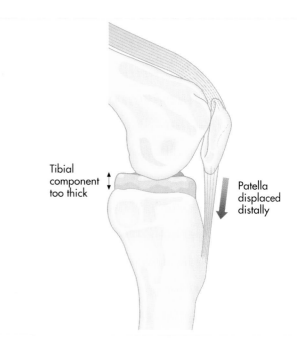

Figure 2.1 – *Stabilising the knee by using too thick a tibial polyethylene component produces a patella infera. (Reproduced from ref. 42 with permission.)*

■ Excessive lateral release from the femur can result in flexor instability. This usually requires a constrained prosthesis, although thicker tibial components can be used.
■ Grossly abnormal femoral rotation.

Occasionally, flexion instability results in posterior tibial dislocation. The management involves revision with thicker tibial polyethylene or the use of constrained prostheses.

Figure 2.2 discusses the management of flexion/extension gap imbalance.

Patellofemoral problems as a cause of pain after TKR

Whilst many surgeons believe that the tibio-femoral articulation in knee replacement surgery is excellent with a high success rate, the patellofemoral joint has historically been 'the problem' with knee replacement surgery, although with recent modifications in prosthetic design these have lessened.

Extensor mechanism complications causing pain after knee replacement surgery include:
■ Fractures of the patella
■ Patellar maltracking

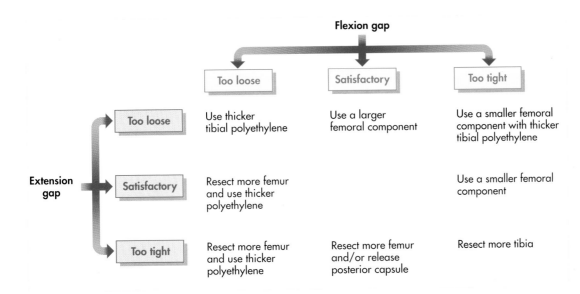

Figure 2.2 – *Management of flexion/extension gap imbalance.*

- The 'patellar clunk'
- Miscellaneous problems.

Fractures of the patella

Fractures of the patella can occur with or without patellar resurfacing, although fractures are more common where the patella has been resurfaced. They can be regarded as a 'complication of success', as they are seen in those who are active with a good range of motion.

Patellar fractures after knee replacement can be either traumatic or fatigue in type.

Traumatic fractures are usually displaced, and can be managed in much the same way as patellar fractures in the normal population. As the extensor mechanism is usually disrupted, they often require open reduction and internal fixation. The fixation can be demanding, as the bone is often osteopenic and the patellar implant (if present) can impede fixation devices.

Fatigue fractures can be horizontal, vertical or comminuted. The possible causes include patellar maltracking (especially in horizontal and some comminuted fractures), a large patellar button hole and avascularity of the patella.

- *Horizontal fractures* – with this type, the patella splits, with one portion retaining the implant and remaining in a normal position whilst the second fragment displaces laterally. This fracture type presents acutely and is often secondary to patellar maltracking. If the extensor mechanism is violated, operative repair is necessary.
- *Vertical fractures* – nearly all pass through the buttonhole. The extensor mechanism is usually intact, even if the fracture fragments are widely displaced. This fracture type often presents subacutely with mild pain and swelling, or may even be asymptomatic. The majority can be treated conservatively, although a fibrous rather than a bony union is more often than not the end result.
- *Comminuted fractures* – these are the most common type of fatigue fracture seen after knee replacement surgery. The fracture pattern is a combination of horizontal and vertical fractures, and the fragments are often widely displaced. It is often asymptomatic, although it may be associated with a minor extensor lag. No active treatment is needed in most instances.

Patellar maltracking – subluxation and dislocation

These problems are usually due to surgical error, and occur especially in the valgus knee. The symptoms can be debilitating and include pain, weakness, limited range of movement, extensor lag and difficulty in managing stairs.

Patellar maltracking can be affected by the depth of the femoral sulcus, the rotation of the femoral and tibial components, valgus alignment and a tight lateral retinaculum. The patellar component should be medialised if possible [16]. However, over-medialising can cause pain between the exposed lateral facet of the patella and the femoral component [17]. The use of lateral release appears to have decreased in recent years with newer components, although it may be necessary. Proper orientation of the femoral and tibial components minimises its need. There is little doubt that lateral release results in an increased complication rate after knee replacement surgery [18].

The necessity to maintain the anatomical joint line in primary knee replacement surgery is controversial. Whilst it is helpful to restore the joint line as much as practicable, less emphasis is placed upon this factor as a cause of patellofemoral maltracking than previously.

In the management of anterior knee pain, if there is maltracking after a knee replacement, the results of revision are in general good, whereas if there is no maltracking the results of revision for anterior knee pain are poor [19]. Extensive surgery may be necessary to correct any underlying anatomical abnormality.

Bocell [20] has described the 'tethered patella syndrome', where there is patellofemoral dysfunction with painful popping, catching, grinding and jumping of the patellar component. Bands can prevent the patella from sitting in the femoral sulcus and tether the patella laterally. Arthroscopic removal of the bands is said to resolve the symptoms very well.

The 'patellar clunk'

This term refers to a collection of fibrous tissue between the patella and the femoral component (usually within the quadriceps tendon) during active knee extension (Fig. 2.3). The patient experiences a painful 'clunk' or snap on extension, and the problem usually presents within 4–12 months after surgery. It is more common in posterior stabilised designs [21], and is probably due to designs with a shallow femoral sulcus and a sharp transition into the femoral box. The fibrous tissue becomes entrapped at the transition area. Arthroscopic debridement is generally successful in relieving symptoms [22,23].

Other extensor mechanism complications

- Tibial tubercle avulsion is an avoidable intraoperative complication, but is often not recognised at the time of surgery. The problem usually occurs in stiff knees with difficult surgical exposures. The problem may also occur during manipulation under anaesthetic, and for this reason a muscle relaxant should ideally be given during any manipulation. Once the problem has occurred, surgical repair is very difficult and long-term morbidity with extensor lag is inevitable.
- Patellar ligament rupture is fortunately rare. It is said to be associated with excision of the patellar fat pad at the time of surgery. Repair, as in the normal

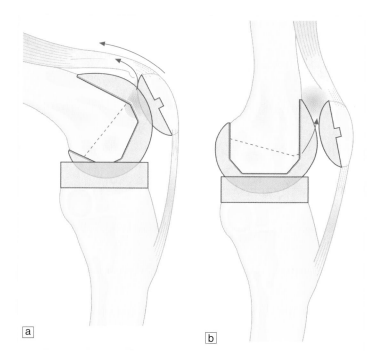

Figure 2.3 – *The 'patellar clunk'. (a) A nodule of fibrous tissue impinges between the patella and the femoral component during knee extension, (b) causing an unpleasant 'clunk' and occasionally locking of the knee. The lesion can be excised arthroscopically. (Reproduced from ref. 42 with permission.)*

population, is difficult. Krackow [24] has used quadricepsplasty with hamstring augmentation to treat the problem, whilst Emerson *et al.* [25] have used patellar tendon allografts. The end results are often disappointing.

- Avascular necrosis of the patella.

To resurface or not to resurface the patella?

Cementless patellar implants can have unique problems, such as stress shielding of the patella causing unexplained knee pain. Such stress shielding can be difficult to diagnose on plain X-ray, whereas with cemented implants the diagnosis may be more obvious.

There is ongoing debate as to whether the patella in osteoarthritic knees should be resurfaced during total knee replacement.

- Murena [26] has stated that patellar resurfacing may offer better clinical results.
- Bourne [27] demonstrated that unresurfaced joints were superior in terms of pain but had similar knee scores to unresurfaced joints.
- Braakman [18] and Keblish [28] were of the view that there were no differences in terms of pain, range of

movement, stability, flexion or extension deficit, stair ability or walking aid usage between resurfaced and unresurfaced patellofemoral joints.

- Enis [29] documented that patellar resurfacing was better in terms of pain relief, whilst Smith [30] showed that patellar resurfacing fared worse than non-resurfacing.
- Barrack [31] stated that there was no difference between the two groups.

There is broad general agreement amongst orthopaedic surgeons and in the literature that the patella should be resurfaced in rheumatoid arthritic patients undergoing knee replacement surgery, and this view has recently been supported by Kajino [32].

Neuropathic causes of pain after TKR

Not all pain after knee replacement surgery is due to mechanical or infective problems. Chapter 12 is devoted to the problem of reflex sympathetic dystrophy or complex regional pain syndrome of the knee.

Neuropathic pain can be both sympathetic and non-sympathetic. Pharmacological diagnosis and treatment is valuable in this type of pain, using alpha blockade (e.g. phentolamine, bretylium Bier block, clonidine patches) or direct blockade (e.g. lumbar sympathetic blocks, calcium channel blockers).

Although Nicholls and Dorr [33] have found success in surgical revision of stiff and painful knees in reflex sympathetic dystrophy, Insall [7] has not.

Miscellaneous causes of pain after TKR

- *Alternative original diagnosis* – it is not unknown for a knee replacement to have been performed where an alternative diagnosis was the cause of the knee pain. Examples include:
  - Hip pathology
  - Vascular claudication
  - Neurological problems, e.g. spinal stenosis, lumbar disc prolapse or common peroneal nerve pain
- Thrombo-embolism
- Vascular complications

- Metal allergy – never proven but suspected by many surgeons. Skin allergies to cobalt have been noted in patients with early and painful loosening.

No diagnosis for pain after a TKR

This is an important group of patients, in whom, despite extensive investigation, no diagnosis can be made for their knee pain after apparently successful surgery. An important principle is that these patients should not undergo revision surgery unless absolutely necessary, as the results of such surgery are in general very disappointing, and often worsen the outcome for the patient.

In such cases, the patient may have unrealistic expectations. Look back at the preoperative X-ray; many do not have advanced disease prior to their replacement. A thorough review of personal psychological and family factors is crucial in the management of this difficult group of patients.

Insall [7] has noted that in his experience, 1 in 300 knee replacements have pain associated with a lack of movement where the components appear to be well seated and positioned. There may be an overlap with reflex sympathetic dystrophy, especially in those with restricted movement [34].

Causes of a stiff TKR

There are several causes for a knee replacement which is stiff but not necessarily painful:

- *Limited preoperative range of movement* – this is the most common cause of a stiff knee after replacement surgery. Most knee systems only provide as much flexion as the soft tissues will allow. Body shape and motivation are also important factors.
- *Inaccurate tensioning* – especially in cruciate-sacrificing prostheses.
- *A tight posterior cruciate ligament (PCL)* – a tight PCL will result in abnormal rollback and early failure.
- Retention of posterior cement.
- *A residual flexion contracture* – this is a surgical error which should be avoided.
- *A tight lateral retinaculum* – may prevent full flexion.
- *An aggressive fibrous tissue response* – some patients inexplicably stiffen after knee replacements following production of excessive fibrosis during the recovery phase from surgery.

Investigation plan for knee pain after TKR

Always assume that a painful knee replacement is infected until proven otherwise. However, revision surgery for unexplained pain is generally unsuccessful and disappointing. A diagnosis should be made prior to revision. Investigation of pain after knee replacement surgery might include the following:

- History and physical examination
- Plain X-rays
- Bone scanning – technetium, gallium, indium
- Aspiration
- Arthroscopy
- Biopsies, including intraoperative frozen sections, for microbiological and histological analysis
- Sinography – not diagnostically useful as, where there is a discharging sinus, it should always be assumed that infection is present
- Selective local anaesthetic injections and sympathetic blocks
- Ultrasound can be used to diagnose polyethylene wear [35].

Arthroscopy of painful TKRs

Arthroscopy can be a useful diagnostic tool in the evaluation of painful knee replacements.

Diduch *et al.* [23] reviewed 40 arthroscopies on 38 patients with symptomatic knee replacements. Complaints were of pain, soft tissue impingement or stiffness. The arthroscopy successfully diagnosed the cause of the symptoms in all but one case. There was no morbidity or subsequent infection as a result of the arthroscopy. Prophylactic antibiotics were given after cultures were taken. Diagnoses included:

- Impinging soft tissues under the patella consistent with the 'clunk' syndrome (43%)
- Impinging hypertrophic synovitis elsewhere in the knee (15%)
- Impinging PCL stump (10%)
- Prosthesis loosening or wear (10%)
- Arthrofibrosis (20%)

Arthroscopic treatments include removal of impinging soft tissues or loose bodies. The authors concluded that arthroscopy was a safe and effective tool for managing problem TKRs, especially 'clunks', and may help to avoid revision TKRs or arthrotomies.

Arthroscopy can also be used to diagnose component wear or damage, occult infection [20] and problems with patellar tracking [36].

Arthroscopy can be used therapeutically for lysis of adhesions in arthrofibrosis [20] and for debridement of soft tissue impingement lesions, e.g. the 'clunk' under the patella. In contrast to Diduch *et al.* [23], Markel *et al.* [37] found the results of arthroscopic treatment of peripatellar fibrosis to be disappointing and variable. Johanson [38] maintains that arthroscopy is successful in removing loose bodies, correcting patellar subluxation via a lateral release, excising a symptomatic pseudo-meniscus and releasing intra-articular adhesions.

Insall [7] is of the view that a preliminary arthroscopy should be performed prior to arthrotomy in patients with 'unexplained pain' after knee replacement surgery.

Treatment options for infected TKRs

This is not fully considered in this chapter. However, the treatment options include:

- Antibiotic suppression – there are no conclusive benefits from this treatment and the treatment may prevent accurate microbiological assessment of the infection.
- Debridement with the prosthesis left *in situ*.
- Removal of the prosthesis in one or two stages, with or without a cement spacer.
- Conversion to a pseudarthrosis – these are rarely satisfactory and are more painful and less functional than a pseudarthrosis at the hip joint.
- Arthrodesis.
- Amputation.

Wilde [39] held that antibiotics alone are ineffective. Debridement with preservation of the prosthesis and intravenous antibiotics were effective in 18–40% of cases. Resection arthroplasty was poor functionally. Arthrodesis was found to give good results, but the patient was left with a stiff knee. Two-stage revision was found to be superior to one-stage revision, with success rates of 80–97%.

Amputations are necessary on some occasions after a TKR. The common factors leading to an amputation are multiple revision operations in the presence of chronic infection, severe bone loss and intractable pain. Isiklar [40] feels that early consideration of arthrodesis rather than multiple revision operations is more likely to avoid amputation.

Denervation procedures

Dellon *et al.* [41] treated persistent knee pain with partial denervation. Aseptic loosening, sepsis, ligamentous instability, malalignment and polyethylene wear were excluded. The procedure was performed after a successful nerve block. Of these patients, 86% were satisfied by the procedure. Denervation is perhaps an option in the treatment of intractable pain after TKR where structural and infective aetiologies have been excluded.

Key points

1. Do not revise a painful knee replacement unless there is a clear diagnosis, as the results of revision for undiagnosed pain are often disappointing.

2. A painful TKR is infected until proven otherwise.

3. The most important determinant of good outcome, especially in terms of range of movement, is the preoperative function of the knee.

4. Do not prescribe antibiotics after knee replacement surgery in the absence of a definitive diagnosis.

5. When taking samples to diagnose infection, samples from the bone–cement interface and cement–prosthesis interface are essential.

6. There is no rationale for the use of oral antibiotics in the management of established infection of a knee replacement.

7. Early arthrodesis is preferable to multiple revision surgeries for painful knee replacements.

8. Beware of the patient with unrealistic expectations following primary knee replacement surgery.

CHAPTER 3

Management of the acutely injured knee

R. L. Allum

Introduction

The knee is the largest synovial joint in the body and the most frequently injured. Injuries occur predominantly in young active patients and the morbidity is not insignificant (Fig. 3.1). In recent years increasing attention has been paid to the management of trauma in the UK. This was highlighted by the publication of the Royal College of Surgeons Working Party Report in 1988 [1] on the Management of Patients with Major Injuries. This Report highlighted the inadequacies in the care of trauma in the UK and made several recommendations for improvements in the delivery of care. Techniques in fracture surgery have advanced considerably in the last few years and much progress has been made in the surgical management of long bone fractures, intra-articular fractures, pelvic fractures and spinal fractures.

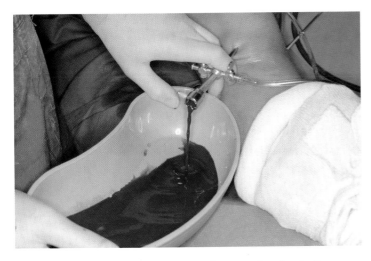

Figure 3.1 – *Acute traumatic haemarthrosis indicates a significant injury.*

To a certain extent, the management of the acutely injured knee has not received the attention that it deserves, and relatively little attention is paid to this problem in undergraduate and early post-graduate training. There is a particular problem with regard to diagnosis. In 1978, Noyes *et al.* [2] reported that only 4% of patients who were subsequently found to have laxity of the anterior cruciate ligament (ACL) were diagnosed correctly at the time of the initial injury. There seems to have been little improvement over the years and in 1996 Bollen and Scott [3] in a UK study reported on the diagnosis of a ruptured ACL in 117 patients with 119 injuries. Of these, 89.9% gave a typical history of injury. The diagnosis was made by the primary treating physician in only 9.8% of cases and by 1 month after the injury, only 32 cases had been diagnosed. The average delay between the first medical consultation and diagnosis was 21 months. Thirty percent of patients had been seen by an orthopaedic surgeon and the diagnosis missed. Thirty-six patients had undergone 51 invasive investigations; in 14 procedures the diagnosis had been established, but in 37 the results were unhelpful or misleading, in that the knee was described as normal. It became apparent during the study that a common sequence of events following injury was a visit to the local casualty department and a normal knee X-ray and, on this basis, the patient was discharged with a Tubigrip bandage. This survey emphasises the importance of a clear and detailed history, particularly of the precipitating injury, and a careful clinical examination. Over the last 20–25 years, there have been significant improvements in the diagnosis and management of knee problems, and the developments in arthroscopy and more recently magnetic resonance imaging (MRI) have increased our understanding of these injuries considerably.

Increasing leisure time inevitably leads to an increase in the incidence of sporting injury, and patients' expectations are forever increasing. As well as the traditional contact sports, other activities place considerable stress on the knee, e.g. skiing, racquet sports, jumping sports such as basketball and netball and all forms of gymnastics. Ironically, improvements in equipment may increase the stress on the knee. Improvements in ski boots and bindings stabilise the ankle but at the expense of the knee. Artificial surfaces increase the adhesion of the boot, again protecting the foot and ankle but increasing the stress on the knee. The knee is said to be an engineer's nightmare, consisting of a joint which must be freely mobile and weight-bearing at the end of the long lever arms of the tibia and the femur. A UK study on the epidemiology of sports injuries [4] estimated that there was a total of 9.8 million substantive injuries a year in the age group 16–45 years and that 16.1% of all injuries affected the knee. Kujala *et al.* [5], reviewing 54,186 sports injuries, reported that the knee was the most common location for injuries resulting in permanent disability. Population surveys have been carried out in both the US and Scandinavia. Miyasaka *et al.*, from San Diego, California [6], reported an incidence of ACL rupture of 0.38 per 1000 population each year. In a similar study in Denmark, Nielsen and Yde [7] found an incidence of 0.3 ACL injuries per 1000 population each year. If these figures were extrapolated to the UK, there would be approximately 17,000 ACL injuries per year, giving approximately 100 injuries per year in a population of 300,000 typically served by a district general hospital.

Clinical considerations

History

Firstly, it is important to make an overall assessment of the patient's age, level of activity, recreational or sporting aspirations and expectations. The plan of treatment partly depends on this; for example, the management of a 20-year-old professional footballer with a torn ACL will be different from that of a 45-year-old executive who skis once a year and takes no other exercise. Different injuries occur in different age groups. Osteochondral fractures and patellar dislocations are more likely to occur in the adolescent, and ligament injuries are less common in this age group than in adults, although they

do occur and can be very demanding to treat. Rupture of the quadriceps or patellar tendon is more likely to occur in the middle-aged and elderly, and these injuries are frequently missed.

The patient must be questioned in detail about any previous injury, no matter how far in the past. A significant injury may have been forgotten or assumed not to be of importance, but on close questioning the patient may recall a previous ligament injury or an injury in which the knee was painful and swollen for a period of time, following which the knee had never really been as good as before the incident.

The history of the mechanism of injury is of prime importance and frequently provides the diagnosis. The ACL is most commonly injured by the following mechanisms, often in combination – change of direction, deceleration, angulation, rotation and landing awkwardly after a jump. The foot is usually anchored and in the case of skiing, the bindings fail to release or release late. The injury is predominantly non-contact, as very high forces are transmitted through the knee joint by the injury mechanisms described. This fact can mislead the inexperienced practitioner; when the patient states that no other player was involved, the assumption may be made that the injury must be an innocuous one, but this is often not the case. Contact with another player may accentuate the injury. Angulation of the knee also puts the collateral ligaments at risk. The medial ligament will be torn by a valgus force and the lateral complex by a varus force. The posterior cruciate ligament (PCL) is more commonly injured by a direct blow to the flexed knee, e.g. a dashboard injury in a road traffic accident or a hyperextension injury. Soccer goalkeepers seem to be particularly prone to this injury. A subluxation or dislocation of the patella is caused by a rotational or angulation stress, and is common in teenage girls following activities such as dancing and gymnastics. A sudden twist and valgus strain to the extended knee may cause an osteochondral fracture of the lateral femoral condyle in the adolescent or young adult [8]. Isolated meniscal injuries are normally caused by a less vigorous injury mechanism, predominantly rotation of the flexed knee under load, e.g. twisting when getting up from a kneeling or crouching position. Rupture of the quadriceps tendon is caused by a sudden violent reflex contraction of the quadriceps against the weight of the body, as when trying to avoid falling after a trip or a stumble. This most commonly occurs in the 6th and 7th decades of life when there is pre-existing weakness of the quadriceps tendon. Certain medical conditions predispose towards this injury; rupture has been reported in association with diabetes mellitus, nephritis, gout and hyperparathyroidism. The patient will describe a sudden severe pain after a typical injury. Following this, the pain may well settle and, although the knee is unstable, the patient and clinician may be lulled into a false sense of security by the lack of pain. Rupture of the patellar tendon occurs by a similar mechanism, but it is much less common and tends to occur in younger individuals than the ruptured quadriceps tendon. There is an increased incidence after patellar tendon harvest for ACL reconstruction.

Fractures of the intercondylar eminence of the tibia occur in children and adolescents following a fall and the most common cause is a bicycle accident. Indeed, it has been stated that if a child is admitted with a painful, acutely swollen knee following a fall from a bicycle, the diagnosis should be assumed to be a fractured intercondylar eminence until proven otherwise [9].

Pain at the time of acute knee injury is variable and not always an accurate guide to the severity of injury. A complete ligamentous tear may disrupt nerve fibres to the extent that pain is reduced. Following an acute ligamentous disruption at sport, pain is normally so severe that the competitor has to leave the field of play immediately. There may be an attempt to continue with the game, with the knee collapsing the first time it is stressed.

An acute rupture of the ACL is often accompanied by a 'popping' sensation in the knee. This does not seem to occur with other intra-articular injuries. A patient or onlooker may well describe an acute crack which at the time will often be thought to be a fracture.

The timing of the onset of swelling gives important information as to the nature of the injury. The only structures in the knee with a blood supply are synovium and bone. Articular cartilage and meniscal fibrocartilage are avascular, apart from the periphery of the meniscus, and therefore will not bleed but will produce a reactive effusion in the joint if injured. Bleeding in the knee will usually produce swelling fairly quickly. An intra-articular fracture will produce swelling almost immediately, and bleeding from a torn ACL will usually produce swelling within an hour or two (Fig. 3.2). Swelling developing overnight is more likely to be due to a reactive effusion in the joint as a response to an injury to an avascular structure. If there is a complete capsular or collateral ligament disruption, then the intra-articular swelling

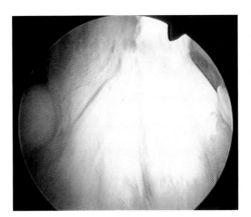

Figure 3.2 – *The vascular synovium overlying the anterior cruciate ligament. When torn, oozing occurs from these vessels causing a clinically detectable haem-arthrosis within 1–2 h.*

may be reduced by the leakage of fluid out of the joint. This must be borne in mind in the initial assessment.

The injury mechanism should be defined as clearly as possible and this may require direct questioning. These injuries occur quickly and at first the patient may find it difficult to recall the exact details, but with patience on the part of the clinician, adequate information can nearly always be obtained.

Examination

Examination of the acutely injured knee is not easy and demands skill and patience if useful information is to be obtained. Pain, swelling and muscle spasm may well obscure physical signs. Every attempt should be made to make the patient comfortable and relaxed.

As well as the injured knee, the overall fitness of the patient must be assessed. Gait and mobility, the use of crutches or a stick and the patient's level of pain are important elements of the overall assessment. On inspection, the degree of swelling and the position taken up by the leg and knee are noted. Fixed flexion may be due to muscle spasm or a true mechanical block such as a fragment of meniscus or an osteochondral fragment at the front of the intercondylar notch. The tibia may appear to 'drop back' on the femur in the flexed knee when the PCL is ruptured or the posterior capsular structures are damaged (Fig. 3.3). An area of visible swelling or bruising may help to localise the site of injury. Skin damage or bruising over the front of the knee or upper tibia implies a direct blow, which should alert the examiner to the possibility of damage to the posterior structures. If possible, the patient should carry out a straight leg raise to confirm that the extensor mechanism is intact, as injuries to the quadriceps and patellar tendons are easily missed.

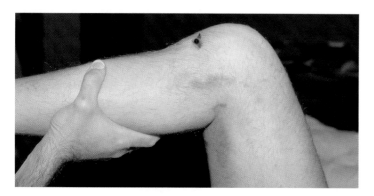

Figure 3.3 – *Posterior cruciate and posterolateral corner injury. The tibia is 'dropped back' on the femur in flexion. Note also the bruising posterolaterally and the abrasion on the front of the knee, evidence of direct trauma likely to lead to damage to the posterior structures.*

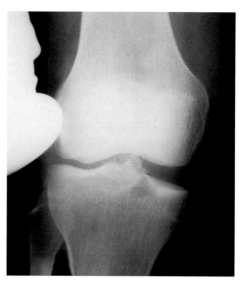

Figure 3.4 – *Stress X-ray of medial collateral ligament rupture. There is also a fracture of the intercondylar eminence of the tibia.*

Palpation of the joint should be carried out in a gentle and systematic manner with particular reference to local tenderness. Tenderness localised to one or other joint line suggests a meniscal lesion; collateral ligament injuries will usually be most tender above or below the joint line, depending on the level of injury. The quadriceps and patellar tendons should be carefully examined for local tenderness; a gap in continuity will indicate a rupture. The patella should be carefully palpated and moved, looking particularly for signs of apprehension on lateral displacement in cases of dislocation or instability. The medial patellar retinaculum will be damaged or torn in acute dislocation and this may lead to visible bruising or tenderness and a palpable gap. The joint should be put carefully through a full passive range of movement, paying particular attention to any fixed flexion, hyperextension or abnormal movement.

The next step is the assessment of instability. Firstly, the uninjured knee is examined to assess what is a normal range of movement and stability for the individual patient.

The collateral ligaments are best assessed at neutral, 20° of flexion and hyperextension if present. By placing the patient's foot on the examiner's hip, the leg is supported and an angulation stress is applied, partly by the hip and partly by the hands, the hands being free to palpate the joint. An objective measurement of laxity can be obtained by a stress X-ray (Fig. 3.4). Comparison with the uninjured side may help if there is doubt as to the degree of instability. The classification using the International Knee Documentation Committee (IKDC) is as follows with the knee at 20° of flexion:

■ Grade A Normal   0 – 2 mm
■ Grade B Nearly Normal   3 – 5 mm
■ Grade C Abnormal   6 – 10 mm
■ Grade D Severely Abnormal   > 10 mm.

Laxity in extension or hyperextension suggests ACL or PCL injury (or both) as well as collateral damage.

There remains considerable confusion regarding the terminology of instability related to the ruptured ACL due to the plethora of tests that have been devised, all with a slightly different name, suggesting differing patterns of instability. The instability is one of anteroposterior translation (demonstrated by the Lachman's test) and also internal rotation/subluxation of the tibia on the femur (demonstrated by the pivot shift test). This has been termed antero–lateral rotatory instability (ALRI), but a much better term to describe the clinical syndrome and all that it encompasses in symptoms and physical signs is ACL deficiency. The most sensitive indicator of a damaged ACL is the Lachman's test at 25° of flexion (Fig. 3.5). With the patient relaxed and comfortable and the femur stabilised, the tibia is gently but firmly drawn forward on the femur. The end point should be graded as hard or soft; a soft end point suggests an ACL rupture with restraint by the more elastic secondary stabilisers. Lachman's test at 25° of flexion is graded by the IKDC with the same values as the collateral ligaments. The pivot shift test originally described by Galway *et al.* [10] can be difficult to implement in the conscious patient, but under anaesthetic it is a very reliable indicator of disabling instability in the knee. The test relies on the

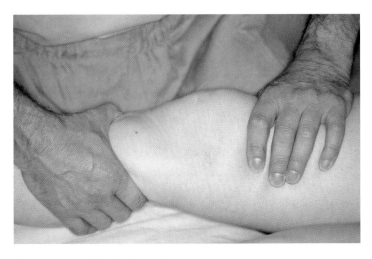

Figure 3.5 – *The Lachman's test.*

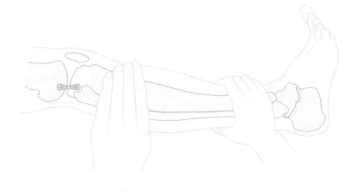

Figure 3.6 – *Diagrammatic representation of the pivot shift. A valgus force is applied over the head of the fibula and the tibia is internally rotated at the ankle while the knee is flexed and extended.*

jerking instability of subluxation predominantly of the lateral tibial plateau. A valgus and internal rotation force is applied to the tibia and as the knee is brought into full extension, the lateral tibial plateau subluxates anteriorly with a clunk (Figs 3.6–3.9). The knee is then flexed and the tibia relocates again with a clunk. Although the subluxation is predominantly lateral, the medial tibial plateau also moves forward, but to a much lesser extent. Therefore the abnormal motion has an element of tibial translation as well as rotation. The degree of jerking instability is also partly dependent on the configuration of the lateral tibial plateau, which varies from individual to individual. In patients with marked convexity of the plateau, the jerk will be more pronounced and the episodes of giving way will therefore be more disabling. The pivot shift test is more difficult to grade than the Lachman's test. The IKDC grading is as follows:

- Grade A Normal   -ve or equivalent to the opposite side
- Grade B Nearly Normal   1+ or glide
- Grade C Abnormal   2+ or clunk
- Grade D Severely Abnormal   3+ or gross.

Assessment of the integrity of the PCL also requires careful assessment of the posterolateral stabilisers, as they are commonly involved and significantly affect the prognosis. Straight posterior laxity is measured by anteroposterior translation at 70° of flexion, the quality of the end point is noted and the instability graded by the IKDC as for the collaterals and the Lachman's. Posterior sag or drop-back of the tibia on the femur at 70° of flexion is best assessed with the two knees flexed

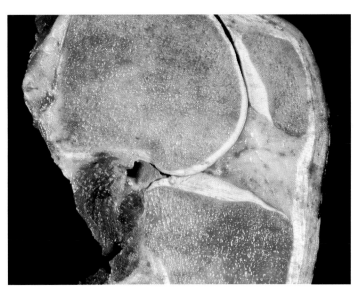

Figure 3.7 – *The pivot shift. At full extension the lateral tibial plateau is subluxated anteriorly on the tibia. It can be readily seen that the lateral meniscus is very vulnerable to damage, as it is squashed between the lateral femoral condyle and the lateral tibial plateau.*

together, so that a direct comparison can be made between the two sides. The reverse pivot shift test, if positive, implies that there is damage to the posterolateral stabilising structures also. A fuller description of these diagnostic tests is given in Chapter 6 on the PCL.

X-ray

Plain X-rays in four planes are essential, particularly in the detection of loose bodies and the examination of the patellofemoral joint. AP, lateral, tunnel and patellar

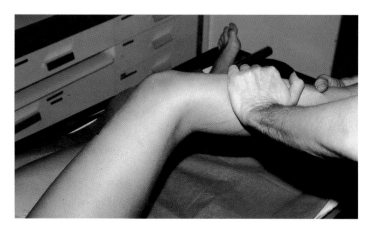

Figure 3.8 – *The pivot shift. Valgus, internal rotation force – tibia reduced.*

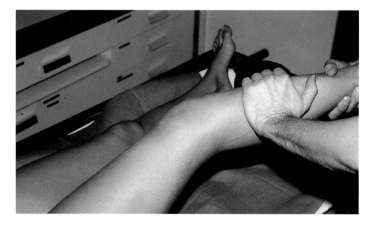

Figure 3.9 – *The pivot shift. Valgus, internal rotation force, knee being extended – subluxation of the tibia, predominantly the lateral tibial plateau.*

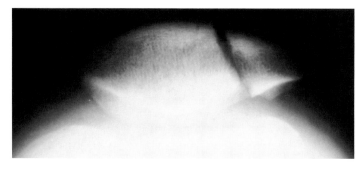

Figure 3.10 – *Intra-articular fracture of the patella visible only on the skyline view.*

skyline are the standard views (Fig. 3.10). The presence or absence of degenerative change is noted. Early changes suggesting pre-existing instability include intercondylar eminence spurring and intercondylar notch narrowing.

The Segond fracture is an avulsion fracture of the lateral tibial condyle and has been described as being frequently associated with an ACL rupture. Computed tomography (CT) scans have shown that the fragment arises from a point midway between Gerdy's tubercle and the head of the fibula [11]. Segond [12] pointed out that the lesion may exist by itself and Irvine *et al.* [11] reported in 1987 that the injury is usually an isolated one and not associated with significant instability.

The lateral notch sign has also been described in ACL insufficiency. There is a normal indentation of the lateral femoral condyle at the junction of the lateral femoral condyle and the patellofemoral joint. An accentuation of this lesion in ACL deficiency has been likened to the Hill–Sachs lesion seen on the posterolateral aspect of the proximal humerus in recurrent anterior shoulder dislocation. If the notch is greater than 2 mm on the lateral X-ray, it is felt to be suggestive of chronic ACL deficiency.

The radiographs must be carefully checked for intra-articular fractures. Fracture of the intercondylar eminence of the tibia commonly occurs in children between the ages of 8 and 15, often due to a fall from a bicycle. The classification by Meyers and McKeever [9] is based on the degree of displacement of the avulsed fragment. In type I fractures there is relatively minor displacement and the knee fully extends. In type II fractures the fragment is attached posteriorly but detached anteriorly, so that it is unstable and hinges upwards and may cause a block to extension. In the type 3 injury, the entire fragment is displaced proximally, detached from its bed and often rotated so that the cancellous surface is pointing anteriorly. This fragment of course has the ACL inserted into it. Similarly, the tibial insertion of the PCL may be avulsed and it is important to remember that this is below the level of the joint line posteriorly.

Osteochondral fractures occur predominantly in adolescents and arise usually from the medial facet of the patella at the time of patellar dislocation, the lateral femoral condyle or more rarely the medial femoral condyle. It may be very difficult to identify an osteochondral fracture on plain X-rays, particularly if the bony element of the fragment is small in comparison with the cartilaginous element. The loose body may well be obscured by overlying bone in the femoral condyles. Patellar skyline and tunnel views are essential, as the fragment may well lie in the suprapatellar pouch or in the intercondylar notch and not be visualised by the AP and lateral views. Other hiding places for loose bodies away from the X-ray beams are the medial and lateral gutters, and the posterior compartments, particularly in relation to the popliteus tendon on the lateral side.

Management considerations

As in any surgical condition, there will be definite and relative indications for surgery.

There is a clear indication for surgery under the following circumstances.

Rupture of quadriceps or patellar tendon

This severe injury will cause a major disability if missed or inadequately treated. As has been previously stated, and it does no harm to repeat this, it is important to be aware of this injury when assessing and examining the patient. Middle-aged and elderly people are prone to ruptures of the quadriceps tendon; rupture of the patellar tendon is much less common and tends to occur in the younger individual. Prompt surgical repair followed by adequate immobilisation in extension and rehabilitation are necessary to obtain a good result in these difficult injuries. The tendons may well be degenerate and some form of reinforcement may be necessary. For the quadriceps a triangular flap of tendon can be turned down distally or the patellar tendon repair can be protected by a Bunnell pull-out wire. The medial and lateral retinacula will also need to be carefully inspected and repaired if necessary.

The locked knee

In a knee that is locked due to a true mechanical block at the front of the intercondylar notch, a definite abnormality will be present in over 90% of cases [13] (Fig. 3.11). If the fixed flexion is not corrected, then a posterior capsular and soft tissue contracture develops and, as time goes by, it becomes increasingly difficult to correct the deformity, even if the intra-articular lesion is dealt with. It is important to differentiate between true mechanical locking and fixed flexion due to hamstring muscle spasm following injury. With a careful and patient examination technique, ensuring that the patient is comfortable and relaxed, the knee that is held in fixed flexion by muscle spasm can usually be coaxed into full extension.

Loose body on plain X-ray

In the acute situation, this will usually be due to an osteochondral fracture. This predominantly occurs on the lateral femoral condyle [8] or from the medial facet

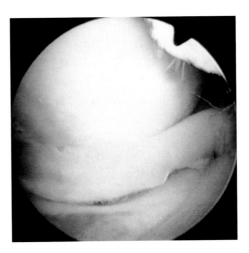

Figure 3.11 – *A displaced 'bucket handle' tear of the medial meniscus causing a mechanical block to full extension.*

of the patella at the time of lateral dislocation. The haemarthrosis is washed out arthroscopically. If the osteochondral fragment is of sufficient size and the diagnosis is made promptly, then it may be possible to reduce and internally fix the fragment with a Herbert screw. If the fragment is small or comminuted, then the loose bodies are removed and the base of the lesion is curetted, cleaned and drilled.

Displaced or unstable intra-articular fractures

A fracture of the tibial spine is essentially an avulsion injury due to the pull of the ACL and if left displaced will cause a mechanical block to extension and instability (Fig. 3.12). Displacement may be due to the anterior horn of one of the menisci (usually the lateral) becoming trapped underneath the fragment. It may be possible to reduce the fragment arthroscopically, although this may

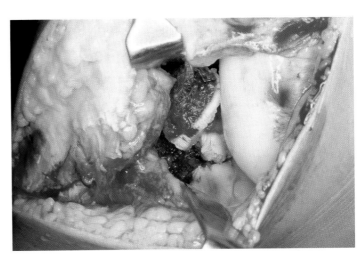

Figure 3.12 – *A displaced comminuted fracture of the tibial spine with the main fragment rotated and pulled proximally by the ACL causing instability and a mechanical block.*

be difficult if there is interposed soft tissue. Once the interposed tissue is cleared away, it is usually relatively simple to reduce the fracture by pushing down and extending the knee. The need for fixation is open to debate. There is some concern that a screw crossing the epiphysis may interfere with growth. The fragment may be fixed with a loop of wire or strong suture passed through drill holes anteriorly proximal to the growth plate. If the fragment is stable in extension once reduced, then some authors feel that fixation is unnecessary and that a period of immobilisation in plaster, in extension, with check X-rays is adequate. In the adult, fixation with a screw is the treatment of choice (Fig. 3.13).

The tibial insertion of the PCL may in a similar way avulse a fragment of bone, and again this will lead to significant instability.

The results of bone fixation are of course better than those of ligament repair, but even after satisfactory bony union has occurred, there may still be a degree of residual instability due to stretching of the involved ligament.

Under other circumstances, the indications for surgery are more open to debate. In the past, these injuries have tended to be treated along expectant lines without a definitive diagnosis being made, and it has been difficult to make a rational plan of treatment. With the development of arthroscopy for chronic knee problems, it is logical that the arthoscope has found a place in the management of acute injury. Early work in

this field was carried out in Scandinavia and North America, predominantly by Gillquist *et al.* [14], Noyes *et al.* [15] and DeHaven [16]. Perhaps the most widely quoted article is that of Noyes, who reported on a prospective series of 85 knees in 83 patients with an acute traumatic haemarthrosis and no or negligible instability on the initial clinical examination [15]. He concluded:

- Acute traumatic haemarthrosis indicates a significant injury.
- Examination under anaesthetic (EUA) plus arthroscopy allows a more accurate diagnosis of injury to joint structures.
- Such data are required for a rational treatment programme to be outlined.

The author has carried out a similar prospective review [17]. Fifty consecutive patients presenting with an acute traumatic haemarthrosis apart from those with significant collateral ligament injury, patellar dislocation or fracture were submitted to EUA and arthroscopy within 2 weeks of injury. The results are summarised in Table 3.1. It can be

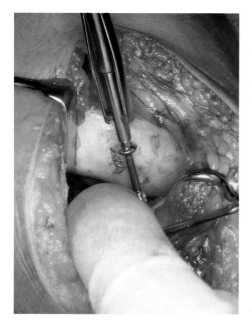

Figure 3.13 – *Reduction and screw fixation of the fragment shown in Figure 3.12.*

Table 3.1 – Injuries in prospective review of 50 cases [17]

	(%)
■ Torn ACL	66
Total rupture	40
Partial rupture	26
■ Torn medial meniscus	10
Peripheral lesion	4
Combined with ACL rupture	6
■ Torn lateral meniscus	12
Peripheral lesion	4
Combined with ACL rupture	8
■ Chondral and osteochondral fracture	8
■ Fractured osteophyte	2
■ Ruptured posterior cruciate ligament	6
■ Capsular or synovial laceration	24
Isolated lesion	14
Combined with ACL rupture	10

seen that these are very significant injuries, with long-term implications regarding the function of the knee if not diagnosed and treated appropriately. Casteleyn *et al.* [18] investigated a prospective series of 100 patients with an acute traumatic haemarthrosis of the knee. All patients had normal X-rays and underwent early EUA and arthroscopy. Only one patient had no serious pathology; in the other 99, a total of 193 lesions was recorded. Thirty knees had only one isolated lesion and 69 knees had combined lesions. Maffuli *et al.* [19] carried out a prospective arthroscopic study of 106 sportsmen presenting with an acute traumatic haemarthrosis of the knee, excluding dislocations of the patella, fractures, extra-articular ligament injuries and significant previous injury. The predominant injury was to the ACL, which was completely ruptured in 43 patients and partially disrupted in 28. There was a plethora of other injuries in the patients with a ruptured ACL, including 17 with meniscal tears, six with cartilaginous loose bodies and 14 with osteochondral fractures. Isolated injuries included osteochondral fractures of the patella, partial and total disruptions of the PCL and cartilaginous loose bodies. In only five patients was no injury detected. The authors concluded that an acute traumatic haemarthrosis indicates a serious ligament injury until proven otherwise, and that arthroscopy is needed to complement careful history and clinical examination. They recommended that all cases with a tense effusion developing within 12 hours of injury should have an aspiration and, if a haemarthrosis is confirmed, then urgent admission and arthroscopy are indicated.

What then are the risks and benefits of EUA and arthroscopy in the acutely injured knee?

The risks
There are, of course, minor risks present in any operative procedure under a general anaesthetic and there will inevitably be a recovery period which will cause a degree of inconvenience to the patient.

If there is a significant collateral ligament injury or capsular disruption, then there is a risk of leakage of irrigation fluid into the fascial compartments of the calf and thigh, which may cause a compartment syndrome. Clearly, it is important to carry out a preliminary EUA.

The benefits
Firstly, it is very important to emphasise that it is EUA and arthroscopy that are being considered here, not just arthroscopy.

EUA allows a full and accurate assessment of the pattern of instability. It can be very difficult to obtain a valid assessment when examining the conscious patient, as pain and muscle spasm may well obscure abnormal motion patterns, particularly the pivot shift or reverse pivot shift tests, and it is on these tests that the plan of management frequently relies.

The joint can be thoroughly irrigated and all the blood washed out; this reduces pain and synovitis and facilitates early rehabilitation, particularly regarding range of movement. Complete removal of the haemarthrosis or effusion can never be achieved by aspiration alone.

Intra-articular damage is evaluated by arthroscopy and appropriate arthroscopic surgery carried out. There may well be more than one lesion, and clinical assessment alone will not be able to give a comprehensive diagnosis.

A clear prognosis and treatment plan can be determined.

Each patient is an individual and should be treated as such, with the treatment tailored to individual needs and circumstances.

The role of MRI
MRI gives a non-invasive picture of intra- and extra-articular injury and has become increasingly used, particularly in the management of chronic joint disorders. As with every investigation, there are advantages and disadvantages. In the acutely injured knee, the MRI gives a static assessment of what is a dynamic problem (Fig. 3.14) and although there is an accurate anatomical image of soft tissue injury, the degree of instability in the joint cannot be fully assessed; only an EUA will do this. MRI has other drawbacks; it can be difficult to judge the extent of the ACL injury, there are false positives in the posterior horn of the medial meniscus, it can be difficult to image articular cartilage damage and a peripheral detachment of the lateral meniscus can cause confusion [20]. There is also the practical problem in many areas of obtaining urgent scans in Health Service practice.

Tips and pitfalls of EUA/arthoscopy in the acutely injured knee
EUA and arthroscopy in the acutely injured knee is not easy and there are pitfalls. Unless the surgical and nursing staff are experienced in arthroscopic techniques and there is adequate equipment, it may be very difficult

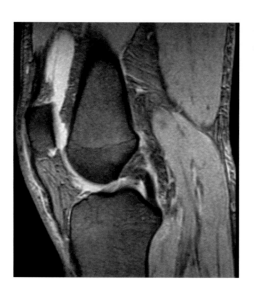

Figure 3.14 –
Ruptured ACL.

to visualise the interior of the knee joint adequately. This is clearly not a true surgical emergency and ideally should be carried out on a consultant-led trauma list during the daytime. There is a high demand on skill, experience, equipment and technology and it is quite wrong for inexperienced staff to be carrying out this type of surgery out of hours or at weekends. If appropriate facilities are not available then the knee can be aspirated under sterile conditions and an MRI carried out.

The EUA should be carried out after aspiration of the haemarthrosis, as a large quantity of blood in the knee may obscure the instability pattern. Also, it should be carried out before the tourniquet is inflated, as this tends to stabilise the knee by tethering the fascia lata and thigh muscles and can lead to a false impression of stability. As stated previously, if there is significant collateral instability, then either a decision should be made not to proceed to arthroscopy or great care should be taken to minimise and monitor the flow of irrigation fluid and observe the calf and thigh for signs of increasing compartment pressure. After the EUA, arthroscopy is carried out. It is necessary to wash out all the blood and this may require some degree of patience on the part of the operating surgeon. It is better initially to irrigate the knee through the sheath of the arthroscope without the telescope inserted, as the inflow down the empty sheath will be much greater. Once the knee has been filled with fluid, it is squeezed empty and again it is better to empty the knee through the empty sheath, particularly as blood clots may block up the outflow cannula and drainage tubes. A pump is helpful but not essential; adequate inflow can usually be obtained using a 3-litre bag with the stand as high as possible. It may be necessary to wash

2–3 litres of fluid through the knee before a clear view is obtained. If there is continued bleeding, then a pump is useful or a second 3-litre bag with a separate inflow cannula can be set up. There should be free drainage through an adequate outflow cannula. If this is connected to suction, then the synovium around the cannula may be sucked into the cannula itself and obscure the outflow. All intra-articular structures must be carefully visualised and probed systematically. The posterior horns of the menisci must be fully visualised and carefully assessed for instability, looking for peripheral detachments when a haemarthrosis is present, particularly if there is no other obvious cause for the bleeding. The ACL is examined for evidence of complete or partial rupture (Figs 3.15, 3.16). Again, probing is essential, the ruptured ligament may be covered by an intact synovial sheath or pseudosheath and the pathology only becomes apparent when the overlying tissue is separated with a probe (Fig. 3.17).

A situation which may cause diagnostic confusion occurs when the ACL has been previously torn at its femoral origin and the proximal end of the stump has become adherent to the PCL. At first glance, the ligament appears to be intact but on closer inspection it is

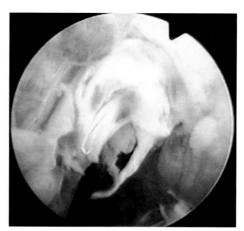

Figure 3.15 –
Complete rupture of ACL.

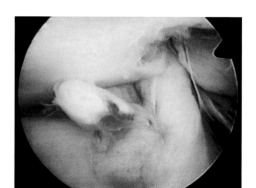

Figure 3.16 –
Partial rupture of ACL.

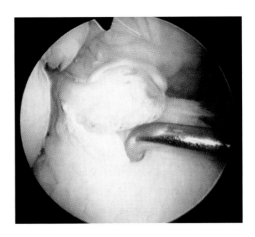

Figure 3.17 – *Ruptured ACL initially obscured by intact synovial sheath. Sheath being opened by a probe.*

apparent that the posterolateral wall of the intercondylar notch is empty and also the PCL is clearly visible at its femoral origin, as it is no longer obscured by the ACL (Fig. 3.18).

The articular cartilage must be carefully examined, particularly in areas vulnerable to osteochondral fractures – the lateral femoral condyle and the medial facet of the patella.

It is essential that documentation is accurate and thorough, as this is an invasive procedure which therefore must provide valid information. Also, once the arthroscope has been taken out of the knee and the patient woken up, there is no chance of a second look to check on things. Everyday diagnostic and investigative procedures such as X-ray and MRI produce a hard copy of the findings for future reference, and video printers are now available which produce an excellent record of the TV image. This is useful not only for the surgeon, but also for explaining the nature and effects of the injury to the patient.

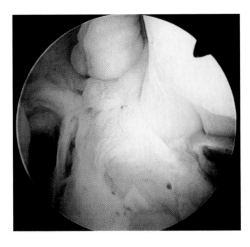

Figure 3.18 – *Ruptured ACL at the femoral attachment. The stump has become adherent to the PCL. The posterolateral intercondylar notch is empty and the femoral origin of the PCL is no longer obscured by the normally sited ACL.*

The management of individual lesions

A detailed description of the complete spectrum of knee injuries is beyond the scope of this chapter, but some general principles can be considered.

Clearly, any loose or unstable intra-articular lesions should be dealt with by either removal or repair. Only fragments of meniscus or articular cartilage that are demonstrably loose or unstable should be removed [21,22] and the surgeon should err on the side of conservatism.

Meniscal repair is carried out if indicated (see Chapter 10) (Figs 3.19, 3.20).

The management of the torn medial collateral ligament (MCL) has changed in recent years. Traditionally repair was recommended for a complete (Grade D) injury, but it is now widely accepted that a satisfactory result will be obtained with non-operative treatment in the form of functional bracing and appropriate rehabilitation [23–25]. This is the case for both isolated MCL ruptures and ruptures in association with ACL injuries [26].

Treatment of lateral complex injuries is considerably more challenging, particularly when these occur in association with a torn PCL. As well as the lateral collateral ligament injury, the other supporting structures are frequently damaged. The popliteus, popliteofibular ligament and arcuate complex may be torn. The fascia lata may be stretched or damaged and the biceps tendon may be avulsed from the head of the fibula. The lateral head of the gastrocnemius may be damaged. Primary repair of these injured structures may not be successful because of the extent of the soft tissue damage. If adequate stability is not obtained with a primary repair, then some form of augmentation will be required. No one procedure is accepted as providing all the answers. Hughston and Jacobsen [27] described an advancement of the arcuate ligament, together with the lateral collateral ligament and popliteus tendon. The soft tissue complex is advanced with a bone block on the distal femur. In the rare cases where the lesion is distal, the attachment of the arcuate ligament to the tibia and fibula is stabilised. Clancy *et al.* [28] have described a procedure whereby the biceps femoris tendon is rerouted and inserted into the lateral femoral condyle with a screw after careful identification and protection of the lateral popliteal nerve. This has the effect of eliminating the deforming pull of external tibial rotation by the biceps femoris muscle, and the transfer into the femur has the static effect of recreating the fibular collateral ligament. Also, because the biceps fibres are inserted into

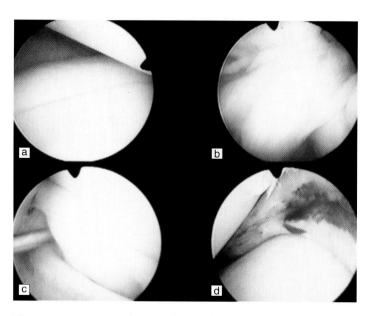

Figure 3.19 – *Acute haemarthrosis. (a) Normal medial meniscus; (b) normal ACL; (c) displaced peripheral detachment of lateral meniscus and (d) site of detachment with bleeding.*

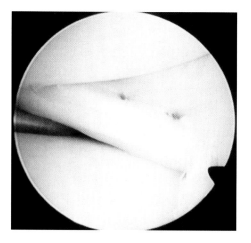

Figure 3.20 – *Peripheral detachment in Figure 3.19 repaired. Probe testing stability.*

the deep inferior posterolateral arcuate complex, moving the tendon forward tightens the fibres and thus strengthens the posterolateral capsule. More recently there has been enthusiasm for recreating the posterolateral corner with either autograft or allograft [29]. The reconstruction may also need to be supplemented by a valgus tibial osteotomy. Clearly, this is a very serious injury and a difficult problem, to which there is no definite surgical answer at the present time.

There is of course continued debate regarding indications for and timing of surgery for acute ruptures of the ACL. Risk factors are age, the degree of instability, particularly the presence or absence of a positive pivot shift, the extent of participation in level 1 and 2 sports

and the presence or absence of repairable meniscal lesions. Level 1 sports involve jumping, pivoting and hard cutting such as in basketball, soccer or American football. Level 2 sports involve lateral motion with less jumping or hard cutting than level 1, such as in racquet sports, skiing or baseball. These factors must be carefully weighed up in the decision making. In current practice, reconstructive surgery is normally recommended primarily in the young, active patient who wishes to continue in level 1 or 2 sport if the pivot shift is positive. A repairable meniscal lesion requires a stable knee for a satisfactory result and is therefore a strong indication for reconstruction.

When the problem of limitation of motion following ACL reconstruction was first addressed, it was felt that early surgery, before the inflammatory reaction from the injury had settled down, predisposed towards this problem. Mohtadi *et al.* [30] reviewed 527 ACL reconstructions in which 37 patients had problems with limitation of motion. There was a statistically significant association between loss of motion and early surgery; the odds of getting knee stiffness were 2.85 times higher if operations were performed within 2 weeks, with a corresponding trend for patients operated on within the first 6 weeks following injury. Shelbourne *et al.* [31] carried out a retrospective study of 169 acute ACL reconstructions. The patients undergoing reconstruction within a week of injury had a statistically significantly increased incidence of arthrofibrosis compared with patients whose reconstruction was delayed for 21 days or more. It was concluded that it was unwise to compound the trauma of the injury with the trauma of surgery, and the knee should be allowed to recover from the injury and regain a satisfactory range of movement with full passive extension, together with early muscle control. Harner *et al.* [32] also reported a statistically significant increase in loss of motion in patients having early surgery, 37.2% in the early group (before 4 weeks) and 5.5% in the late group (after 4 weeks). More recently, this view has been challenged. Marcacci *et al.* [33] reported on two groups of patients having ACL reconstructions, 23 patients were treated within 15 days of injury and 59 patients were treated more than 3 months after injury. They found that the patients who had early reconstructions returned to sporting activities quicker and overall had better results. Following an early aggressive rehabilitation programme, there was certainly no increase in loss of motion problems in the patients having early surgery. Majors and Woodfin [34] reviewed 119 consecutive ACL reconstructions and concluded that the time from injury to surgery had no effect on range of motion; in fact, the only patients in this series with slight decrease in range of movement had late surgery. Twenty-one patients had early surgery and all obtained 0° of knee extension or better and 135° of knee flexion or better. In a prospective comparison of three techniques for reconstruction of the ACL, O'Neill [35] reported that there was no significant difference in outcome between the patients having surgery early (within 3 weeks of injury) and those having surgery at a later date.

There is a more conservative approach to the treatment of ruptures of the PCL. This is described in more detail in Chapter 6 on PCL injury. Essentially, displaced bony avulsions are treated with open reduction and internal fixation. When the PCL rupture is combined with a lateral complex injury, then surgery is advisable. An isolated rupture of the PCL is usually treated conservatively initially, reserving surgery for cases of significant long-term instability.

Summary and conclusions

The acutely injured knee usually occurs in the young active individual. Problems remain in the UK regarding the diagnosis and early management of these injuries and if untreated or inadequately treated, there is the potential for significant long-term disability. It is important to secure an early diagnosis and then embark upon a rational programme of treatment. As with every other medical and surgical condition, history and examination are the cornerstones of diagnosis and further measures often serve only to confirm the clinical diagnosis. Frequently the injury is non-contact, which may lull the primary treating physician into a false sense of security regarding the magnitude of the injury. As in other surgical problems, there are clear indications for surgery. However, in the majority of patients a rational decision regarding treatment needs to be made based on an overall assessment of the patient and the nature of the injury. Surgical management should be carried out by a surgeon experienced in these problems with appropriate backup and facilities.

Key points

1. Acute traumatic haemarthrosis implies a significant injury usually in a young, active patient.
2. Untreated or inadequately treated, these injuries can lead to a long-term disability.
3. It is important to secure a full and early diagnosis.
4. History and examination are the cornerstones of diagnosis.
5. Most injuries are non-contact.
6. There are definite and relative indications for surgery.
7. Decision making depends on careful assessment of the patient and the injury.
8. Arthroscopy and reconstructive surgery require an experienced surgeon, experienced theatre staff and adequate equipment.

CHAPTER 4

The stiff knee following anterior cruciate ligament reconstruction

R. L. Allum

Introduction

As one of the prime functions of a joint is mobility, any loss of movement following injury or surgery is bound to lead to a significant disability. Patients requiring anterior cruciate ligament (ACL) reconstruction are almost invariably involved in significant athletic activity and will therefore need maximum flexibility in the knees. Even if the knee is perfectly stable postoperatively, a patient with significant limitation of motion may well be unable to return to his or her sport. Loss of extension causes particular problems, not only during sport but in normal gait and function. Knee flexion less than 125° interferes with functional activities such as sitting, squatting, stair climbing and more vigorous activity such as running. Loss of motion, particularly extension, also leads to other problems. There is an increased incidence of patellofemoral problems with anterior knee pain and painful patellofemoral crepitus. Rehabilitation is obviously slower, and return to physical activity both at work and on the sports field will be delayed. The gait pattern never returns to normal and muscle function recovers slowly and incompletely.

In the literature, the definition of loss of extension varies between 5° and 10°, while loss of flexion varies between 125° and 130° [1–5]. The incidence of problems therefore varies depending on the definition, but loss of motion problems have been reported in up to 24% of cases [3]. Sachs *et al.* [3] carried out a survey of 50 prominent knee surgeons who had published in the field of ACL reconstruction. From the 40 who replied, flexion contracture was the most common complication following ligament surgery. This condition is associated with a high level of patient dissatisfaction and it is also

very frustrating for the surgeon and physiotherapist. Treatment is difficult, requiring a lot of hard work on the part of the patient, and progress is usually painfully slow. Shelbourne *et al.* have devised a classification of arthrofibrosis based on a review of 72 patients [6]. Four types are described:

- Type 1 is < 10° extension loss, normal flexion.
- Type 2 is > 10° extension loss, normal flexion.
- Type 3 is > 10° extension loss, > 25° flexion loss with a tight patella.
- Type 4 is > 10° extension loss, 30° or more flexion loss and patella infera with marked patellar tightness.

Predisposing factors

The problem is multi-factorial and a number of possible risk factors have been identified.

Age
Inevitably, the older patient will recover less quickly from reconstructive surgery due to age-related changes in connective tissue, such as increased stiffness and decreased elasticity. There may be a greater risk of loss of motion in the middle-aged patient when compared with the younger patient.

Sex
A higher incidence of loss of motion has been reported in men [5], but there is no obvious explanation for this and it is not a consistent finding in the literature.

Early surgery
A number of authors have reported on the increased incidence of loss of motion following surgery in the

acute stage following injury. Harner *et al.* [5] reported that 16 of 43 patients (37.2%) undergoing reconstruction within 4 weeks of injury developed loss of motion, whereas only 11 of 201 patients (5.5%) developed this problem when surgery was delayed. This was statistically significant with a *p* value of < 0.001. Mohtadi *et al.* [7] demonstrated a statistically significant association between ACL reconstructions performed less than 2 weeks after injury and limitation of motion. The odds of loss of motion were 2.85 times higher if surgery was carried out within 2 weeks of injury, and there was also a trend for patients having surgery within 6 weeks of injury to develop problems with loss of motion. Similarly Shelbourne *et al.* [8], in a retrospective review of 169 acute ACL reconstructions, found that patients whose ligaments were reconstructed within the first week after injury had a statistically significant increased incidence of loss of motion when compared with patients who had their ACL reconstructions 3 weeks or later post-injury. The patients who had their ACL reconstructions between 8 days and 3 weeks post-injury had a similar incidence of stiffness to the early group when they followed a conventional rehabilitation programme, but only a small percentage of cases developed motion problems when they followed an accelerated rehabilitation programme.

ACL reconstruction, even when carried out arthroscopically, remains a major intra-articular surgical procedure which will inevitably set up an inflammatory and healing reaction in the joint. It has therefore been felt that if the joint is already inflamed from the effects of the acute injury, then recovery from surgery is likely to be slow and there will be a much greater risk of stiffness and associated problems. However, this line of thinking has more recently been thrown into question. Majors and Woodfin [9] presented a retrospective series of 111 arthroscopic intra-articular reconstructions and showed that the time from injury to surgery (early versus delayed) did not make a difference in obtaining a full range of motion; indeed, only patients with late surgery had a slight decrease in range of motion. Marcacci *et al.* [10] reported similar findings, and O'Neill [11], in a prospective randomised analysis of three techniques for ACL reconstruction (two incision hamstring grafts, two incision patellar tendon grafts and single incision endoscopic technique patellar tendon grafts) stated that with the numbers available there was no significant difference in outcome between acute reconstructions performed less than 3 weeks after the injury and later ones, regardless of the technique used.

It would seem wise, however, to ensure that preoperatively the knee was in an appropriate condition for surgery with minimal swelling and a satisfactory range of movement, particularly full extension, and it would seem to be of importance to follow an early and aggressive rehabilitation regime.

Concomitant injury

Inevitably, there will be an increased incidence of loss of motion when other injury has occurred to the joint. Meniscal injury may require partial meniscectomy or meniscal repair. Collateral ligament injury may require a surgical reconstruction or conservative measures with a period of immobilisation. Capsular and soft tissue contracture may occur as a result of these injuries, particularly in the posteromedial capsule following injury to the medial collateral ligament (MCL).

Additional surgery

If the intra-articular procedure is supplemented by an extra-articular procedure, such as a fascia lata tenodesis or a meniscal repair which may in itself require a period of immobilisation, then there will be an increased risk of loss of motion. It has been suggested that patients having an ACL reconstruction carried out through an arthrotomy are more likely to develop range of movement problems than those having arthroscopically assisted surgery, but there has been no conclusive proof of this.

Errors in graft placement and impingement in ACL reconstructive surgery

It is obviously of prime importance to replace the ACL anatomically so that its function can be accurately reproduced. If the graft is sited wrongly, then not only will the stability be compromised, but the range of movement of the knee will be affected. The inexperienced surgeon is likely to site the femoral tunnel too far forward in the intercondylar notch and this will lead to restriction of flexion. Because this creates an anatomical block to movement, flexion can then only be regained by either stretching or rupture of the graft with consequent loss of stability. If the tibial tunnel is placed too anteriorly, then the intra-articular portion of the graft is likely to impinge on the roof of the intercondylar notch and this will limit extension. Inadequate notchplasty will have a similar effect, particularly if a bulky construct such as a four-strand hamstring graft is used. Howell *et al.* [12] carried out an MRI study to analyse the relationship between tibial tunnel placement and impingement. The tibial insertion of the ACL is nearly twice as deep in the sagittal plane as the proximal half of the ligament; it fans out to accommodate the undulating contour of the intercondylar roof. This broad tibial insertion means that the drill hole position may be incorrect if imprecise. Because of the discrepancy between the size of the graft emerging from the drill hole and the insertion of the original ligament, a compromise must be made in siting the tunnel. Positioning the graft within the centre of the ACL insertion would require resection of 2–3 mm of bone from the roof of the intercondylar notch in order to avoid impingement, according to Howell's study. If the tunnel was sited eccentrically, more anteriorly, then up to 5–6 mm of bone would need to be resected. Positioning the graft within the bulk of the ACL fibres 3 mm posterior to the centre of the original insertion would require little or no bone resection to prevent impingement. If the knee hyperextends preoperatively, then it may be necessary to resect more bone. The need for notchplasty is not universally agreed and the size of the graft is also a factor, but this study illustrates the importance of correct positioning of the tibial tunnel, particularly avoiding too anterior a position, despite the fact that the drill appears to be emerging through the stump of the ACL. In a further study, Howell and Barad [13] have shown radiologically that there is a variability in the slope of the intercondylar roof. The more vertical the slope of the intercondylar roof, the more likely impingement will occur. The combination of a vertical intercondylar roof and a knee that hyperextends is defined as an 'unforgiving knee', and in these cases it is particularly important to position the tibial tunnel as far posteriorly as possible.

A build-up of scar tissue may occur at the front of the intercondylar notch. Jackson and Schaefer [14] have described the so-called 'cyclops' lesion. This is a fibrous nodule that forms anterior to the ACL graft and the intra-articular opening of the tibial tunnel. It has a head-like appearance with a vascular colouration (Fig. 4.1). Venous channels on the surface may appear as 'blue eyes' at arthroscopy. Histologically, there is vascular granulation tissue in the centre surrounded by a mature well-organised fibrous capsule. Occasionally cartilaginous or bony tissue may develop. It is usually associated with a clunk on terminal extension. Clinically, four different patterns have been described. In type 1, there is a clunk at terminal extension only; in type 2, there is associated loss of extension that resolves after

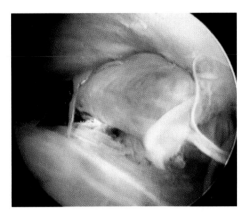

Figure 4.1 – *The 'cyclops' lesion.*

warm-up exercises. A more advanced lesion causes a degree of fixed flexion (type 3) and in the most severe lesions (type 4), there is a more global restriction of movement and extensive fibrous proliferation in the intercondylar notch with associated more widespread knee arthrofibrosis. The lesion is produced by excessive scar tissue at the front of the intercondylar notch, this may be residual scar tissue from the ACL stump or tissue and other debris produced by drilling the tibial tunnel. The cannulated drill enters the knee obliquely and this tends to produce a flap or trapdoor of cartilage. Drilling debris may remain attached to the anterior horn of the lateral meniscus and the joint surface. When the drill is withdrawn from the tunnel, the trapdoor of tissue tends to flap back, preventing debris from being washed out of the knee. As the graft is then pulled through the knee, the flap of tissue is pushed back into the joint and this acts as a potential nidus for the build-up of scar tissue.

Infection
Postoperative infection will inevitably lead to an increased incidence of stiffness.

Inadequate rehabilitation programme
Obviously an adequate and appropriate rehabilitation programme is of prime importance in regaining function following major knee surgery. A number of authors, notably Shelbourne and Nitz [15], have stressed the importance of early aggressive rehabilitation and the avoidance of prolonged immobilisation. It is particularly important to regain full extension immediately following surgery, and it has been postulated that an early fixed flexion deformity will create a potential space at the front of the intercondylar notch which will allow the formation of scar tissue, such as the cyclops lesion. It is therefore of fundamental importance to ensure that

full extension is achieved and maintained following surgery and similarly that a satisfactory range of flexion is achieved and maintained.

In addition to the above risk factors, two other conditions occur which can cause disabling post-operative knee stiffness and are difficult to manage.

The infrapatellar contracture syndrome

Paulos *et al.* [16,17] have reported on a group of patients with a combination of pain, significant loss of movement and reduced patellar mobility following anterior cruciate ligament reconstruction. All patients demonstrated a significant lack of extension ranging from 7 to 35° of fixed flexion. Knee flexion ranged from 60 to 139°. Other physical signs included moderate to severe quadriceps atrophy, an antalgic gait and patellofemoral crepitus. The patellar tendon shelf sign was described. A shelf appeared at the distal attachment of the patellar tendon due to induration around the tendon creating a step off at the tibial tubercle. There was significant loss of patellar mobility. There was shortening of the patellar tendon with obvious patella infera in 16% of cases. On X-rays, there was disuse atrophy in the patellofemoral joint in most cases. Patella infera was usually associated with joint space narrowing and osteophyte formation. O'Brien *et al.* [18] reported that following ACL reconstruction, 55% of the knees had an average of 20% shortening of the patellar tendon (range 10–50%). This had a bearing on patellar pain; 10% shortening was associated with an 18% incidence of patellar pain, 20–30% shortening with a 30% incidence and 40% shortening with a 50% incidence. Dandy and Desai [19] have also described changes in patellar tendon length after ACL reconstruction, using both the medial third of the patellar tendon as a free graft and the Leeds–Keio ligament. It was concluded that surgical exposure with dissection and retraction of the patellar tendon was partly responsible for the contracture. Clearly, the patellar tendon and tissues adjacent to it, including the anterior capsule and fat pad, are vulnerable to the trauma of graft harvest and intra-articular surgery. Management of this condition is difficult, and the natural history of an ACL-deficient knee appears to be more benign than the natural history of a knee that develops the infrapatellar contracture syndrome.

Complex regional pain syndrome I (formerly reflex sympathetic dystrophy)

This condition should always be kept in mind when a knee is failing to progress satisfactorily following injury or surgery. Its occurrence is not specifically related to ACL reconstruction. The predominant problem is pain out of proportion to the injury or operation, together with hypersensitivity or vasomotor disturbances. Stiffness may also be a feature, particularly fixed flexion. For a more detailed description of this problem, see Chapter 12.

Management of the patient with loss of motion

Prevention

Management of the established case can be a very difficult clinical challenge. Prevention is in many ways better than cure; it is easier, requires much less time and considerably less in the way of resources. Each individual patient must therefore be carefully assessed pre-operatively for possible risk factors and preventative measures taken as follows.

Age

The older patient may be more susceptible to loss of movement. This should be considered when the risks and benefits of surgery are being discussed. Special attention needs to be given postoperatively to ensure that a full range of movement is restored at as early a stage as possible in this group of patients.

Timing of surgery

Although the evidence in the literature is not entirely conclusive, it would seem to be wise to wait until the inflammatory reaction in the joint has settled down following the injury. It is difficult to give a precise length of time, as the rate of recovery varies from patient to patient. The knee should be pain free and any effusion present should have settled. There should be virtually a full range of movement, particularly full extension. The knee is then said to be 'quiet'. This usually takes between 3 and 6 weeks. Often work and other commitments mean that early surgery is not feasible, and in National Health Service practice in the UK there is almost always a delay. RICE (rest, ice, compression, elevation), non-steroidal anti-inflammatories (NSAIDs) and appropriate physiotherapy will accelerate the return of the joint to normality. Shelbourne and Foulk [20] have shown that delaying surgery in this way also has the advantage of a more rapid return of quadriceps muscle strength. The patient can also be prepared psychologically for what is a major surgical procedure, even when carried out arthroscopically. Preoperative instruction in exercises and the rehabilitation regime will facilitate the postoperative rehabilitation.

Concomitant injury

In addition to the ACL rupture, there may also be injury to the menisci, the collateral ligaments, the posterior cruciate ligament (PCL), the patellofemoral joint and the articular cartilage of the knee. The force required to rupture the ACL is a severe one and it is not surprising, therefore, that other structures are vulnerable. The occurrence of the bone bruise as a frequent magnetic resonance imaging (MRI) finding following ACL injury is confirmation that the joint itself is subject to significant trauma.

There is no evidence that delaying meniscal surgery has a harmful effect, and the results of repair are probably not prejudiced by delay. Indeed, a proportion of acute peripheral meniscal tears occurring at the time of injury to the ACL may well have the capacity to heal spontaneously. The haemarthrosis and inflammatory response to the acute injury creates an ideal environment for healing. An aggressive attitude towards meniscal repair at an early stage may result in unnecessary procedures being carried out, and it has been noted that some acute peripheral tears have healed when the arthroscopy is repeated at the time of ACL reconstruction. Fitzgibbons and Shelbourne [21] have shown that certain types of lateral meniscal tear can be left alone at the time of ACL reconstruction without causing later symptoms. These are posterior horn avulsion tears, vertical tears posterior to the popliteus tendon and stable longitudinal tears usually of one surface only. This may, of course, partly explain the success of meniscal repair at the time of ACL reconstruction. It may be that stabilising the knee reduces the stress on the meniscus and the tear then either heals or remains mechanically stable. The only situation where early surgery must be seriously considered occurs when the knee is locked due to a displaced bucket-handle meniscal tear. The mechanical block needs to be dealt with before a fixed flexion deformity develops. Shelbourne and Johnson [22] have recommended a two-stage procedure with a partial meniscectomy or meniscal repair, followed by ACL reconstruction when the knee has recovered from the initial surgery. This is reported as giving several advantages – the more aggressive use of repair, the prevention of problems in regaining range of movement,

a second look to judge the success of the meniscal repair and time for the patient to prepare for ACL reconstruction physically, academically, mentally and socially. Certainly, a major surgical reconstruction carried out in a locked knee carries a significant risk of limitation of motion. Care should be taken when carrying out an 'in-to-out' meniscal repair not to tie the sutures with the knee flexed, particularly on the medial side, as this will cause restriction of extension due to tethering of the capsule.

MCL injuries not uncommonly occur in association with the ruptured ACL. In recent years, the approach to this injury has become more conservative. There appears to be no advantage in surgical repair of the MCL in association with an ACL rupture [23,24]. Certainly, there is a risk with open surgery to the MCL and the posteromedial capsule that postoperative scarring may lead to difficulty in regaining a full range of movement, particularly extension.

There are few reports in the literature regarding combined ACL and PCL injuries and ACL and lateral complex injuries. In these more severe injuries, recurrent instability is more likely to be a problem than limitation of motion, and the advantages of early repair may outweigh the risks of limitation of movement.

An extra-articular lateral tenodesis has been used by some authors to supplement an intra-articular graft, but there is no firm evidence that this confers any additional stability to an appropriate intra-articular graft, positioned anatomically and isometrically. At the present time, given the risk of postoperative stiffness, there does not seem to be a specific indication for this procedure.

Surgical technique

It is essential that the ACL graft is sited in the correct position. In recent years, there has been hot debate regarding the issue of isometric positioning of the graft. As the graft is usually at least 9 or 10 mm in width, there is no one single isometric position. It is, however, important to position the graft as near as possible to the isometric points on the tibia and femur.

The most common fault in the learning curve is too anterior a placement of the femoral tunnel. The architecture of the intercondylar notch may well be altered by osteophytes and scar tissue which have formed as a response to instability, particularly in UK practice, where a significant proportion of patients present at a relatively late stage following injury. It is essential to determine without question the back of the intercondylar notch. The so-called 'residents ridge' approximately 1 cm in front of the posterior edge of the intercondylar notch may cause confusion to the inexperienced; this is a ridge of bone which initially appears to represent the back of the intercondylar notch, but on probing it becomes clear that there is more bone posteriorly. Defining the anatomy is easier with modern arthroscopic equipment and certainly there are advantages over conventional open surgery. If the notch is narrowed, then an arthroscopic osteotome passed from the medial portal will open up the front of the intercondylar notch (Fig. 4.2) on the lateral side. The posterior part of the fat pad can be removed with a shaver, so that the arthroscope can be backed up for a clearer panorama of the intercondylar notch. Using a combination of hand instruments, soft tissue shavers and bony burrs, the lateral wall of the intercondylar notch is cleared until a probe can be passed over the back without any doubt (Fig. 4.3). As in all arthroscopic surgery, observation must be reinforced by palpation and there is no substitute to feeling the probe pass out over the back of the notch. This feels completely different from the probe passing over the resident's ridge. A

1–2 mm bridge of bone only should be left at the posterior edge of the femoral tunnel and commercially available drill guides can be used for this important step (Figs 4.4, 4.5). The tunnel is drilled at the 11 o'clock position in the right knee and the 1 o'clock position in the left knee. Failure adequately to visualise the posterior end of the intercondylar notch may result in too anterior a position of the femoral tunnel, which will restrict flexion or lead to graft stretching and rupture.

Less emphasis in the past has been placed on the site of the tibial tunnel, but it is of equal importance. The reference points for the intra-articular opening of the tibial tunnel are the PCL, the anterior horn of the lateral meniscus and the ACL stump. The tip of the guide wire should emerge level with the posterior edge of the anterior horn of the lateral meniscus, which is 5–7 mm anterior to the anterior attachment of the PCL. The hole should be drilled through the posterior part of the ACL stump if still visible (Fig. 4.6). If the drill hole is anterior to this point, then impingement may occur on the roof of the intercondylar notch, causing limitation of extension. Again, commercially produced drill guides are available. Care must be taken to ensure that the tip of the drill guide is placed far enough posteriorly; commonly the guide is designed so that the guide wire hits the 'axilla' of the intra-articular portion rather than the tip, and this may produce a tunnel that is too far anterior.

It is important to clear away all soft tissue from the anterior end of the intercondylar notch at this stage. Drilling the tibial tunnel will usually produce a trapdoor

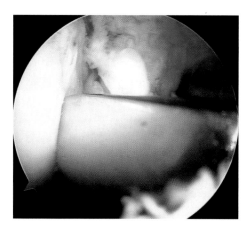

Figure 4.2 – *Osteotome from medial portal opening up the front of the intercondylar notch.*

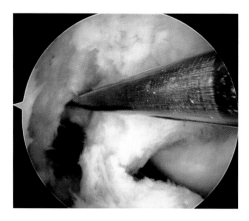

Figure 4.3 – *Defining the back of the intercondylar notch with a probe, feeling the probe dip down over the back of the notch.*

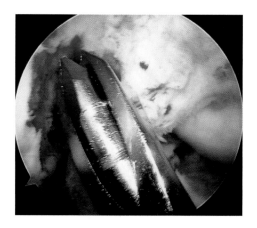

Figure 4.4 – *Femoral drill guide positioning the guide wire in the correct position at the back of the intercondylar notch; the guide hooks over the back of the notch and the channel for the guide wire is offset at a variable distance, usually 5–7 mm, to leave a bridge of the bone when the hole is drilled, usually 9–11 mm.*

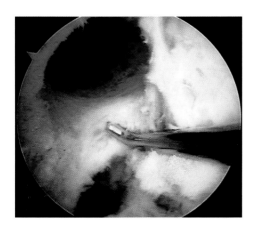

Figure 4.5 – *Femoral tunnel with 1 mm bridge of bone posteriorly. A small cuff of soft tissue remains posteriorly; the probe defines the bony margin.*

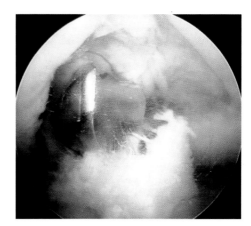

Figure 4.7 – *Tibial drill breaking through into the joint, showing a trapdoor of tissue being raised.*

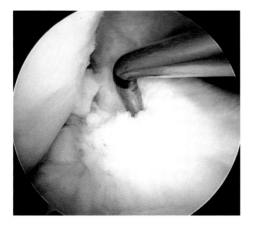

Figure 4.6 – *Tibial drill guide in posterior part of ACL insertion. The posterior edge of the anteior horn of the lateral meniscus is seen in the bottom left-hand corner and the guide wire must emerge level or posterior to this.*

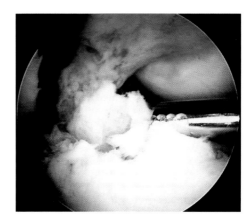

Figure 4.8 – *Removing the trapdoor with a shaver. Punches can also be used and the instruments can also be passed up the tibial tunnel.*

of tissue (Fig. 4.7). This needs to be carefully removed (Fig. 4.8). The edges of the tibial· tunnel should be probed to check that there are no loose fragments of tissue. A cyclops lesion may result if this tissue is not adequately cleared. To prevent a build-up of debris when the tibial tunnel is being rasped, the shaver can be parked in the intercondylar notch with the blade open and the suction on to clear any debris formed (Fig. 4.9). Once the graft has been inserted, it is important to view the graft arthroscopically while the knee is put through a full range of movement, to check that full extension and flexion can be achieved without impingement or compromise of the graft.

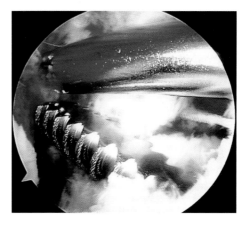

Figure 4.9 – *Shaver with blade open on suction removing debris during rasping.*

Infection

Although there is no definite statistical evidence from controlled trials, prophylactic antibiotics are advisable as in implant surgery. Firstly, fixation hardware is present. Secondly, the graft is initially avascular because it is a free graft and therefore vulnerable to bacterial colonisation.

Any evidence of infection in the postoperative period must be treated promptly, adequately and vigorously with appropriate antibiotics and early arthroscopic washout if indicated. Particular attention should then be given to restoring mobility in the knee at an early stage.

Rehabilitation

As surgical techniques have improved with more reliable graft positioning and fixation, the trend has been towards more aggressive rehabilitation, avoiding the prolonged periods of immobilisation necessary when positioning and fixation were less adequate. To this end, it is important to ensure that as well as satisfactory graft positioning at the time of operation, fixation is also satisfactory. The rehabilitation of the patient with an ACL reconstruction begins before surgery. The patient must be physically and mentally prepared for the surgery and the demanding postoperative rehabilitation programme. The three most important considerations are reduction of swelling, range of movement and the preservation of muscle strength, and these factors are particularly important if surgery is being carried out in the acute rather than the chronic situation. Swelling is reduced by active movement, NSAIDs if not contra-indicated and ice or a cryocuff (Air Cast Inc., Summit, NJ, US), which combines cryotherapy with a degree of compression. As full a range of movement as possible must be regained following injury and retained prior to surgery. This will reduce the likelihood of range of motion problems postoperatively. Full extension or hyperextension equal to the opposite knee is regained through passive exercise (Fig. 4.10). Full passive extension in the supine position is assisted with a towel placed underneath the heel; the towel needs to be high enough to elevate the calf and thigh adequately above the level of the table or couch when the knee is hyperextended. In the supine position a weight may be applied to the proximal tibia (Fig. 4.11). Prone hanging with the mid-thigh positioned over the end of the table to act as a fulcrum, together with weights placed over the Achilles' tendon, is a very effective way of regaining and maintaining full extension and hyperextension (Fig. 4.12). Flexion should not be neglected, and specific active and passive measures are used to achieve as full a range of flexion as possible, preferably equal to the uninjured side. Wall slides facilitate the return of both flexion and extension (Fig. 4.13). It is important that muscle wastage is minimised, although in the patient with significant instability, a full range of activity may not be possible. Cycling, both outdoor and on an indoor machine (Fig. 4.14), swimming and other activities which do not involve jumping, turning, cutting, acceleration, deceleration and change in direction are recommended, as the better the quality of muscle control preoperatively, the quicker the recovery from surgery. The patient also needs to be mentally prepared and familiar with the postoperative exercise programme and goals.

The postoperative rehabilitation programme begins immediately following the surgery. Indeed, it is important to check that there is a full range of movement in the knee at the time of graft insertion. The first 72 hours is a critical period and the patient's early response to surgery may well determine progress long-term.

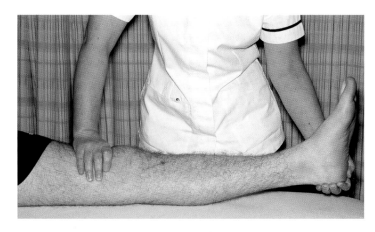

Figure 4.10 – *Passive extension or hyperextension equal to the opposite side is obtained by elevating the heel with one hand, at the same time stabilising the femur by placing the other hand above the patella.*

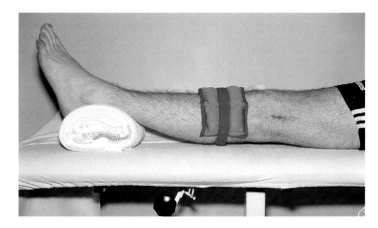

Figure 4.11 – *Full extension (or hyperextension) equal to the opposite side with a heel prop, usually a rolled towel; a weight is applied to the proximal tibia.*

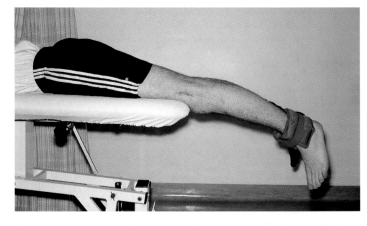

Figure 4.12 – *Prone hanging with a weight over the Achilles' tendon.*

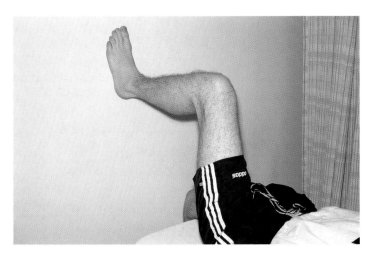

Figure 4.13 – *Wall slides facilitate return of range of movement.*

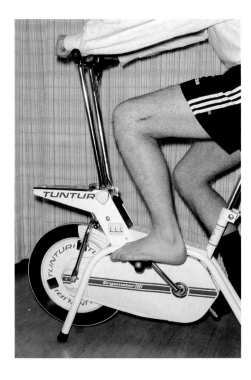

Figure 4.14 – *Exercise bicycle. Invaluable for both range of movement and return of muscle strength.*

It is vitally important to abolish or minimise postoperative pain. If the patient wakes up in the recovery room free of pain, then their mental and physical recovery from the surgery will be significantly better than if pain is their first impression on regaining consciousness. The fact that this is immediately perceived as a painful experience will have a discouraging effect on their recovery and rehabilitation. Various options are available for pain control: 3-in-1 femoral, obturator and lateral cutaneous nerve block, local infiltration of the knee with local anaesthetic and morphine, patient-controlled analgesia, supplementary analgesia and NSAIDs. Swelling is minimised by early elevation and the use of the cryocuff. The patient should not be allowed to sit out with the leg dependent, as this will increase the risk of swelling. It is vital to achieve full extension equal to that in the unoperated limb in the immediate postoperative period. The position of the knee must be closely monitored. If pain is not controlled, then there is a tendency to hold the knee in a flexed position, which is the position of comfort, and the patient or a well-meaning observer may place a pillow underneath the knee to maintain this position of flexion. A fixed flexion deformity will very quickly develop; to prevent this, pain must be controlled and pillows should not be placed under the limb. A knee immobiliser in extension may help, particularly at night. As with the preoperative rehabilitation programme, active and passive supine extension exercises are carried out with a heel prop, with or without a small weight on the proximal tibia, as are prone hangs with or without a weight over the heel. Active flexion is commenced immediately. To aid this, the bulky postoperative dressings are removed after 24 hours. Flexion is initially within the limits of pain and if the pain increases, this may be indicative of excessive activity and the patient should be advised to rest. The role of continuous passive motion (CPM) in the early postoperative period in the uncomplicated case is debatable. There is certainly no definite evidence in the literature that CPM has any effect on the long-term range of movement in the knee, but some believe that it helps reduce postoperative pain and it also serves to elevate the knee and leg. Quadriceps and hamstring muscle wastage occurs almost immediately, and it is important to commence static quadriceps and straight leg raising exercises at as early a stage as possible to minimise the muscle wasting. Open chain exercises (with the exception of straight leg raising) should be avoided initially, as these will result in excessive strain on the ligament graft. It is important to pay attention to the donor site, particularly if the patellar tendon has been harvested. Gentle manipulation of the patellofemoral joint or gentle hamstring stretching should commence on day 1 to minimise the risk of donor site adhesions and stiffness. The patient is mobilised with the aid of elbow crutches initially, once there is a controlled straight leg raise, and is instructed to weightbear as much as is comfortable; weight-bearing will not harm the graft. At the time of discharge, ideally the patient should have full extension in comparison with the uninjured limb and approximately 80° of active flexion. During the first 2 weeks until the sutures are removed, it is important to continue with the above measures, but in general terms the knee should be allowed to recover from what is after all a major surgical procedure. The patient should be instructed to rest and elevate the limb; over-zealous activity at this stage is likely to be counter-productive, with increased pain and swelling, and potentially this may slow down later rehabilitation. Weight-bearing is gradually increased so that ideally full weight is being taken by the third week. There is no evidence that bracing influences the result of surgery, and indeed bracing for a prolonged period may hinder recovery and rehabilitation. During the first 2 weeks, the patient may find that it helps to use a knee immobiliser in extension for support.

Once the sutures have been removed and the normal postoperative swelling and bruising has settled, then the accelerated rehabilitation programme can begin in earnest. The patient undergoes a supervised and graduated exercise programme. All patients are different and progress is variable between individuals, but the goals are to restore a full range of movement, improve muscle strength and regain normal gait. The patient can return to such activities as cycling and swimming as soon as he or she is able and should be encouraged to do so. The patellofemoral joint must not be neglected and the aim of treatment is to restore all flexibility to the joint. The patella is passively moved superiorly, inferiorly, medially and laterally, and a patellar tilt lifting the lateral border of the patella is also carried out to maintain length and flexibility in the lateral retinaculum. Ideally, by 6 weeks postoperatively there should be full extension and 120° of flexion. At times the knee may become over-stressed in a rapid rehabilitation regime and if persistent pain, erythema and swelling develops, it may be wise to slow down the rehabilitation programme for a period of time until the knee has settled down.

The approach to the problem in the patient with established loss of motion

If the patient fails to regain movement satisfactorily in the early postoperative phase, despite adequate conservative measures, then a decision will have to be made regarding more active intervention. Timing is difficult. If an invasive procedure is carried out when the knee is still inflamed from the surgery, then the problem may be aggravated. If there is undue delay, then an established contracture may occur which will be difficult to alleviate. With modern techniques of accelerated

rehabilitation, the literature would now suggest that manipulation under anaesthetic (MUA) and arthroscopy are indicated between 6 and 12 weeks if there is 10° or greater of fixed flexion [15,25]. Regarding flexion, there is less agreement. Ideally, the patient should achieve 120° of flexion by 6 weeks postoperatively, and failure to achieve this target or to progress satisfactorily indicates that further measures may be necessary. Each patient must be individually assessed and several factors may have to be taken into consideration in the decision making. On occasion, it may be better to rest the knee and stop active rehabilitation for a short period to let the dust settle, so to speak, particularly if the patient has been working the knee very vigorously. Certainly if the knee is tender, swollen and inflamed, excessive manipulation or physiotherapy may make matters worse.

If a decision is made to proceed to arthroscopy and MUA, the patient needs to be counselled regarding the risks and benefits of the procedure.

A thorough arthroscopy is carried out with removal of any adhesions. These are found predominantly in the suprapatellar pouch and also in the intercondylar notch, particularly anteriorly. The surgery is carried out with a combination of hand instruments, particularly punches and a powered shaver using a synovator blade, or a more aggressive resector for fibrous tissue. The graft and other intra-articular structures are inspected and any other intra-articular lesions are dealt with. The position of the graft is checked and the knee is moved into full extension to make sure that there is no mechanical block at the front of the intercondylar notch; if there is, an appropriate notchplasty will need to be carried out. The instruments are removed from the joint and a gentle manipulation is then performed. Adequate postoperative analgesia is very important. Intra-articular bupivacaine and morphine can be of benefit combined with adrenaline to reduce the bleeding following this quite extensive intra-articular surgery. A 3-in-1 nerve block helps if the pain is severe and consideration can also be given to a continuous epidural infusion. CPM may be useful in maintaining the range of movement in the early postoperative period. If the predominant problem has been fixed flexion, then the knee can be immobilised in extension in plaster for 7–10 days. The cast can then be removed and bivalved to be worn at night. An extension board is useful to maintain full extension. These are commercially available, but can be readily made by the hospital carpenter or the occupational therapy department (Figs 4.15, 4.16). The surgical

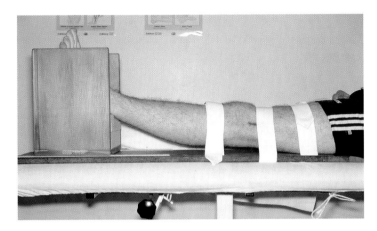

Figure 4.15 – *Extension board.*

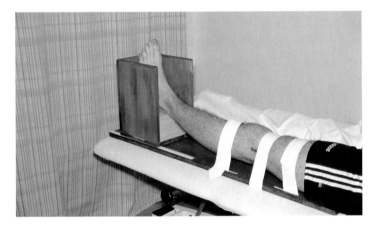

Figure 4.16 – *Extension board.*

procedure is then followed with an appropriate rehabilitation regime tailored to the patient's individual needs, again avoiding over-aggressive treatment if the knee is inflamed.

If the failure to regain full extension is associated with an audible or palpable clunk then a cyclops lesion should be suspected. Early surgery is advisable, as it is unlikely that the lesion will resolve spontaneously and the longer the knee remains in fixed flexion, the more difficult correction will be. The junction between the cyclops and the ACL graft is carefully defined by probing and the lesion itself is removed with a combination of hand and powered instruments with due respect to the graft immediately posterior to it. A characteristic 'fibrous fluff' appearance has been reported following resection of the lesion. In Jackson and Schaeffer's series, all ACL grafts were intact when this lesion was present [14].

Patients presenting with range of movement problems at a later stage in their rehabilitation or patients with recalcitrant range of movement problems may require more intensive initial investigation. Impingement is an important cause of failure to regain full extension after adequate rehabilitation, and it must be remembered that if the normal knee hyperextends then impingement may exist if the operated knee extends to 0°. Clinically, the patient typically presents with a block to extension together with effusions, particularly on activity, due to irritation of the graft by the roof of the intercondylar notch. Anterior knee pain may also occur as a consequence of the fixed flexion deformity. If the impingement is severe with an anteriorly placed tibial tunnel and/or a vertically sloped intercondylar notch, then the graft may be guillotined as it enters the joint, leading to graft failure and recurrent instability. Watanabe and Howell [26] have described typical X-ray, MRI and arthroscopic appearances of impingement. The diagnosis can be confirmed by plain X-rays. A lateral X-ray of the knee in maximum passive extension is taken; if a portion of the tibial tunnel lies anterior to the tibial intersection of the slope of the intercondylar notch then impingement is said to be present. An objective measurement can be made. The distance between the intersection of the anterior border of the tibial tunnel with the tibial plateau and the intersection of the line of slope of the intercondylar roof and the tibial plateau is measured. This figure is then divided by the width of the tibial tunnel and the result expressed as a percentage. If fixed flexion is not correctable, then impingement may still be present if the anterior edge of the tibial tunnel is in line with the roof as the tunnel would move forward relative to the intercondylar notch as full extension is reached. In fact, the graft may well be filling the gap between the tunnel and notch, preventing terminal extension.

MRI gives a specific appearance of high signal in the distal two-thirds of the graft and there may be visible evidence of direct compression of the graft. The high signal represents an area of mechanical weakness of the graft and this area can appear quite extensive. This appearance takes between 6 and 12 weeks to develop and persists for at least 3 years postoperatively.

Arthroscopically, Watanabe and Howell describe four distinct patterns of graft injury as well as the fibrous nodule or cyclops lesion. These are:

- Partial rupture of the graft at its mid-section with visible fractured bundles.
- Short graft fibres distally at the entrance of the tibial tunnel indicating guillotined fibres.
- Parallel fragmentation indicated by multiple lax parallel uninterrupted bundles.

■ Moulding of the graft by the distal end of the notch indicating extrusion.

It can be difficult to assess the degree of impingement arthroscopically, as the view of the graft at the front of the intercondylar notch tends to become obscured as the knee comes into terminal extension and hyperextension.

As in other aspects of the problem of stiffness following ACL surgery, prevention is better and easier than cure and it is important to ensure that the tibial tunnel is placed correctly as outlined earlier in this chapter, with special attention to posterior placement in the patient with hyperextension and/or a vertical type of intercondylar roof. Appropriate tibial drill guides which operate in extension and impingement rods utilising measurements made on the preoperative lateral X-rays are commercially available to address this problem if necessary.

Treatment of the established case is by arthroscopic notchplasty, taking care not to extend the bone resection too far proximally, as this may encroach upon the patellofemoral articulation. In severe cases, debridement of the anterior part of the graft may have to be considered.

In established limitation of motion problems due to incorrect femoral tunnel placement, the fault is commonly too anterior a position, in which case it will be flexion rather than extension which is limited. Again, in severe cases consideration will have to be given to debridement of the anterior part or even all of the graft, and under these circumstances a formal revision procedure with correct tunnel positioning may have to be carried out if disabling instability recurs.

Often in the late case there is a more global problem with widespread arthrofibrosis, and the adhesions may well be firmer and more difficult to divide than in the earlier cases. The cyclops lesion may be present together with extensive fibrosis in the anterior part of the intercondylar notch. Visibility at the front of the knee may be difficult due to the inflexibility of the joint and scar tissue. If this is the case, a more proximal portal such as the lateral mid-patellar or lateral suprapatellar portal may well give a better view, and the shaving and cutting instruments can be passed into the knee through the anterolateral and anteromedial portals. Following division of adhesions, the knee is manipulated and an appropriate programme of immobilisation and rehabilitation is carried out. It can be extremely difficult to bring this problem under control, particularly in the later cases, and great patience is required on behalf of the surgeon, physiotherapist and patient, as inevitably progress will be slow.

Shelbourne *et al.* [6] reported on the management of the 72 patients with established arthrofibrosis who formed the basis for the classification system described at the beginning of this chapter. Arthroscopic surgery was carried out at a mean of 12.5 months following ACL reconstruction. Patients with type I arthrofibrosis had an arthroscopic resection of scar tissue from the front of the intercondylar notch, including the cyclops lesion if present, so that full extension was possible without impingement. This was followed by appropriate postoperative physiotherapy. In the type II patients, extra-synovial scar tissue anterior to the proximal tibia required excision as well as a full clearance of the anterior part of the intercondylar notch. An extension cast was applied for 24 hours, followed by extension exercises and prone hanging with further casting on a daily basis for 2–3 days if full extension could not be achieved. Patients with type III problems required resection of scar tissue from between the fat pad and the patellar tendon, into the fat pad and proximally as far as the insertion of the vastus medialis obliquus and vastus lateralis muscles. If the ACL graft was too anterior, then the anterior fibres were resected together with a notchplasty. A similar procedure was carried out in the type IV patients, with a more extensive scar resection medial and lateral to the patella. More radical graft resection was also carried out, if indicated. An MUA was carried out in all type III and IV patients followed by serial casting usually for 3–4 days, physiotherapy and a bivalved cast at night. Once full extension was achieved and maintained, then flexion exercises were introduced. Using this regime at a mean follow-up of 35 months, type I patients gained an average of 7° extension, type II patients 14° of extension, type III patients 13° of extension and 28° of flexion and type IV patients 18° of extension and 27° of flexion. No patients in any group developed problems with instability symptomatically or on objective testing, despite partial resection of the graft in 10 and complete resection in four. In the type IV patients, the mean patellar tendon length increased from 42 mm preoperatively to 45 mm postoperatively.

Management of the infrapatellar contracture syndrome is very difficult. Paulos *et al.* [16] described three stages. First is the prodromal stage (stage 1), with diffuse oedema and a painful range of movement with restricted patellar mobility. Patients fail to gain the expected postoperative range of movement during this stage. Stage 2, or the active stage, follows with restriction of movement, quadriceps atrophy and patellofemoral crepitus. At this stage, vigorous physiotherapy or manipulation will only aggravate the problem. In the residual stage or stage 3, there is patella infera and evidence clinically and radiologically of patellofemoral osteoarthrosis. The key to the diagnosis clinically is reduced patellar mobility. A zero or negative passive patellar tilt and superior or inferior patellar glide less than 2 cm confirms the diagnosis [17]. If the diagnosis is confirmed, then it is important to determine whether the problem is predominantly suprapatellar or infra- and peripatellar. Suprapatellar entrapment with adhesions in the suprapatellar pouch usually responds to arthroscopic debridement and manipulation. If the pathology is infra- and peripatellar, then all vigorous rehabilitation should cease. The patient is placed on a gentle exercise programme with NSAIDs. If these measures do not resolve the problem, then open surgery is indicated. This consists of intra- and extra-articular removal of adhesions, release of the patellar tendon and a lateral retinacular release. If patella infera of 8 mm or more is present, a tibial tubercle osteotomy may be advisable moving the tubercle proximally and anteriorly. The postoperative regime consists of CPM and graduated range of motion with extension splintage if necessary. A further arthroscopic procedure may be required. However, the overall outcome in terms of function was only fair, indicating the recalcitrant nature of this condition.

Complex regional pain syndrome I (formerly reflex sympathetic dystrophy) may also be a cause of limitation of movement following ACL reconstruction. As well as restriction of movement, there will be a constant burning type of pain out of proportion to the physical findings, hypersensitivity and vasomotor disturbances. Plain X-ray may show osteoporotic changes locally in and around the knee joint and an isotope bone scan may show diffuse increased uptake.

Summary and conclusions

Loss of motion is a serious complication of ACL surgery and it may well negate any benefit from the procedure. Under certain circumstances, e.g. the infrapatellar contracture syndrome, the condition may be more disabling than ACL insufficiency itself.

Prevention is better than cure, and a number of factors have been identified which predispose towards this problem. These must be eliminated as far as possible and the majority are under the control of the surgeon. It is essential that technical errors are avoided, particularly with regard to the site of the bony tunnels. There is a very small margin of error in this operation and very minor errors may lead to an unsatisfactory result. If the graft is incorrectly positioned, then no amount of postoperative physiotherapy will regain full movement and function in the knee. Of equal importance to the quality of the surgery is the quality of the rehabilitation programme which starts preoperatively. The principles of accelerated rehabilitation concentrating on the early return of motion, particularly full extension, are now firmly established. Control of postoperative pain and swelling is also of fundamental importance. It is important, however, to be aware of the knee that is failing to progress because it is being pushed too hard, and at times a short respite may be in the patient's and the knee's best interests.

Treatment of the established case is difficult, particularly where infrapatellar contracture syndrome or complex regional pain syndrome I is present, and a careful and logical plan of treatment must be followed. Progress is inevitably slow and there are no quick and easy answers. There has certainly been a reduction in the incidence of this complication as the various predisposing factors have been recognised, and it is to be hoped that with continuing experience and advances in surgical techniques, the occurrence of this difficult condition will be further reduced.

Key points

1. Prevention is better than cure; management of the established condition is very difficult.
2. Operate when the knee is 'quiet' with no significant inflammation or restriction of movement.
3. Avoid technical errors. Tunnel placement must be correct; anterior positioning of both tunnels is the usual mistake.
4. Postoperative analgesia must be effective to allow early return of movement.
5. The rehabilitation programme should be adequate, stressing the immediate return of full extension.
6. Consider the infrapatellar contracture syndrome or complex regional pain syndrome I if the disability is severe.

CHAPTER 5

The patient with the failed anterior cruciate ligament reconstruction

N. P. Thomas

Introduction

The 'Holy Grail' of substituting a non-functioning part of the weight-bearing locomotor system with one that is as good as the original continues to elude orthopaedic surgeons. In an elderly population, total arthroplasty of the hip and knee has achieved uniform durable functional success, but in younger and more physically demanding patients the results are not as good and the same is true for anterior cruciate ligament (ACL) reconstruction in this age group [1].

The immense volume of literature surrounding the ACL over the last 15 years bears testament to this struggle and though significant progress has been made especially in areas such as the graft selection [2,3], anatomical placement [4,5], fixation [6] and rehabilitation [7], there remains a paucity of published material on how to manage a patient with a failed ACL reconstruction [8].

In the UK, approximately 5000 ACL reconstructions are performed per year. This may be viewed as low, as the US boasts up to 75,000 [9]. In the best centres, a success rate of 75–90% means there may be at least 1000 patients per year in this country whose reconstruction has failed. Provided these are not infected, they may be no worse off functionally than they were preoperatively, accepting a restricted level of activity whilst experiencing a slow progression of degenerative change, especially in compartments where there has been previous meniscal surgery. Not all failed primary procedures give such benign results; intra-articular prosthetic ACL reconstructions can be particularly troublesome both in their synovial and bony reactions.

The important stages in assessing a patient with a failed ACL reconstruction include the history, patient selection, physical examination and investigations, choice of graft, surgical technique and rehabilitation.

History

This is usually undervalued as both an investigative and a therapeutic force. The patients are usually very apprehensive and sometimes blame themselves for their 'failure'. Despite a varying amount of 'knowledge' usually gleaned from articles, the general practitioner, physiotherapists and more recently the internet, they have often failed to understand their basic problem, i.e. the biology of reconstruction, the impact of their injury on other intra-articular structures and the likely functional outcome with regard to their knee. This first meeting with the patient is an opportunity to re-establish their trust in the medical profession and also extract key pieces of clinical information.

Current symptoms should be elicited with care to distinguish between true symptoms of instability, which may be due to a ligamentous or meniscal pathology, and those of degenerative disease. It is not uncommon for all three aetiologies to co-exist in the same knee. The position of the knee when it gives way can be important and the patient should be encouraged to stand up and demonstrate this and any 'trick manoeuvre'. I have seen patients demonstrate manoeuvres due to associated laxities at this stage in the consultation which have been hitherto undiagnosed.

The original injury should be revisited in detail : clues about associated injuries can be present, e.g. if it was a high velocity or dashboard injury, more than the ACL may have been damaged.

The original clinical notes, including the operating note, can yield useful information. Details of peroperative problems encountered, delayed wound healing and most importantly the postoperative X-ray help provide a complete picture of the previous treatment and with it the patients' attitude to his or her experience: was he or she compliant or a difficult non-attender?

Patient selection

Knowledge of the natural history of the ACL-deficient knee is important for both surgeon and patient [10–16]. Historical papers have usually been of uncontrolled series or a skewed population, though today a controlled randomised prospective trial of surgical versus non-surgical treatment is unlikely to be performed. A reduced activity level or excellent natural proprioception may result in no symptoms of instability. Such patients should not be offered a reconstruction unless they wish to increase their activity level to include activities which involve twisting or a sudden change of direction. They should be informed of the gradual progression of osteoarthritis, however they are managed. After instability, the commonest problem experienced by this group of patients is pain. It should be carefully explained that this is likely to be caused by degenerative disease or a torn meniscus, and that a revision ACL reconstruction is unlikely to be the answer to this problem.

A full history of occupational and future recreational activities is mandatory and unless expectations are realistic, the resultant stabilised knee, usually in a middle-aged athlete with degenerative disease, will not result in a contented patient.

There has been much emphasis on patient compliance with a structured postoperative rehabilitation regime. The most universally accepted programme evolved from patient non-compliance [7], and it is hard to believe that some patients never perform forbidden activities in the early post-operative weeks, though reported graft damage at this time is rare. Revision patients should be warned that biological healing may be delayed and the emphasis is on regular and controlled rehabilitation as with the ACL primary graft.

Physical examination

A thorough general examination to include the lumbar spine, hip, leg lengths and leg alignment should be

Table 5.1 – Clinical examination

- Gait, leg alignment
- Thigh wasting
- Full range of movement documented in degrees
- Lachman's (clinical and/or instrumented)
- Pivot shift
- Medial collateral ligament (MCL)
- Lateral collateral ligament (LCL)
- Posterior sag (medial tibial plateau step-off sign)
- Posterolateral laxity*

*Use the feet as goniometers in the prone position with the knees at 20° and 90° of flexion.

made. Clinical gait analysis, looking for lateral thrust which when combined with increased genu varum increases the forces on the ACL and the lateral structures, may indicate the need for correction with a tibial osteotomy as a preliminary or a concomitant procedure. Generalised ligamentous laxity should be noted, as the graft should be inserted so that it does not impinge in physiological hyperextension.

Great care is needed to assess the ligamentous laxity of the knee. The patient should be relaxed and time should be spent examining the normal knee, using the tests described in Table 5.1.

Investigations

The most useful is the plain X-ray series of anteroposterior (AP) standing, lateral in full extension, tunnel and skyline views. These will show both the type of primary graft (in the absence of other information, the fixation is usually the best clue), and whether the bone tunnels are in an optimal position. The commonest cause of primary graft failure is anterior positioning of the tibial and/or femoral bone tunnels, and the lateral X-ray in full extension is the best view to elicit this information (Figs 5.1, 5.2). The Rosenberg view (posterior–anterior (PA) 45° standing) is informative about joint space narrowing and the possible degenerative changes [17].

Modern software reduces metallic interference and it has been my practice to obtain a magnetic resonance imaging (MRI) scan. However, this has rarely provided

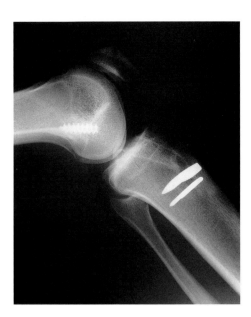

Figure 5.1 –
Anterior tibial tunnel placement. Acceptable femoral tunnel position.

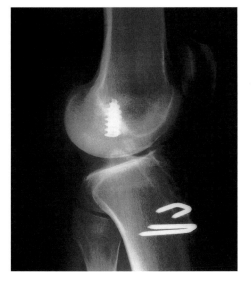

Figure 5.2 –
Anterior tibial tunnel placement and anterior femoral tunnel placement.

Table 5.2 – Serological test in cases of suspected infection

- FBC
- ESR
- CRP
- Anti-staph titres
- ASO titres

Table 5.3 – First stage

- EUA and arthroscopy
- Meniscal surgery
- Articular cartilage assessment and treatment
- Old graft removal and notch assessment
- Metalwork removal
- Graft expanded bone tunnels
- Rule out infection

- Could the patient cope with a change in plan brought about by unexpected findings during the EUA and arthroscopy which would significantly alter the time spent off work?

If the answers to all the above are positive, then consider a one-stage procedure, but in the majority of cases and certainly when starting revision ACL surgery I would recommend a two-stage approach.

The checklist of a first-stage procedure is shown in Table 5.3. The importance of the EUA cannot be over-emphasised, with the other (normal) side being examined first. The presence of associated laxities which may need surgical correction is noted at this stage: the commonest ones are posterolateral corner, posterior cruciate ligament (PCL) or lateral collateral ligament (LCL) laxities. The extent of meniscal surgery needed depends on the time from primary graft failure, the number of episodes of giving way and the experience of the initial surgeon. Partial meniscectomy rather than meniscal suture is the norm, as this is an older population than primary ACL patients and with repeated giving way the usual pathology is a chronic or complex

useful clinical information that was unavailable after an examination under anaesthetic (EUA) and arthroscopy. Bone scanning should be performed in suspected cases of infection, together with the usual serological tests (Table 5.2). If no reason for primary failure has been elicited, then re-examine the knee for a complex or missed laxity.

One- or two-stage procedure

Ask the following questions:
- Do you know why the primary ACL failed?
- Have you obtained the full diagnosis?
- Can you deal with whatever is found peroperatively?
- Has the patient been fully counselled?

white–white meniscal tear. Articular cartilage assessment usually reveals more changes than previously seen or discovered on a weight-bearing plain X-ray or MRI scanning. Notoriously hard to quantify meaningfully, the changes should be documented [18] with regard to depth, size and position, loose flaps removed and overhanging edges bevelled. The finding of exposed bone is not a contra-indication to a revision ACL procedure. These lesions should be dealt with as per the surgeon's usual practice.

The intercondylar notch is usually full of scar tissue and ruptured or incompetent graft. A combination of power and hand tools clears autologous graft efficiently, whereas prosthetic graft usually takes longer as the material is tougher, more fibrosis has been stimulated and if the 'over the top position' was used for the femoral placement, a large 'wadge' of lax swollen graft is seen situated posteriorly exiting the joint superolaterally. Care should be taken to identify the edge and then the whole of the PCL and remove all other structures from the notch. A small curette usually identifies the femoral screw edge; the AP and lateral preoperative X-ray will indicate the position, depth and angulation of this screw.

Complete clearance of bone and soft tissue from around the end of the screw is recommended before attempted removal. The screwdriver must be placed in the exact position to engage the recessed head. This is usually achieved by having the knee at a precise degree of flexion and often an accessory portal is necessary to achieve the necessary medial/lateral angulation. Before cutting this, a long percutaneous needle is useful to gauge accuracy of attack angle. Once the screw is out of the bone, a mosquito clip with straight arms with one arm in the cannulated centre and one around the edge of the screw can be used to 'unscrew' it and withdraw it through the soft tissues and exit from the portal.

Tibial or femoral fixation devices can be time-consuming to remove if they are buried, and very occasionally X-ray localisation is needed. It is only strictly necessary to remove them if they interfere with the revision procedure, but an argument could be made for their removal if they may interfere with future surgery, e.g. total knee joint replacement.

If the tibial tunnel is expanded (more than 12 mm) and in the correct position or impinging upon it then consideration should be given to drilling it out and filling it up with bone graft (Fig. 5.3). The clearing out procedure is performed with a combination of hand and

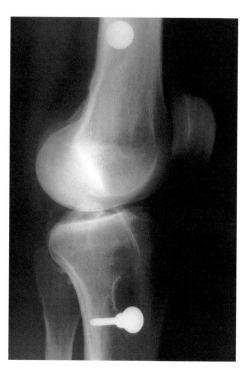

Figure 5.3 – *Lateral X-ray showing expanded tibial bone tunnel after a prosthetic ACL reconstruction.*

power instruments and results are checked with the arthroscope in bone in an air medium (osteoscopy) (Figs 5.4, 5.5). Bone in the form of dowel grafts taken from the iliac crest can be conveniently fitted into the canal. It is less common to need to perform this procedure with the femoral tunnel. Either the screw and graft is too anterior, when the screw can be removed, the graft ignored and the tunnel will be in virgin bone, or frequently as so little of the graft is within bone, little expansion of the tunnel will have occurred. Often the prosthetic grafts were used in the 'over the top' position so no femoral tunnel was used. The carbon fibre ACL reconstruction shown in Figure 5.6 failed within a year of insertion. The hook is seen indicating the correct tibial tunnel position. The graft emerged 2 cm anterior to this.

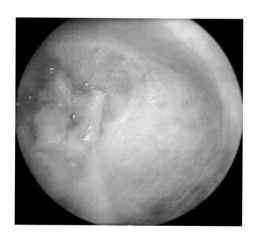

Figure 5.4 – *View during osteoscopy of the tibial tunnel once the prosthetic ligament debris has been removed.*

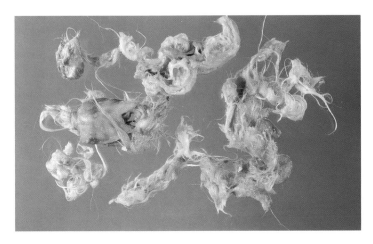

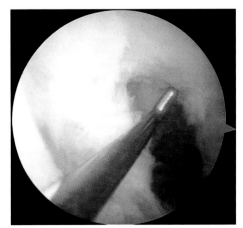

Figure 5.8 – *Hook showing the correct position of ACL graft insertion at the 1 o'clock position on the lateral femoral condyle.*

Figure 5.5 – *Prosthetic material removed from the expanded tibial tunnel.*

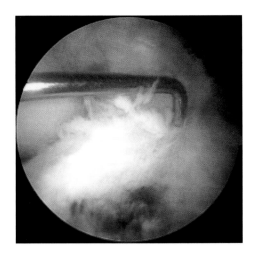

Figure 5.6 – *Hook showing correct position on tibia of ALC insertion. Black area in foreground is ruptured carbon fibre graft (too anterior).*

Table 5.4 – Second stage

- Repeat examination under anaesthetic and arthroscopy
- Meniscal surgery
- Articular cartilage assessment and treatment
- Graft harvest and preparation (if using autologous material)
- Revision ACL reconstruction

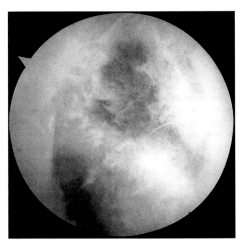

Figure 5.7 – *Femoral insertion of ruptured carbon fibre graft is shown and is far too anterior.*

It is a prudent precaution to send biopsy specimens to the laboratory during the first stage of a revision procedure to rule out infection.

The steps of the second stage of a revision ACL reconstruction are shown in Table 5.4. If there is no significant delay from the first stage and episodes of giving way are avoided, then this is usually straightforward. The revision part is similar to a primary ACL reconstruction, and great care must be taken in anatomical placement of the tibial and femoral tunnels. As the landmarks are often less distinct than in a primary case, the tibial tunnel should be referenced off the PCL on the medial side of the mid-intercondylar point and the femoral tunnel referenced from the over-the-top position using proprietary jigs. Peroperative imaging using an image intensifier may occasionally be necessary to ensure optimal placement.

The femoral position is likewise 2 cm too anterior; the carbon fibre is seen very anteriorly on the lateral femoral wall (Fig. 5.7) and the hook is seen indicating the correct position of the femoral tunnel (Fig. 5.8).

The choice of graft is shown in Table 5.5. This reflects my preference for autologous over allograft material,

Table 5.5 – Choice of graft

Primary graft	Revision graft
■ Bone–patellar tendon–bone	Four-strand hamstring or contralateral bone–patellar tendon–bone
■ Four-strand hamstring	Bone–patellar tendon–bone or contralateral four-strand hamstring
■ Prosthetic	Choice of autologous graft
■ Other	Choice of autologous graft

though this is acceptable if host material is scarce. I am opposed to prosthetic constructs except in exceptional circumstances, and then in an extra-articular position.

Initially, the weakest part of an ACL reconstruction (primary or revision) is the fixation. After 6–12 weeks, failure will be mid-substance [19]. When dealing with bone-to-bone fixation, the interference screw first popularised by Kurosaka [6] has stood the test of time. Data are now available on its length [20], diameter [21], angle [22] and bioabsorbable options [23,24]. Soft tissue fixation to bone, as well as suture fixation, has shown equal ultimate tensile strength to interference screw fixation [25]. Various methods of fixation are therefore available to the surgeon which will cope with current rehabilitation regimes [19], but recent studies have questioned the stability of fixation of hamstring constructs [26,27].

Rehabilitation remains an area which has been led by enthusiasts and the patients themselves [28], with most clinicians following at a safe distance, not wishing their own patients to be the first to try out the new regime. The weakest link is the fixation and knowledge of these values which will assist in the planning. In revision cases, the biology of both intraosseous and intra-articular healing may be delayed but we have no finite proof in the human. With such sparse information it would seem wise to progress at the primary rate if there are no reasons to delay, and in my own series we have had no failures in any revision case due to rehabilitation problems.

The main points in rehabilitation are:
■ Full extension and early movement are recommended to avoid intra-articular adhesions.
■ Avoid active flexion from 30° to 0°, as this places significant stress on the graft.
■ Isometric hamstring and quadriceps exercises at knee flexion angles of 60° or more do not adversely stress a well positioned graft construct.

■ As the graft is weakest from 6 to 12 weeks, protection from anterior translation forces is recommended.
■ Closed kinetic chain exercises lead to more axial force orientation and are safe.
■ Open kinetic chain exercises produce maximum shear and minimal muscular contraction and should be avoided.

Revision ACL reconstruction will become more frequent, and in common with other revision procedures meticulous preoperative planning is required. This should concentrate on the mechanism of failure and information, e.g. damage to articular cartilage and menisci, should be available to the surgeon so that an accurate prognosis be given to the patient. Too often, revision ACL reconstruction is salvage surgery with less than 50% being pain free, as was found recently in a series of 133 revisions [29]. The choice of graft and type of fixation are important, and the surgeon should be familiar and proficient with the best and commonly used procedures. The surgery is time-consuming and technically demanding [30,31], and the concept of a reduction in the patient's envelope of activity can be useful [7]. The future cannot be predicted [32,33], but the application of the principles outlined above, together with realistic patient expectations is the cornerstone on which to base the management of this difficult problem (Fig. 5.9).

Key points

1. In the UK, 1000 patients a year may have a failed ACL reconstruction.
2. Finding the cause of failure is of utmost importance.
3. A detailed history is one of the most helpful aspects of the assessment.
4. a. Anterior positioning of the femoral and/or tibial tunnels is the commonest cause of failure.

b. Other undiagnosed instabilities are another cause of a poor result.

5. The majority of cases should be managed by a two-stage approach.

6. The surgery is technically demanding and the surgeon should be familiar with a range of grafts and fixation techniques.

7. Patients should be counselled so that their expectations are realistic.

CHAPTER 6

The patient with a torn posterior cruciate ligament

G. S. E. Dowd

Introduction

Over the past 10–15 years, significant advances have been made in the management of knee ligament injuries. An increased knowledge of basic science and anatomy has improved our understanding of the function of the various ligaments and ligament complexes. New procedures, including arthroscopy, have improved surgical techniques, and results for some specific injuries have improved considerably. Along with the surgical procedures, instrumentation including jig systems has simplified the vexed problem of graft placement with the aim of having a reproducible result of a supple but stable knee joint.

Ligament augmentation or substitution has evolved over the years, with some graft materials being discarded while others have become the 'gold standard' by which other materials are judged.

Postoperative rehabilitation has also advanced dramatically. Very few ligament reconstructions require plaster immobilisation resulting in prolonged stiffness. The aim is to allow strong fixation of grafts and early mobilisation. Early movement with partial to full weight-bearing and muscle strengthening exercises has contributed to a lower morbidity compared to prolonged immobilization, allowing the knee joint to return to full function at a much earlier stage than previously.

Despite these improvements, optimal management of certain ligament injuries continues to be debated. While management of anterior cruciate ruptures has improved considerably, accompanied by a huge volume of research and clinical investigation, very little has been written about injuries of the posterior cruciate ligament (PCL) and associated structures.

There are perhaps several reasons for this situation developing. Isolated posterior cruciate injuries are relatively uncommon compared to anterior, and are frequently overlooked in the acutely injured knee. The incidence of posterior cruciate injury varies depending on the mechanism of injury. Bergfeld [1] found about a 2% incidence in routine examination of pre-draft American footballers, whereas Fanelli [2] reported an incidence of 42% in patients arriving in a trauma centre with a haemarthrosis of the knee. In the chronic case, the clinical signs and symptoms are often vague and ill defined, again making the diagnosis difficult for the unwary. The percentage of patients with a posterior cruciate injury who complain of giving way or buckling is probably very small, and probably the commonest symptom is aching pain [3].

Added to the problems of diagnosis, the history of posterior cruciate reconstruction has been littered with failed surgical procedures. Despite major surgery and prolonged rehabilitation, the degree of posterior sag of the tibia on the femur has perhaps improved by only one grade, or not at all. A further problem with successful management of the isolated posterior cruciate tear is to be sure, following a careful and detailed examination, that the injury is indeed isolated. It has been argued by many experienced knee surgeons that isolated tears are not as frequent as believed, and that many have a degree of posterolateral instability together with true posterior sag of the tibia. Besides replacing the posterior cruciate, any significant posterolateral laxity must also be addressed by surgery. There is little doubt in the author's experience that, in the early days, the degree of posterolateral laxity was often overlooked from lack of clinical judgement, leading to a poor result when only a posterior cruciate reconstruction was performed.

Until recently, surgical reconstruction of the PCL required a posterior approach to the knee in order to visualise the tibial insertion of the ligament. While the procedure was possible, it usually required the patient to be turned from the supine to the prone position, compromising sterility and also prolonging the operating time. With the development of arthroscopic techniques to replace the ligament, a posterior approach has been obviated, although the operating time may not have been improved because of the technical difficulties involved in the arthroscopic procedure.

In regard to graft substitution, much of the knowledge from anterior cruciate substitution has been applied to the posterior. Grafts available include autografts (patellar tendon, hamstrings, quadriceps tendon), allografts (os calcis) and prosthetic grafts. Despite these many options, the ideal graft has not yet been identified.

Controversies still exist over graft placement. Should the graft have one or two tunnels in the femur to mimic the two bands of the posterior cruciate? What is the ideal positioning of the knee to apply tension on the graft before fixation? What form of rehabilitation is ideal for the patient having undergone posterior cruciate reconstruction? Is early weight-bearing beneficial? Does the patient require a brace and for how long after the operation?

Besides the so-called 'chronic isolated tear', injuries in combination with structures of the posterolateral corner, including the fibular collateral, popliteus tendon and arcuate ligament, which result in posterolateral instability, may have to be addressed. Various procedures are available to reduce the rotational laxity, but again none are ideal. Further evaluation is necessary to identify which, if any, is most beneficial to the patient.

In the acutely injured knee joint with relatively isolated injuries, early rehabilitation and delayed reconstruction for at least a month is advised for an anterior cruciate rupture, to avoid knee stiffness and accelerate rehabilitation. Very few isolated posterior cruciate ruptures will require acute reconstruction. However, what about complex acute knee ligament injuries, including the dislocated knee? Many authorities believe early suture and replacement of damaged ligaments offers the patient the best opportunity of a successful outcome. However, the problems of residual stiffness are not inconsiderable. The alternative policy is

a more conservative approach, similar to that for the anterior cruciate ligament (ACL) with graduated movement and bracing followed by reconstruction of residual laxity at a stage where the knee is fully mobile and rehabilitated. Again, no definite conclusions have been drawn. Too few such injuries occur and are seen by too many surgeons to obtain meaningful long-term studies on the problem.

Basic anatomy of the PCL and the posterolateral corner

The PCL is the primary restraint to posterior translation of the tibia throughout the full range of knee flexion. Girgis *et al.* [4] stated that the average length of the ligament was 38 mm with an average width of 13 mm. Functionally, it is divided into two components, the anterolateral portion which forms the bulk of the ligament and the posteromedial portion which is small and runs an oblique course to the back of the tibia. The anterolateral bundle runs from the anterior aspect of the intercondylar surface of the medial femoral condyle posterolaterally to insert into the lateral aspect of the posterior tibial fossa. The posteromedial component arises from the posterior part of the femoral insertion and passes obliquely to insert into the medial aspect of the tibial insertion. The menisco-femoral ligaments travel in close proximity to the PCL. They attach to the posterior horn of the lateral meniscus and insert into the lateral facet of the medial femoral condyle. Of the two ligaments, the ligament of Humphrey runs anterior to the PCL whereas the ligament of Wrisberg runs posterior to the PCL. The anterolateral bundle is taut in flexion, whilst the posteromedial component is taut in extension (Figs 6.1a,b). It should be emphasised that the anterolateral bundle of the PCL provides most of the ligament's strength.

The posterior cruciate tibial insertion is attached to a depression approximately 1 cm below the articular surface posteriorly between the two tibial condyles, and extends a few millimetres onto the posterior surface of the tibia to blend in with the posterior capsule. The femoral insertion is to the lateral face of the medial femoral condyle in a fan-shaped fashion. The most vertical of the PCL fibres attach to the summit of the intercondylar notch. As the fibres fan out, they attach a few millimetres behind the articular cartilage on the lateral face of the medial femoral condyle.

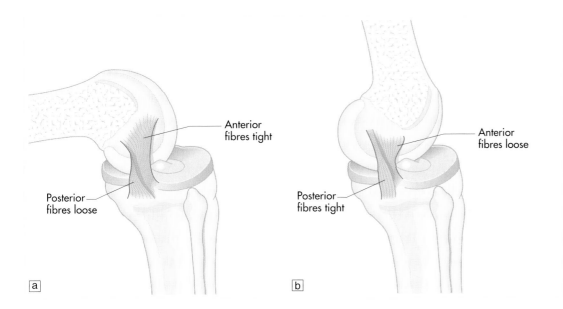

Figure 6.1 – *(a) In knee flexion: the posteromedial fibres of the posterior cruciate are slack and the antero-lateral fibres are tight. (b) In knee extension: the posteromedial fibres are tight and the anterolateral fibres are slack.*

In patients with posterolateral instability, not only is the posterior cruciate usually ruptured but also the structures comprising the arcuate complex. This consists of the lateral collateral ligament, the popliteus tendon, the lateral head of the gastrocnemius and also the arcuate ligament [5]. The arcuate ligament is a variable-sized structure, usually consisting of several bands passing from the popliteus tendon and fascia to the capsular structures below the lateral head of the gastrocnemius muscle. There may be slips passing to the lateral meniscus, lateral femoral condyle and the posterior capsule (Fig. 6.2).

The popliteus muscle originates from the posterior surface of the upper tibia and passes, as the popliteus tendon, to insert into the lateral meniscus through the popliteal hiatus, and also by another large slip to the lateral femoral condyle. Nielsen and Helmig believe that it is a significant contributor to posterolateral joint stability [6].

There is a frequent association between posterior cruciate instability and posterolateral instability [7]. Posterior cruciate rupture and posterolateral complex ruptures can therefore be combined, the former being, in practical terms, a milder form of the latter.

Mechanism of injury

Rupture of the PCL is caused by either high velocity accidents, such as motor vehicle accidents and competitive skiing, or athletic accidents during football, rugby and recreational skiing. Cross and Powell. [8] observed a more favourable outcome in sporting injuries, and Torg *et al.* [9] observed fewer complex ligament injuries in sporting accidents compared to

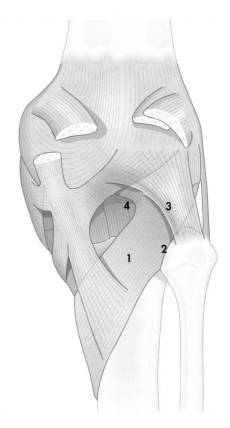

Figure 6.2 – *The posterior aspect of the knee showing the structures around the posterolateral corner of the knee (Reproduced from ref. 28 with permission, courtesy of PD Dr H-U Stäubli). 1 = popliteus muscle; 2 = popliteofibular fascicle; 3 = arcuate popliteal ligament; 4 = posterosuperior popliteomeniscal fascicle.*

other mechanisms of injury. Often motor vehicle accidents are associated with complex knee ligament injuries and other injuries, including fracture. It should be emphasised that knee ligament injuries can easily be missed in patients with ipsilateral femoral fractures, and a careful examination of the knee joint is an essential part of assessment in patients with femoral fractures.

Several mechanisms of injury have been reported to cause rupture of the PCL. A blow to the front of the tibia with the knee flexed, producing a posteriorly directed force, is a common mechanism of injury (Fig. 6.3) [10,11] and includes the typical dash-board injury described by Insall and Hood [12]. A similar mechanism of injury is caused by landing on a hyperflexed knee, with the downward force through the thigh producing a posteriorly directed force on the tibia (Fig. 6.4). Simple hyperflexion of the knee was found to be the cause of posterior cruciate ligament rupture in 46% of Fowler's patients [11] with sports-related tears, and only 15% reported a pre-tibial blow. Hyperextension of the knee resulting in PCL rupture with or without posterior capsular rupture may also occur [4]. It was observed in 20% of Dandy's patients [10], but in only 8% of Cross's patients [8].

Tears of the PCL associated with damage to the posterolateral or posteromedial structures may occur with excessive external rotational forces on the tibia,

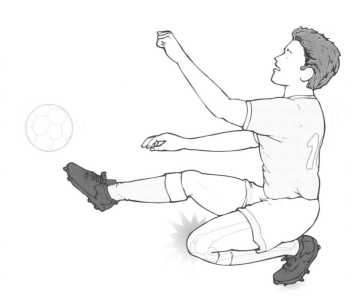

Figure 6.4 – *Hyperflexion of the knee may produce an isolated tear of the posterior cruciate ligament. (Reproduced from ref. 21 with permission.)*

with or without a varus component in the former and a valgus force with posterior in the latter.

In chronic PCL injuries presenting for the first time, it is not too uncommon to find that the patient cannot remember a specific knee injury causing the rupture.

Symptoms and signs

Acute injuries

In the acute stage of injury, many patients with an isolated PCL rupture may have very little in the way of symptoms. While they may be able to relate the history and type of injury, they may notice only mild swelling and discomfort in the knee. They may also notice bruising over the front of the tibial tubercle and at a later stage bruising over the popliteal fossa. Many patients will tell their surgeon that their knee does not 'feel right', but the ligament injury may well be missed because of only a cursory examination and low index of suspicion.

In complex tears, the knee may be obviously dislocated or swollen. Often, the seriousness of the ligament injury may not be obvious, since the knee will not be swollen due to extravasation of blood through the torn capsule. A completely torn ligament may not be as painful as a partial tear, since all the pain fibres have been disrupted.

Chronic injuries

In patients with chronic isolated PCL injuries, presenting symptoms will vary. It is possible to have an almost asymptomatic knee despite the physical signs of a torn PCL.

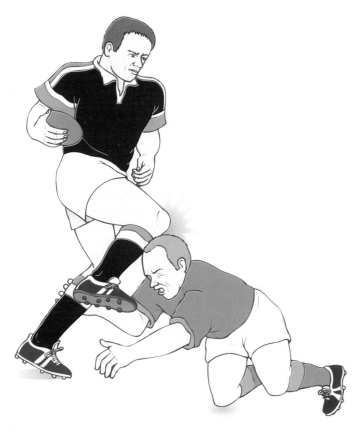

Figure 6.3 – *A direct blow to the front of the flexed knee may produce a posterior cruciate rupture.*

Up to 90% of patients may complain of some degree of pain in the knee, ranging from mild intermittent aching to more significant symptoms. Some, with time, will develop the typical pain of osteoarthritis which will affect the medial compartment and or the patellofemoral joint and finally generalised osteoarthritis [3,13]. In a variable number of patients, their symptoms will be sufficient to limit their activity level.

A true feeling of instability and giving way is uncommon, but the feeling that the knee does not feel normal is frequent [14–16].

In patients with more severe injuries, including the posterolateral structures, instability is a more frequent complaint together with pain. Patients tend to present earlier than most of those with an isolated posterior cruciate tear.

Physical signs

There are many physical signs associated with PCL and posterolateral structure rupture. Many are minor modifications of another. Individual surgeons will find some tests very useful; others will find different tests useful. The ones described are used by the author, but it should be emphasised that this does not necessarily mean that they should be the only tests used to assess posterior cruciate instability.

The posterior drawer test

The posterior drawer test remains the most useful method of assessing whether the posterior cruciate is intact (Fig. 6.5). The knee is flexed to about 80° and the examiner sits on the patient's foot to obtain stability. Often the posterior sag of the tibia on femur will be obvious. In more subtle changes, the position of the tibial plateau compared to the femur should be observed, comparing the injured to the uninjured side. Normally, the tibial plateau lies in front of the femoral condyle when viewed from the side. In acute rupture, this test may be impossible to perform since the patient cannot flex the knee because of pain and swelling.

In the patient with only a slight sag, the examiner's hands over the proximal tibia should actively push the tibia back on the femur. In cases with rupture, this may reveal a more significant sag than first observed. A grading of posterior cruciate laxity from 0 to 3 is useful to assess the degree of laxity [17]. In 90° of knee flexion, grade 1 is where the tibial plateau remains anterior to the femoral condyles, grade 2 where the plateau is flush with the femoral condyles and grade 3, where the tibial plateau is

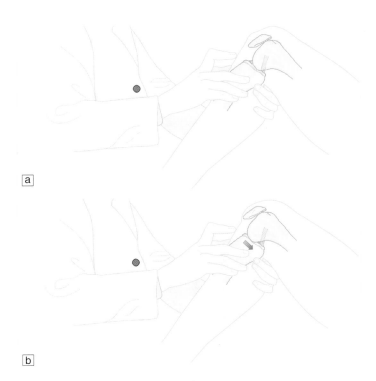

Figure 6.5 – *(a) The posterior drawer test: The examiner's fingers palpate the tibial plateau on the medial joint line to assess its relationship with the femoral condyles in the normal knee. (b) Note the posterior sag of the tibial plateau in relation to the femoral condyles in a ruptured posterior cruciate.*

behind the femoral condyles. A second part of the posterior drawer test is to rotate the tibia externally on the femur with the examiner's index finger on the fibular head. In cases of posterolateral laxity, the degree of external rotation will be greater on the affected side and also the extent of the posterior sag will be increased. When the tibia is internally rotated, the sag will become less.

The Godfrey test is similar to the posterior drawer test, but with the hips and knees flexed to 90° while the patient lies on the couch. This test also allows the increased external rotation of the tibia to be observed from the end of the examining couch (Fig. 6.6).

The reverse pivot shift test

This test has been described by Jakob et al. [18] to assess posterolateral instability. The patient lies supine with the examiner on the side of the injured knee. The examiner's hand holds the foot and rotates the tibia externally, resulting in posterior subluxation of the lateral tibial plateau on femur. The other hand is placed over the lateral aspect of the knee with the thumb over the fibular head. A valgus force is applied to the knee with the knee flexed and as the knee straightens, the lateral tibial

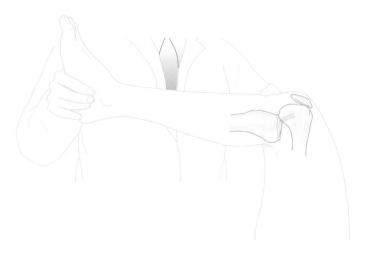

Figure 6.6 – *The Godfrey test with the hips and knees in flexion of 90°.*

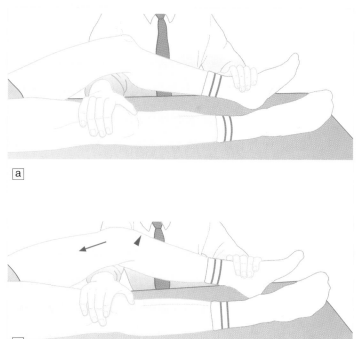

Figure 6.7 – *(a) The affected knee lies flexed and relaxed over the examiner's arm. The posterior sag can be observed. (b) As the quadriceps contracts the tibia can be seen to move forward on the femur.*

plateau reduces with a painful clunk at about 20° short of full extension. As in the pivot shift test, the reverse test may be positive in normal lax individuals; therefore, the injured side must be compared to the normal side.

The active quadriceps test
The patient's knee is flexed to about 30° with the thigh over the examiner's forearm (Fig. 6.7). As the patient attempts to lift the foot off the ground by contracting the quadriceps, the tibia can be seen to move forward on the femur. The examiner should assess the relationship of the tibial tubercle and the patella during this procedure. It should be emphasised that in mild cases of laxity, it may be difficult to identify whether the movement of the tibia is anterior to the tuberosity, as in an anterior cruciate rupture, or whether the tuberosity is moving from a point behind the neutral position forward, as in a PCL rupture.

External rotation recurvation test
If the extended knees are lifted by the toes by the examiner, the injured knee will move into hyperextension and increased varus and external rotation of the tibia compared to the normal side [19]. This test will only be positive in severe injuries of the posterior cruciate and posterolateral structures.

Investigations

X-rays
Routine anteroposterior and lateral X-rays may show an avulsion fracture of the posterior tibial plateau (Fig. 6.8), or of the tip of the fibula or Gerdy's tubercle in cases of

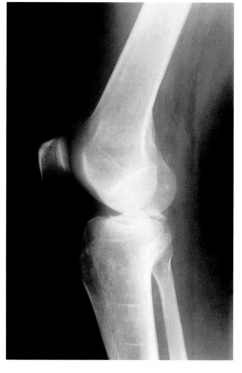

Figure 6.8 – *Lateral X-ray of the knee showing bony avulsion of the origin of the cruciate from the tibia.*

posterolateral instability. Standing films will aid the assessment of degenerative change in long-standing posterior cruciate ruptures.

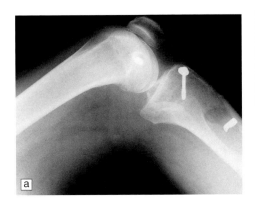

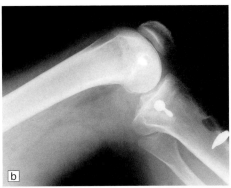

Stress views may show the excessive posterior glide of the tibia on the femur when compared to the normal knee. Adding external rotation of the tibia on the femur to the posterior drawer may show a more dramatic subluxation of the tibia on the femur (Figs 6.9a,b).

Magnetic resonance imaging

Magnetic resonance imaging (MRI) may or may not be useful in evaluation of the posterior cruciate laxity, but it should be emphasised that a normal PCL shows a curved image compared to the straight ACL (Fig. 10). A break in the continuity of the image may support rupture of the ligament (Fig. 6.11). With a posterior sag of the tibia, the anterior cruciate may give the false impression of laxity, which will be reduced on a forward pull of the tibia from the posteriorly subluxed position of the femur on the tibia.

The PCL can be identified on all three conventional MRI planes. It is uniformly of low signal on all fast spin echo sequences, T1 weighted and T2 weighted and fat suppression techniques. On gradient echo images, the signal pattern is usually not uniformly low but the normal PCL is frequently of mixed high and low signal.

Occasionally, the so-called magic angle effect due to the orientation of the PCL within the field may produce some inhomogeneity of signal which may be mistaken for a partial tear.

On sagittal sequences, the PCL is seen as a curved low signal band, usually visible throughout its length on a single cut or more. In a coronal plane, the PCL is cut through obliquely as it runs from the tibial to the femoral insertion.

On axial sequences, the PCL is viewed as a rounded low signal structure. A synovial sheath surrounds the PCL, which is therefore intra-articular but extra-synovial.

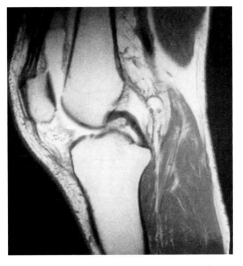

Figure 6.10 – *MRI of a normal PCL.*

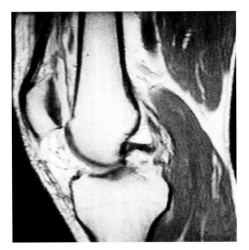

Figure 6.11 – *MRI of a ruptured PCL showing break in continuity of the structure.*

Pathological changes
Acute tears

As the PCL is such a strong structure, isolated tears commonly seen in the ACL are rare with the PCL. Any increase in signal on fast spin echo sequences, be it T1,

T2 or fat suppressed, is indicative of a tear (though note the 'magic angle effect' mentioned previously).

A complete rupture is shown as discontinuity of the PCL which is interrupted by high signal material, though this is a rare finding. More commonly, a complete tear is shown as a diffuse high signal throughout a long length or even the whole length of the PCL, which is also thickened. A partial or intra-substance tear is seen as some thickening of the PCL with oedema separating some of the fibres. This is seen as a striated pattern through a portion, usually the mid-segment, of the PCL. The sagittal plane is the most revealing for PCL damage.

A second form of PCL rupture is an avulsion rupture of the PCL from its tibial attachment. This is normally associated with the avulsion of a bone fragment. Very occasionally, a ruptured PCL is manifest as an inability to identify this structure on MRI.

In a review of 2739 consecutive knee MRI studies, Sonin *et al.* [20] detected 71 tears of the PCL (2.6%), 38% of which were complete, 55% partial or intra-substance and 7% avulsion injuries. The majority of the complete and partial tears were mid-substance. Associated injuries were common. The ACL was torn in 27%, the collateral ligaments in 27%, the collateral ligaments in 27%, meniscal tears in 63% and bone bruising/fracture in 35%.

Chronic tears

Old tears which have healed by fibrosis may return some abnormally low signals along the length of the PCL on all spin echo sequences, but this may be a subtle finding and hard to detect. Eosinophilic degeneration in the elderly may also lead to some high signal change.

Sensitivity and specificity in the identification of complete and intra-substance tears on MRI have been recorded as 100%.

In the author's opinion, in cases where the MRI evaluation is equivocal, the diagnosis of posterior cruciate laxity should be made on the clinical signs. Surprisingly, even at operation, the posterior cruciate may appear in continuity because the posterior cruciate has a greater potential to heal than the anterior, even though it may be effectively lengthened by the injury.

The natural history of 'isolated' posterior cruciate rupture

Despite the fact that many papers have been written about posterior cruciate ruptures and that the basic physical signs associated with the injury can be found in most general orthopaedic textbooks, very little is known about the natural history of 'isolated' PCL tears. Most experienced knee surgeons can provide anecdotal evidence that some patients do well and some may do very well in sporting activities despite a rupture. On the other hand, there are patients presenting in clinic who despite many years of activity and knowing that they have a chronic rupture, develop changes of osteoarthritis. There are others who have pain, a feeling of instability or chronic effusion at a relatively early stage.

One of the main reasons for our lack of knowledge is the relative rarity of the condition. In addition, very few long-term prospective studies are available from the literature. Of the nine papers reviewed by Spindler *et al.* [21], the longest follow-up was about 7 years and many papers presented a retrospective symptomatic series of patients with multiple aetiologies for the injury. The percentage of PCL injuries that may be asymptomatic in the long term is unknown.

Accepting this serious weakness in documentation, Fowler and Messieh [11] reported 100% of patients returning to full daily activities of work and to sport, while Keller *et al.* [14] found that only 45% of patients in their series did the same. Most papers reported a high incidence of a return to sport at the pre-injury level, apart from Keller *et al.*

Pain following posterior cruciate ligament injury varied from 0 to 90% [10,11,14]. In most patients, pain was mild and aching in nature and did not appear to interfere with sport. The incidence of instability also varied from 0 to 40% [11,14]. Most studies could not correlate the degree of posterior laxity with symptoms and functional results. In fact, only Keller *et al.* [11] found a positive correlation. Both Cross [8] and Parolie [22] demonstrated a positive correlation between quadriceps strength and function, while Keller *et al.* found no correlation.

Overall, 80–90% of patients were satisfied with the results of non-operative conservative treatment in the short term according to Dandy and Pusey [10] and Parolie and Bergfeld. [22].

Whilst an isolated tear was associated with a good outcome, combined injuries were associated with a less favourable prognosis. Certainly it would appear in the early years after an isolated PCL rupture, defined as straight posterior laxity of the tibia on the femur of less than 1 cm without varus–valgus laxity in flexion, extension, hyperextension or abnormal external rotation and an intact ACL, the prognosis is good.

However, there do appear to be increasing symptoms and radiological signs of osteoarthritis with time, and the author agrees with the opinion of Dejour *et al.* [13]. Dejour *et al.* described a period of functional adaptation lasting 3–18 months, with discomfort on stair climbing and running. This period merges into a period of functional tolerance in which the patient returns to full activity, including sport. Finally, the third stage of 'functional decompensation' occurs at about 10 years from injury when the patient develops symptoms from early arthritis which may or may not progress. Parolie and Bergfeld [22] noted degenerative changes on X-ray in 36% of patients about 6 years from injury. Clancy *et al.* [16] showed a 31% incidence of radiological change affecting the medial femoral condyle and patellofemoral joints, with 90% incidence of articular damage at surgery in patients with an injury greater than 4 years from surgery (Fig. 6.12).

From this limited information, it would appear that most patients with an isolated PCL tear will do well in the early stages with intensive rehabilitation. A few may be considered for reconstruction for early, more significant, symptoms of giving way or pain, or for symptoms in the chronic stage before arthritis develops. The problem is whether early repair will prevent the possibility of late onset arthritis and the answer to this problem is not known.

Surgical management of the acute injury of posterior cruciate and posterolateral corner

Isolated acute PCL ruptures, apart from those with a bone avulsion, do not in the author's opinion require immediate reconstruction. Early rehabilitation, including ice facilitation, muscle exercises and knee flexion exercises, are the aims of early treatment in order to obtain a strong, supple and mobile knee joint. At a later stage the knee can be reassessed for any symptoms that may indicate surgery.

In patients with a bony avulsion of the cruciate from the posterior aspect of the tibia, early surgery is advised to allow accurate reduction of the fragment with the aim of returning function to the ligament [23]. If the operation is delayed too long, the ligament tends to contract and accurate reduction may no longer be possible.

The posterior approach to the back of the knee joint is made with the patient lying prone. The medial head of the gastrocnemius is divided towards its insertion and is then retracted laterally to allow the posterior capsule to be visualised. The presence of the medial head of gastrocnemius protects the neurovascular bundle during retraction and while dividing the posterior capsule. The approach is simple and safer than dissecting down to the capsule between the two heads of gastrocnemius and working around the neurovascular bundle. The bone fragment can be fixed by a cancellous screw and washer (Fig. 6.13).

Postoperative rehabilitation will depend on how secure fixation has been at the end of the procedure. A strong fixation may permit early mobilisation, while a less firm fixation may require plaster immobilisation for a period of 4–6 weeks.

In patients with a combined rupture of the PCL and posterolateral or posteromedial structures, especially with avulsion of bony fragments, early reconstruction and repair is recommended.

The surgery should only be performed by a surgeon with experience of the difficulties that may be encountered, since the anatomy may well be distorted and surgical options will depend on what is found on exploration. The PCL reconstruction is performed in a

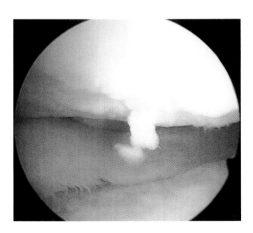

Figure 6.12 – *Medial compartment degenerative change in a patient with a 12-year history of untreated PCL rupture.*

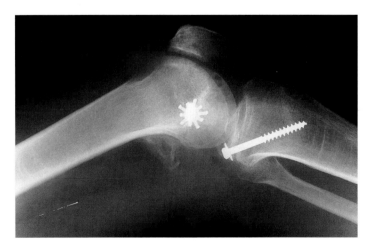

Figure 6.13 – *Screw fixation of a tibial avulsion of the PCL together with fixation of the medial ligament.*

routine fashion, bearing in mind the potential problems of fluid extravasation from capsular damage. Tears of the lateral meniscus can be repaired at the same time, since the lateral meniscus contributes to knee stability and every effort must be made to retain the meniscus. The surgical treatment of the damaged lateral structures will depend on findings, but may include suture of the torn biceps femoris and lateral collateral ligament. Avulsion fractures make this part of the procedure relatively simple. Often the popliteus is ruptured at the musculo-tendinous junction and the lateral head of the gastrocnemius has to be mobilised to allow good visualisation. It is essential that, in all repairs of the lateral ligament complex, the common peroneal nerve is identified and protected throughout the procedure.

The reconstruction should be performed with the knee flexed and the tibia internally rotated in order to repair the structures in a tight position.

In patients with marked varus of the knee, consideration should be made for a valgus tibial osteotomy at some point to offload the tension on the already damaged lateral structures. The indications for osteotomy are not clear but in the author's small experience, it should be strongly considered where there has been a significant injury to the lateral structures combined with a posterior cruciate ligament rupture and a varus knee.

Arthroscopic posterior cruciate reconstruction

As previously mentioned, rupture of the PCL may occur as an isolated injury or as part of a combined injury, including the posterolateral structures or part of a more complex injury such as a complete knee dislocation. Therefore, PCL reconstruction may be performed in isolation or as an integral part of dealing with combined or complex knee ligament injuries.

Recent advances in the 'jig' systems have made an arthroscopic reconstructive procedure possible, however, the ideal type of graft is still being sought. The most commonly used grafts are:

- The middle third of the patellar tendon
- Hamstring grafts (three or four strands)
- Achilles' tendon allograft
- Prosthetic ligaments (including augmentation devices)
- A combination of autograft and prosthetic ligaments.

The author has been disappointed by the stability of os calcis allografts and his preferred graft has been the middle third patellar tendon, using the allograft for the posterolateral reconstruction when indicated.

Posterior cruciate reconstruction using the middle third patellar tendon

The main sequences of the arthroscopic procedure are as follows:

- A routine arthroscopic examination of the knee. Torn menisci may require repair. Osteochondral defects may require treatment. Assessment of any degenerative changes should be made, together with examination of the anterior cruciate and remnants of the posterior cruciate.
- Harvesting of the middle third bone–patellar tendon–bone autograft (or preparation of a suitable alternative graft).
- Clearance of soft tissue, including remains of the posterior cruciate and the ligaments of Humphry and Wrisberg only if they obstruct good visualisation of the back of the knee.
- Drilling of the tibial tunnel.
- Drilling of the tunnel in the medial femoral condyle.
- Passage of the graft.
- Fixation of the graft in the tunnels.

Position of the patient

The patient lies supine on the operating table with a tourniquet applied to the thigh as high as possible. A sandbag is placed onto the table with adhesive tape, so that the heel lies at the proximal edge with the knee in 90° of flexion. The sandbag allows some stability to the knee when carrying out various sequences of the procedure. A fluid pump is ideal to maintain a maximal volume within the knee.

Harvesting the middle third patellar tendon graft

A longitudinal incision is made over the midline of the lower third of the patella along the line of the patellar tendon and onto the upper two-thirds of the tibial tuberosity. The paratenon is then divided longitud-inally and dissected off the tendon. The edges of the tendon are defined with the knee in 90° of flexion and the width measured with a ruler. The tendon is divided into thirds and full thickness incisions are made through the middle third. The patellar bone block is outlined with a scalpel measuring about 1 cm in length. The bone block from the tibial tuberosity is also outlined using a scalpel and may measure up to 4 cm in length.

The patellar bone block is smaller than for the anterior cruciate block, to facilitate the passage of the block through the tibial tunnel and back into the knee joint. The tibial tubercle block is longer, since the tibial tunnel is longer than for the anterior cruciate. The bone blocks themselves are removed using a small end cutting saw blade which cuts through the cortex and then is angulated to the midline to produce a trapezoidal-shaped block when seen on cross-section. The block is levered gently out of its bed with a narrow osteotome. The graft is passed through the circular acufex sizers and usually measures 10–11 mm in diameter.

Both bone blocks are drilled with a 3.2 mm drill bit to allow passage of strong thick sutures which will facilitate passage of the graft at the end of the procedure.

Clearance of soft tissue including the remains of the posterior cruciate

The 30° arthroscope is inserted into an anterolateral portal to the lateral side of the remaining strip of patellar tendon. With the knee flexed to 90°, the anterior cruciate will be lax, since the tibia will sag back on the femur. The arthroscope should pass easily into the back of the knee to the medial side of the anterior cruciate and the lateral side of the medial femoral condyle. In many knees, the posterior cruciate initially appears to be intact, but probing and preoperative clinical examination will show the knee to be lax and the posterior cruciate has either ruptured and healed with lengthening or may have stuck down to neighbouring tissue, giving the illusion of being intact. In these patients, wide strong meniscectomy punches may be used to remove the cruciate up to the insertion and as far down as possible to its origin at the back of the tibia.

Further removal of the soft tissue will require a full radius resector or 5.5 mm alligator power cutter. At the insertion of the posterior cruciate into the medial femoral condyle, a burr should be used to demarcate the area on the bone before completely clearing the ligament. This mark will be helpful when the femoral jig is used.

The most difficult area to clear of soft tissue is the tibial attachment of the posterior cruciate. Angled power tools and the acufex rasps and cutting instruments will be required to facilitate this part of the procedure. Occasionally the power tool may be inserted into a posteromedial portal to allow access to this area. It is essential that the tip of the power tool be seen through the arthroscope at all times. It should be emphasised that the ligament attaches over a wide area of the back of the tibia and the tibial tunnel entrance to the knee must be below the edge of the tibial plateau. An angled probe and image intensifier will help confirm that the surgeon is in the correct area.

In the first few cases, it may be surprising how anterior the probe will be placed on viewing the lateral image. The back of the tibia is a long way back and behind the posterior horn of the medial meniscus. It is worth spending time on clearing the soft tissue, since the ligament remnant is thick and strong and its removal will reduce the risk of 'trapping' the bone plug at a later stage in the procedure.

Drilling of the tibial tunnel (Fig. 6.14)

In order to drill the tibial tunnel, the image intensifier is placed over the knee to obtain a lateral view of the knee joint. The acufex tibial jig is passed through the anteromedial portal to the back of the knee medial to the anterior cruciate. The position of the guard at the tip of the jig is checked on the image intensifier and must be behind and inferior to the tibial plateau surface. The jig is checked in the medial to lateral plane to ensure the tip is in the midline. The jig should be pulled forward after positioning to ensure that it lies against the bone of the tibia. The other end of the jig with the guide wire introducer is placed to the medial side and at the lower edge of the tibial tubercle and locked into position. The line of the guide wire should be checked on the image intensifier. It should be low enough to decrease the angulation of the graft as it passes from the tibia into the medial femoral condyle, but not so low that it may penetrate the posterior tibial cortex in too inferior a position. It must be remembered that the posterior cortex fans out superiorly towards the point where the tibial tunnel opening is situated.

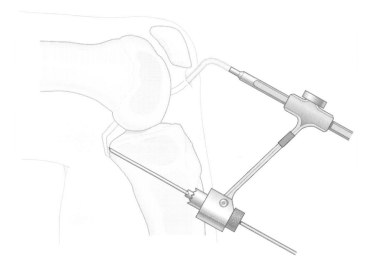

Figure 6.14 – *Lateral view of the knee showing position of Acufex guide with guide wire in place.*

Once in the correct position, a guide wire is passed through the jig under image control. Penetration of the posterior cortex by the guide wire should be avoided for fear of damaging the neurovascular bundle.

A drill bit 1 mm larger than the diameter of the graft is then passed along the guide wire after removal of the jig. As an extra precaution, a drill stop may be fitted on the drill at the point equal to the length of the guide wire within the tibia. Once the drill has passed about half-way along the guide wire, the guide wire may be removed to avoid the complication of it being caught by the drill and being pushed accidentally into the popliteal fossa.

Once the drill approaches the posterior cortex, the back of the knee must be visualised directly by the arthroscope and by the image intensifier. When the drill penetrates the cortex resistance can be felt, the bit can be seen on the image and usually bubbles of air will be seen by the arthroscope. The inner rim of the tunnel is smoothed with a rasp and the tunnel closed with a plastic plug to maintain fluid within the knee.

Drilling of the femoral tunnel (Fig. 6.15)

The knee is flexed to 90° with the foot against the sandbag. The entrance of the femoral tunnel into the medial femoral condyle is high (11 o'clock on the left,

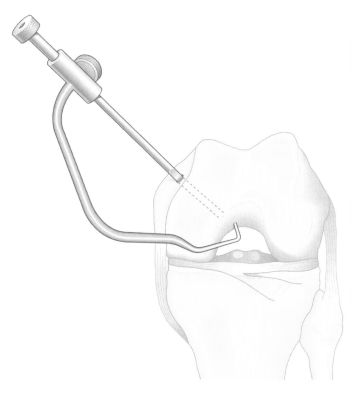

Figure 6.15 – *Anteroposterior view of knee showing position of femoral guide before passage of guide wire.*

1 o'clock on the right) and anterior, about 1 cm behind the anterior articular margin. A rough guide for this point will have been made previously by the burr.

The origin of the femoral tunnel on the outer cortex of the medial femoral condyle is at the mid-point between the medial epicondyle and the anterior articular surface. A small incision is made between the epicondyle and the articular surface and any soft tissue, including the medial vastus. The jig is passed through the medial portal and the point place on the lateral wall of the medial femoral condyle. The distance between the jig and the articular surface must be assessed and measured if necessary with a graduated probe to ensure the distance is more than half the diameter of the drill. Otherwise the tunnel may encroach onto the articular surface.

The outer part of the jig is fixed into position and the guide wire passed through the condyle. Since the area of bone between the guide wire and the articular surface is small, it is safer gradually to enlarge the tunnel starting with a small drill and increasing to the full size, previously measured from the acufex sizers. This will avoid cracking the condyle. The inner edge of the tunnel is smoothed with the rasps and temporarily blocked with a plastic plug.

Passage of the graft (Fig. 6.16)

There are various ways to pass the graft through the two tunnels.

Usually the graft is passed through the tibial tunnel around the back of the knee and into the femoral tunnel. The short bone plug from the patella is attached to a plastic tendon leader using a strong suture. The tendon leader is passed up the tibial tunnel until it is seen at the back of the knee using the 30° arthroscope. Often the leader will catch on the soft tissue, and several attempts to identify the leader may be necessary. Once the tip of the leader is seen, a pair of Leahy forceps is passed through the medial portal and catches the suture, bringing it though into the intercondylar notch.

A second set of forceps is passed down the femoral tunnel and picks up the suture, pulling it through the femoral tunnel. Sometimes the bone plug will catch against the anterior cruciate and may have to be assisted round the corner with the forceps or a probe. Flexion and extension of the knee while pulling on the suture may facilitate passage of the graft.

Without doubt, this part of the procedure can be most difficult, but with patience will be successful.

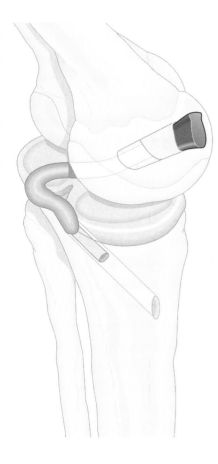

Figure 6.16 – *Position of graft after passage up the tibial tunnel, around the back of the knee joint and into the tunnel in the medial femoral condyle.*

Once the graft is in the tunnels, the femoral bone plug is locked into position with an interference screw of suitable size.

The graft is tensioned by pulling on the strong suture passing out of the tibial tunnel and the tibia is brought forward on the femur in about 70° of knee flexion. At this point, the bone plug is fixed into the tibia with an interference screw or by tying the suture over a staple. The knee is taken through a full range of movement to ensure the joint has not been trapped and the position and tension of the graft checked by direct vision.

A Redivac drain is inserted into the knee and the wounds closed.

Reconstruction for chronic posterolateral instability (the Larson procedure)
Introduction
Symptomatic posterolateral instability can be quite a disabling disorder with pain, apprehension and instability. If the knee shows significant varus angulation on full-length standing films, then an opening or closing wedge valgus osteotomy of the tibia should be considered at an early stage. This is done by the author as an isolated initial procedure, since in some cases this will provide enough stability to obviate any further surgery.

In reconstruction of the soft tissue component of posterolateral instability with an absent posterior cruciate, the cruciate is reconstructed at the same time as the posterolateral corner. Any procedure to the posterolateral corner requires identification and protection of the common peroneal nerve.

Many procedures have been described to restore the posterolateral corner. Bousquet *et al.* [24] describe the use of the middle third of the iliotibial tract, 15–20 cm long based distally or the central one-third patellar tendon. The graft is used in a 'figure of eight' fashion through bone tunnels in the femur and tibia. Advancement of the popliteal insertion and lateral collateral ligament with a bone block antero-superiorly has also been advocated by several authorities including Hughston and Jacobson [25]. The problem with these procedures is that the soft tissues tend to stretch and fail especially when the procedures are performed on their own.

Clancy *et al.* [16,27] have described a procedure in which the biceps tendon is isolated near to its insertion into the fibular head, and is brought up under the iliotibial tract to be fixed into a trough in the lateral femoral condyle over a screw and washer. They state that the procedure eliminates the deforming force of the biceps femoris and that the transfer tightens the posterolateral capsule by tightening the fibres from the biceps tendon which attached to the arcuate complex.

The author's preferred technique at present is the Larson technique, in which an allograft or semitendinosus autograft is passed through the fibular head from front to back and then up to the lateral epicondyle of the femur where it is fixed by a screw and washer. Larson argues that this graft is relatively isometric and acts as a restraint limiting posterolateral rotation [26].

The Larson reconstruction
The aim of the procedure is to reconstruct the absent popliteofibular ligament with or without reconstruction of the lateral collateral ligament. The former is the portion of the popliteus tendon which passes from the posterior aspect of the fibular head to the anterior border of the lateral femoral condyle. Either a 6–8 mm diameter Achilles' tendon allograft or a semitendinosus autograft is utilised for the procedure.

A curved incision based over the lateral epicondyle passes several centimetres proximal and also down over the fibular head. The posterior skin flap is reflected back so that the common peroneal nerve can be identified behind the biceps tendon after dividing the deep fascia longitudinally. The nerve should be traced to the neck of the fibula and protected for the duration of the operation.

The head of the fibula is dissected out, and using some form of guide, a 6–8 mm tunnel is made from front to back of the head of the fibula.

The allograft with the attached piece of bone, a few millimetres wider than the fibular tunnel, is passed through the tunnel from front to back and the bone plug is jammed against the anterior opening in the fibular head. A semitendinosus graft doubled on itself is passed through the fibular head tunnel and fixed with a low profile screw and washer into the tibia anterior to the entrance to the tunnel. A thick guide wire is drilled into the anterior aspect of the lateral epicondyle and the graft is passed over the guide wire. Isometry of the reconstruction can be tested by holding the graft over the wire and passing the knee through a range of flexion and extension. The position of the guide wire can be altered to obtain the best position of fixation. Once the point has been identified, a low profile screw and washer can be fixed into position and the graft locked into place under the washer while the tibia is pulled forward on the femur. It is essential that the graft is held taut while being fixed (Fig. 6.17). If the lateral collateral ligament requires reconstitution, the end of the graft can be brought down and fixed by a screw and washer just in front of the fibular head into the tibia (Fig. 6.18).

The wound is closed in layers. Postoperative rehabilitation is similar to that of the posterior cruciate reconstruction which is often performed at the same time.

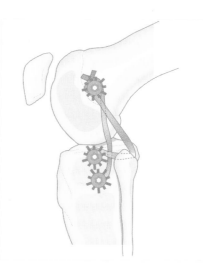

Figure 6.18 – *Combined reconstruction of the popliteofibular ligament and the lateral collateral ligament using a single strand of semitendinosus.*

Rehabilitation following PCL reconstruction

Currently there are opinion differences as to the most effective way to rehabilitate the patient who has had a PCL reconstruction. One of the reasons is the limited number of articles on long-term follow-up following surgery.

The rehabilitation should aim at reducing the swelling, allowing muscular rehabilitation and improving the range of motion without stretching the graft. Several points need to be highlighted here:

- Hamstring muscle contractions produce a significant posterior shear force at the tibio-femoral joint which increases as flexion increases.
- There must be adequate quadriceps muscle strength before closed kinetic chain (CKC) exercises are introduced. It is known, however, that aggressive quadriceps rehabilitation puts much stress on the retropatellar surface. This point is of importance since many PCL deficient knees tend to have patellofemoral irritation signs preoperatively, since the quadriceps has to work at a disadvantage to achieve extension.
- The type of surgical procedure undertaken has a role in determining the pace and type of rehabilitation. If posterolateral rotatory instability has been corrected simultaneously with a PCL reconstruction, it is advisable that the patient does not bear weight for an average period of 6 weeks to prevent stretch of the tissue used. If synthetic material is used for the PCL reconstruction, then immediate mobilisation is possible. Therefore, rehabilitation is tailored to the individual patient.

The rehabilitation protocol is divided into stages. The stages and their objectives are discussed below:

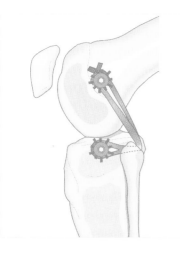

Figure 6.17 – *The Larson technique for posterolateral instability using a double strand of semitendinosus.*

- Stage 1: (0 weeks)
    Reduction of pain and swelling
    Graft protection
    Quadriceps atrophy prevention
- Stage 2: (2–6 weeks)
    Partial to full weight-bearing
    Increase motion range
    Progressive quadriceps strengthening

Bracing and crutches may be used in the first and second stages up to 6 weeks.

- Stage 3: (6–12 weeks)
    End of bracing
    Full ROM (range of motion)
    Hamstring exercise introduction
    Increase dynamic joint stability
- Stage 4: (3–6 months)
    Improve neuromuscular co-ordination
    Increase power, strength and endurance
    Gradual development of sports skills
- Stage 5: (6–9 months)
    Allow return to full sporting activity

Key points

1. This injury is relatively uncommon.
2. Isolated ruptures are rare and associated posterolateral instability should always be suspected.
3. Knowledge of the natural history is incomplete.
4. An isolated tear is often associated with a good initial outcome, whereas combined injuries have a less favourable prognosis.
5. Osteoarthritic changes and functional disability usually develop in time following isolated injury.
6. Isolated injuries apart from bony avulsions do not require immediate reconstruction; surgery is indicated when there is combined instability.
7. It is not known whether reconstruction prevents osteoarthritis.

CHAPTER 7

Complex knee instability

R. W. Nutton

Introduction

The challenging problem of knee instability has stimulated keen interest amongst orthopaedic surgeons and other professional groups who treat patients with this condition. Over the last 10 years, a clearer understanding has emerged of the effects of injuries to individual knee ligaments, particularly the anterior cruciate ligament (ACL). Combination injuries of more than one ligament are less well understood, and unfortunately frequently go unrecognised. O'Brien et al. [1] observed that the poor outcome following ACL reconstruction can frequently be attributed to untreated injuries to other ligaments, resulting in persistent instability and stress on the cruciate reconstruction, and ultimate failure of the graft.

It is perhaps not surprising that knee instability presents such a difficult medical challenge. Our understanding of the function of knee ligaments is based upon mechanical testing in a static, fixed mode by measuring joint displacement to different applied forces, usually after selective, sequential ligament sectioning. Although these experiments provide vital information about the principal role of individual ligaments as the knee stabilisers, they do not reproduce the complex mechanisms interacting in the knee during walking, running, cutting, twisting and all other functional activities demanded of the knee. The knee is stabilised by a complex interaction of many ligament structures working in combination with muscle groups and fine tuned by proprioceptive feedback from nerve endings in ligament, tendon and muscle. In the presence of isolated ligament injuries, the main elements of knee instability are usually effectively treated by repair or grafting of the injured structure. Injuries to more than one ligament result in a far more complex pattern of instability, which can be more difficult to define, but if inadequately corrected, will result in persistent knee instability. It is essential that orthopaedic surgeons and others treating patients with knee injuries should be able adequately to assess the stability of the knee and recognise patterns of instability which may represent complex injuries of the knee ligaments.

Combination injuries are usually caused by high energy forces on the knee, often resulting in concomitant injuries, such as peri-articular fractures, nerve and vascular injuries. The seriousness of the injury may not initially be recognised and many patients will be treated by splinting and rehabilitation, presenting later with persistent and severe instability which is not responding to muscle rehabilitation. Patients with complex knee instability caused by a combination of ligament injuries usually present with a more severe level of knee instability, which impinges on activities of daily living and work. These patients are not having problems during sport, simply because they find it very difficult to run and change direction, and consequently have not managed to return to sport at the lowest level of activity. The principal complaint may be that the knee instability is too severe to manage daily activities without the support of a knee brace, which understandably becomes uncomfortable, as sports braces are not designed for long periods of wear. Overall, the level of disability is greater than for patients with isolated ligament injuries, and the priority in this group of patients may be to regain enough knee stability to manage work and daily activities without a knee brace and to regain more confidence in the affected knee.

It is important to appreciate that these patients represent a small subgroup of all patients presenting with knee instability. The purpose of this chapter is to highlight the main features of the commonest patterns of combined ligament injuries, to assist in the recognition of these injuries and to review the surgical techniques which have been described to address this difficult problem.

Anatomy and biomechanics

Anatomical studies of the structure, alignment and areas of attachment of individual ligaments have improved our understanding of the primary roles of these structures. In addition, meticulous dissection of cadaver knees has demonstrated the complex and variable ligament bundles in the capsule, particularly in the lateral ligament complex. By identifying discrete ligament bundles (e.g. fabello-fibular ligament, arcuate complex, and popliteofibular ligament), biomechanical studies can elucidate the primary and secondary roles of these structures in resisting applied forces. Kinematic studies in particular identify the relative motion of the knee to externally applied loads and, by sequential ligament sectioning, ligaments can be identified as primary or secondary restraints to a particular force applied to the knee [2]. A structure which provides the main resistance to applied force is a primary restraint; secondary restraints have a lesser but significant effect on resisting displacement of the joint. Isolated sectioning of a primary restraint will allow a significant displacement to occur, whereas isolated sectioning of a secondary restraint may have no discernible effect. If, however, the secondary restraint is sectioned after a primary restraint, the magnitude of joint displacement is much greater.

Anterior cruciate ligament

The ACL has a hemispherical attachment to the lateral femoral condyle over an area of 20 mm x 10 mm at its widest point. Two discrete bundles, anteromedial and posterolateral, spiral around one another before attaching slightly medial to the sagittal midline over a length of approximately 30 mm.

Biomechanical studies by Butler [2] reported that the ACL contributed 80% of the resistance to anterior translation of the tibia. This effect is maximum at 30° of knee flexion, indicating the sensitivity of the Lachman manoeuvre for diagnosing isolated tears of the ACL. A secondary role is to resist tibial rotation, particularly when the knee is close to full extension and most significantly internal tibial rotation. The ACL also resists varus–valgus rotation when the knee is in full extension; however, this effect is minimal in the presence of an intact superficial medial collateral ligament.

Posterior cruciate ligament

The posterior cruciate ligament (PCL) is a more substantial structure than the ACL, measuring an average of 13 mm in diameter and arising from an oval-shaped area of the medial femoral condyle of approximately 30 mm in length. Anterolateral and posteromedial bundles have been described [3], which attach to the posterior surface of the proximal tibial, extending 15 mm distal to the surface of the tibial plateau.

The PCL is the major restraint to posterior tibial translation. A less well known, but important, role of the PCL is as a secondary restraint to external tibial rotation, most notable at 90° of flexion. This is the basis of the tibial rotation test at 90° of flexion for posterolateral rotatory instability (PLRI), discussed later.

Medial collateral ligament (Fig. 7.1)

The medial collateral ligament (MCL) arises from the adductor tubercle of the femur, fanning out into a sail-shaped structure towards its attachment to the proximal tibial, deep to the pes anserinus. The ligament has deep and superficial layers, the former attaching to the medial meniscus, which it stabilises.

The superficial (MCL) is the primary restraint to valgus displacement of the knee and internal tibial rotation. A secondary role of the medial collateral ligament and posteromedial capsule is to restrain anterior tibial translation, but this effect is negligible in the presence of an intact ACL. When the ACL is torn, external rotation of the tibia will tighten the posteromedial capsule, which will reduce the degree of anterior tibial translation. When the MCL and posteromedial capsule are torn, the restraining effect is lost and the anterior drawer is positive. This is the basis of the Slocum [4] modification of the anterior drawer manoeuvre.

Lateral ligament complex (Fig. 7.2)

Considerable attention has been focused on this complex of ligaments in the posterolateral 'corner' of the knee [5–10]. The lateral collateral ligament is a cord-like band, approximately 4 mm in diameter, extending from the lateral epicondyle of the femur to the tip of the

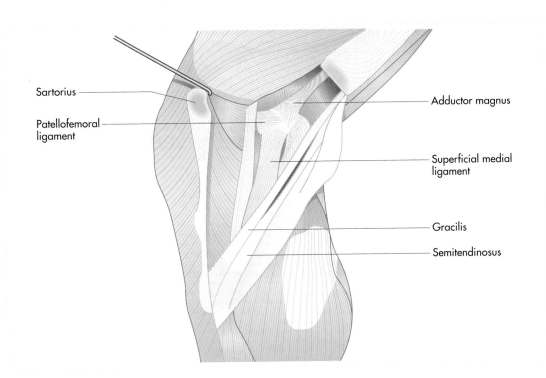

Figure 7.1 – *Dissection of the medial aspect of the knee to reveal the superficial medial collateral ligament beneath the reflected pes anserinus and tendons of gracilis and semitendinosus. (Reproduced from ref. 32 with permission.)*

Sartorius

Patellofemoral ligament

Adductor magnus

Superficial medial ligament

Gracilis

Semitendinosus

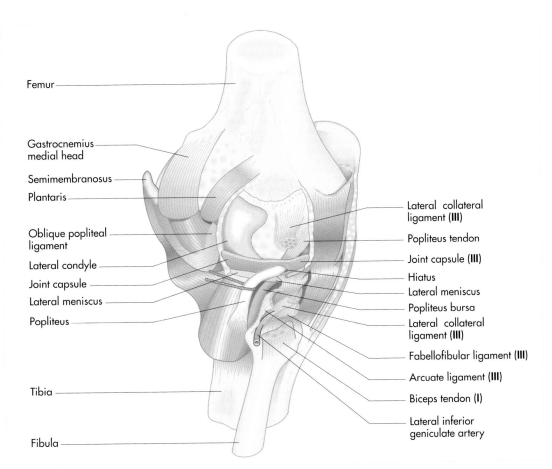

Figure 7.2 – *The posterolateral aspect of the knee. I = first layer; II = second layer; III = third layer. (Reproduced from ref. 6 with permission.)*

Femur

Gastrocnemius medial head

Semimembranosus

Plantaris

Oblique popliteal ligament

Lateral condyle

Joint capsule

Lateral meniscus

Popliteus

Tibia

Fibula

Lateral collateral ligament (**III**)

Popliteus tendon

Joint capsule (**III**)

Hiatus

Lateral meniscus

Popliteus bursa

Lateral collateral ligament (**III**)

Fabellofibular ligament (**III**)

Arcuate ligament (**III**)

Biceps tendon (**I**)

Lateral inferior geniculate artery

fibula. The important capsular structures in this area are often collectively referred to as the 'lateral ligament complex', comprising the arcuate ligaments, the lateral collateral ligament, the popliteus tendon (and popliteofibular ligament) and the fabello-fibular ligament. The fabello-fibular ligament is a variable structure providing a connection between the fabella, lateral head of gastrocnemius and the head of the fibula. The arcuate ligament is a Y-shaped structure arising from the fibular head and blending with the fascia of the lateral head of gastrocnemius. The importance of the arcuate ligament lies in its role of primary stabiliser of varus rotation and external rotation of the tibia, acting in combination with the PCL to restrain posterolateral rotation (external rotation) of the tibia [9,10]. The ligamentous band attaching the popliteus tendon to the head of the fibula, the popliteofibular ligament, is also an important restraint to external rotation of the tibia.

In 1993, Wroble *et al.* [11] demonstrated that in ACL deficient knees, isolated sectioning of the lateral collateral ligament produced a marked increase in varus rotation, but little change in tibial rotation. Combined sectioning of the lateral collateral ligament and arcuate ligament complex produced increased varus rotation, hyperextension and increased tibial rotation at 30° of flexion. If the PCL was sectioned, followed by the lateral collateral ligament and arcuate ligament complex, a significant increase in the magnitude at posterior tibial translation was seen (greater than 20 mm) and varus rotation of the tibia. In addition, isolated sectioning of the lateral collateral ligament and arcuate ligament, when the PCL was intact, produced a significant increase in external tibial rotation at 30° of knee flexion. If the PCL was subsequently sectioned, there was a significant increase in external tibial rotation when the knee was flexed to 90°.

These important biomechanical studies improve our understanding of the complex kinematics of the knee and help to explain important physical signs detected at knee examination. In turn, these physical signs may be used to define the nature of the instability before planning appropriate reconstructive surgery, if this is indicated.

Clinical assessment

It is important to be aware of the potential for combined multiple ligament damage when assessing a patient with a soft tissue injury to the knee. Underestimating the extent of soft tissue disruption can lead to inadequate treatment and continuing instability. In the first instance, a careful history of the cause and mechanism of the injury is essential. Isolated injuries to the ACL may occur without contact forces being applied to the knee, very often due to the knee being forced into hyperextension or over-rotation when the individual is load bearing on

the affected knee. Combined ligament injuries, however, are nearly always associated with physical contact or a blow to the knee, resulting in a higher energy injury. Although combination injuries commonly occur in sports, injuries caused by falls, road traffic accidents and other high energy forces represent a significant proportion of patients in the author's series.

Concomitant injuries to other structures are common. Disruption of the popliteal artery, common peroneal nerve and peri-articular fractures are frequently associated with combined ligament disruption. Knee dislocation can result in different patterns of ligament injury, depending upon the direction and magnitude of the force applied to the knee. Disruption of the ACL and PCL is often seen with knee dislocations, usually combined with either medial or lateral capsular disruption. The management of these catastrophic knee injuries is a major surgical challenge, but most reported series point to a better outcome with surgical repair and augmentation, compared to non-surgical treatment [12–14].

Unfortunately, most patients with combined ligament injuries present late to orthopaedic clinics with established and severe instability in the knee. The clinical history may suggest the possibility of multiple ligament damage. Physical examination seeks to answer three basic questions:

- Which ligaments are disrupted?
- What is the extent and severity of the ligament disruption?
- Has the ligament injury produced a recognisable pattern of instability?

This latter question may, however, seek to simplify a complex problem. Many observers have attempted to classify patterns of knee instability based on the rotatory movement of the tibia on the femur during giving way of the knee. As mentioned earlier, this greatly simplifies the complex mechanisms which interact when the knee gives way. A logical approach to knee examination can isolate the individual elements of a complex ligament injury.

The first stage in a physical examination is to ask the patient to stand and walk at a normal pace across the examination room. A significant abnormality of gait pattern has been reported, particularly hyperextension of the knee, producing recurvatum of the knee during the stance phase of the gait cycle [15]. This is a compensatory mechanism which helps to stabilise the knee by locking it out in extension. Formal gait analysis may be helpful to recognise and correct this abnormal gait pattern. When standing, overall limb alignment, particularly asymmetrical varus alignment of the affected limb, should be noted.

With the patient supine on the examination couch, routine observation of muscle bulk, surface scars around the knee and swelling of the joint should be noted. It is also important to look for any evidence of constitutional ligament laxity by examination of the normal knee, elbows, wrists and fingers. The range of knee movement is assessed, taking into account hyperextension of the knee or flexion contractures. The maximum range of knee flexion is noted and compared to the uninjured knee. Following these standard routine observations, individual ligament groups can be tested.

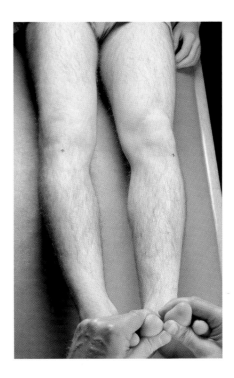

Figure 7.3 – *A positive varus recurvatum sign affecting the right knee.*

Collateral ligaments

Convention requires the knee should be flexed 20–30° to relax the posterior capsule before applying the varus and valgus stresses on the knee to test the integrity of the collateral ligaments. Although this is important, it is also essential to examine the knee in full extension, as joint line 'gapping' in this position usually indicates concomitant damage to either the ACL or the PCL, or both. During this manoeuvre, the examiner should attempt to quantify the amount of joint space opening in the presence or absence of a firm end-point. Joint space opening of greater than 10 mm usually indicates a very significant disruption of the collateral ligament capsular structures.

The varus recurvatum sign (Fig. 7.3) is also an important indicator of damage to the posterolateral capsule in the lateral ligament complex [16], although this sign can be present without ACL injury. When performing the varus recurvatum test, it is also always important to compare the injured limb to the opposite side, as individuals with constitutional ligament laxity may have an apparently positive varus recurvatum sign.

On occasions, it can be very difficult to determine whether the medial or the lateral capsular structures have been damaged, or indeed whether both collateral ligaments are involved. When the neutral position, in terms of varus and valgus, is difficult to identify, stress X-rays will provide valuable evidence of the site of maximum ligament lengthening (Fig. 7.4). Rarely, both medial and lateral collateral ligament structures may be damaged.

Cruciate ligaments

The Lachman manoeuvre is the most sensitive test for anterior cruciate disruption; with the posterior capsule relaxed and the tibia in neutral rotation, the ACL is the only restraint to anterior tibial translation. The drawer test can be confusing if care is not taken to establish the 'neutral' position of the tibia in relation to the femur. In 90° of flexion there is a 10 mm step-off between the front edge of the tibia and the femoral condyles. Any decrease in this obvious step-off suggests posterior tibial 'sag' (Fig. 7.5), indicating disruption of the PCL; an anterior drawer will demonstrate increased anterior tibial translation but only to the neutral position with a firm end-point as the ACL restrains tibial translation. Another useful test for posterior cruciate disruption is the quadriceps 'active' test. The patient is asked to flex the knee to 60° with the foot on the examination couch. The quadriceps are contracted by attempting to slide the foot down the couch against resistance; the pull of the quadriceps acting through the patellar tendon reduces the posterior tibial sag with visible anterior translation of the tibia.

The pivot shift test demonstrates subluxation of the lateral tibial plateau in the presence of an ACL disruption. The test can be crudely graded by the extent of the tibial movement on the femur, as a gliding movement (grade I) or a 'clunk' as the knee is flexed (grade II), or, on occasions, the tibia can be felt to 'lock-out' before the tibial plateau snaps back into position (grade III). A positive pivot shift test, estimated to be grade III, is frequently an indicator of concomitant injury to the posterolateral complex of the knee.

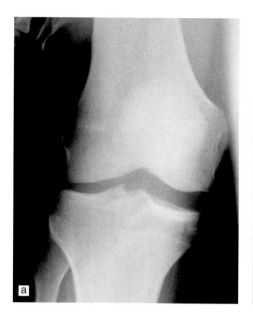

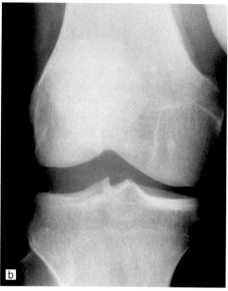

Figure 7.4 – *(a,b) Stress X-rays demonstrating laxity of both medial and lateral capsular structures.*

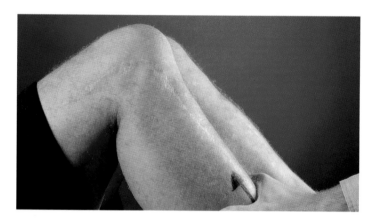

Figure 7.5 – *Posterior tibial sag indicating disruption of the PCL.*

If the posterolateral complex is disrupted in combination with a complete tear of the PCL, a 'reverse' pivot shift test [17] may be demonstrated. In this manoeuvre, the knee is flexed to 90° with the foot held in external rotation and a valgus force applied to the knee. In this position, the tibia is subluxated in relation to the femur, but as the knee moves into terminal extension, a definite glide or jerk is felt as the lateral tibial plateau subluxates posteriorly. As with the varus recurvatum sign, individuals with constitutional ligament laxity may have a naturally positive reverse pivot shift test and it is essential to examine the opposite knee for comparison. A positive unilateral reverse pivot shift test may be an indicator of posterolateral rotatory instability of the knee, usually indicating disruption of the PCL, combined with disruption of the lateral ligament complex. Other positive findings will be a positive tibial sag sign and quadriceps active test and increased lateral joint line gapping on varus stressing of the knee in extension and at 30° of flexion. In addition, there will be an increase in the external rotation of the tibia, compared to the opposite side, when the affected knee is flexed to 90°, indicating disruption to the primary restraints to external tibial rotation, the popliteofibular and arcuate ligaments.

Lateral ligament complex

The lateral ligament complex resists both varus and external rotation forces on the tibia. The lateral collateral ligament stabilises the knee against varus forces only. More extensive injury to the lateral collateral ligament, arcuate ligament, popliteus tendon and popliteofibular ligament will result in loss of control against varus and external rotation forces on the tibia, producing a particularly disabling pattern of instability when in combination with either ACL or PCL tears. It is important to recognise injuries to this ligament complex, as failure to address these at the time of cruciate ligament reconstruction may result in a poor outcome.

The most reliable physical signs for diagnosing disruption of the lateral ligament complex are varus instability of the knee in extension and increased tibial external rotation at 30° of knee flexion. The latter is an important, but poorly recognised, test for knee instability (Fig. 7.6). This test is easier to perform with the patient lying prone with the thighs pressed together and held in this position by an assistant. Both knees are

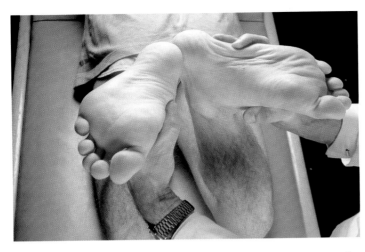

Figure 7.6 – *Tibial external rotation test. Increased rotation of greater than 10° indicates disruption of the primary restraints to tibial external rotation, popliteus tendon, popliteofibular ligament and arcuate ligament.*

flexed to 30° and the foot is maximally externally rotated. The medial border of the foot is used to assess the degree of tibial external rotation, a range of greater than 10° on the affected side indicating significant disruption of the lateral ligament complex. If this test is performed when the knee is flexed to 90°, there should be no difference between the two sides, unless there is combined disruption of the posterior cruciate and lateral ligament complex.

Summary

A careful clinical assessment is the only means by which combined ligament injuries producing complex patterns of instability can be detected and fully evaluated. Clinical assessment aims not only to determine the degree of instability, but also to assess the degree of disability experienced by the patient. As stated previously, these patients experience a degree of instability of the knee which affects daily activities and may prevent the individual from working. Most patients have already been through a long course of physiotherapy with limited benefit, and often use a knee brace throughout the day. On occasions, individuals may have undergone an isolated reconstruction of a damaged cruciate ligament, which has subsequently failed. In these cases, failure of the reconstruction may be attributed to concomitant injuries to other ligament structures, which have not been addressed at the time of surgery, resulting in stresses on the reconstruction, which subsequently resulted in its failure.

Patients with this severe degree of instability may be keen to consider surgery. However, it is important to discuss in detail the indications for surgical intervention, particularly the serious nature of the surgery and the prolonged period of recovery and rehabilitation. It is essential to emphasise to these patients that the principal objective is to obtain a painless, stable knee, which will allow the individual to cope with daily activities and, it is hoped, to return to work. It is essential that both the patient and surgeon have realistic expectations and clear objectives before undertaking this course of treatment.

Surgical reconstruction

An understanding of the detailed anatomy of knee ligaments is essential before undertaking surgery. The anatomical layers and anatomical relations of the medial side of the knee has been described in detail by Warren and Marshall [18]. The lateral ligament complex has also been described in detail, including the anatomical variants of the arcuate ligament complex [5,6,8,19]. Reference to these papers is recommended before undertaking a ligament reconstruction procedure for complex knee instability.

Broadly, ligament reconstruction procedures can be divided into three categories:

1. Advancement or recession of ligament attachments. This procedure may be effective if the substance of the ligament has not been affected and the main injury is an avulsion of the ligament attachment from bone. Ideally, the exact anatomical site of the attachment is identified and the ligament is detached with a block of bone which is countersunk, producing effective shortening of the ligament at its anatomical insertion. This avoids moving the ligament attachment to a non-isometric position, which may restrict knee movement and eventually stretch the ligament reconstruction. This technique can be applied to the MCL and to the posterolateral ligament complex.

2. Augmentation of ligaments with autogenous grafts. It is common to find that the substance of the ligament has been damaged beyond the point that advancement will correct the instability. Autogenous grafts are commonly used to reconstruct injuries to the cruciate ligament, and similarly the collateral ligaments can be augmented by transferring hamstring tendons on both the medial and lateral sides of the knee. In these procedures the tendons are left attached to their point of insertion, but the free

end is released from the muscle belly and rotated towards the anatomical insertion site on the opposite side of the joint. In doing so, the alignment and the insertion of the collateral ligaments are reproduced, resulting in an augmentation of the stretched collateral ligament. It is also possible to augment the collateral ligament by using free tendon graft, usually semitendinosus, to augment the lateral collateral ligament and the popliteus tendon.

3. Augmentation of ligaments with allograft. Severe knee injuries, resulting in multiple ligament disruption, places great demands on the technical skills and ingenuity of the surgeon. Advancement of ligaments and augmentation with autogenous tissue may not be adequate when the injury may involve both cruciate ligaments, in combination with a severe capsular and collateral ligament injury. Allografts and prosthetic ligaments are an additional resource for reconstructing these damaged ligaments, but unfortunately the lack of readily available allograft tissue limits this option. In Edinburgh, tendon allografts have been available through the Scottish National Blood Transfusion Service for 5 years, and have provided an invaluable resource in treating combined ligament injuries. Recipients must be counselled on the implications of receiving allograft tissue, particularly the risk of virus transmission. Achilles' tendon and patellar tendon allografts are available in limited numbers from a small number of tissue banks allied to blood transfusion centres; however, the limited supply of tissue confines its use to reconstructions in the more complex cases.

Ligament advancement and augmentation with either autogenous tissue or allograft are the main techniques used for reconstructing ligaments in combined ligament injuries. Although many combinations of ligament injury may be encountered, in practice four situations occur most commonly:

- Combined injuries of the ACL and MCL
- Combined injuries of the ACL and lateral ligament complex
- Disruption of the PCL, combined with disruption of either the medial or lateral ligament complex
- Combined injuries to both ACL and PCL and collateral ligaments.

An outline description of the surgical techniques used for reconstruction in each of these combined ligament injuries will be described.

Combined injury of ACL and MCL

Patients with this combination of injuries may present after conservative treatment for a knee injury with late, persistent instability, or after isolated ACL reconstruction which has not cured the patient's symptoms. It is important to appreciate the link between the ACL and the MCL in resisting valgus forces on the knee. In addition, the MCL has a small but significant role in resisting anterior tibial translation. When both ACL and MCL are deficient, the knee is unstable to valgus stress and the magnitude of the Lachman and the anterior drawer tests is greater. Physical examination will reveal medial joint line opening to valgus stress at 20–30° of knee flexion. In severe disruption of the MCL and posterior oblique ligament, medial joint line gapping when the knee is in full extension will also be present. Gapping of the medial joint line at 30° of flexion greater than 10 mm usually requires reconstruction of the medial structures. Gapping of between 3 and 5 mm will usually improve with ACL reconstruction alone. When gapping is between 5 and 10 mm, other factors should be taken into account, including the quality of the 'end point' on valgus stressing of the knee and the effect of placing the tibia in maximum external rotation when performing the anterior drawer test. Stress X-rays may also be helpful in quantifying the degree of medial ligament insufficiency.

Under anaesthetic, a further careful examination of the knee is undertaken. If a medial ligament reconstruction is to be performed, the knee will be approached through a medial para-patellar skin incision. The individual surgeon will decide whether the cruciate ligament reconstruction will be performed by the arthroscopically assisted method, or by an open technique. However, in all cases preliminary arthroscopy of the knee is performed before proceeding with the ligament reconstruction.

The author's preference is to use a central third patellar tendon bone–tendon–bone graft of 10 mm diameter for reconstruction of the ACL, when combined with a disruption of the MCL. The hamstring tendons may be required for augmentation of the medial collateral ligament. The patellar tendon is exposed for harvesting the graft and the intercondylar notch is prepared, either arthroscopically with a power shaver, or through the tendon defect after harvesting the graft using gouges and a curette. An ACL guide system is used to insert guide wires through the tibia and femur for drilling the tunnels. Reconstruction of the ACL may be performed either by the single incision technique using a blind-ended femoral tunnel and interference screw, or alternatively by the two-incision technique where the femoral tunnel is drilled externally and interference screws are also used proximally and distally. When the MCL requires advancement or augmentation, the ACL graft is inserted but fixed on the femoral side only until the collateral ligament reconstruction has been completed.

The medial side of the knee is exposed by turning down the crural fascia to expose the superficial medial collateral ligament. At this stage, it is important to examine the integrity of the ligament and its attachments proximally and distally. The fibres of the ligament may be attenuated, with firm attachments proximally and distally, but the incompetent ligament fibres stretch on valgus stressing. The posteromedial capsule should also be inspected, particularly the obliquely orientated fibres which receive a contribution from semimembranous tendon sheath, creating the so-called posteromedial corner of the knee.

Occasionally, the medial collateral ligament and capsule are well preserved and the laxity is principally due to detachment of either the proximal or distal insertion of the ligament. Avulsion of the medial collateral ligament from the femur is the most common avulsion injury [20] of the collateral ligament and, in these cases, recession of the femoral attachment into the medial femoral condyle may be possible. The femoral attachment, however, is very sensitive to proximal or anterior displacement and this reconstruction must be performed at the anatomical attachment site of the medial collateral ligament adjacent to the adductor tubercle. The medial collateral ligament is outlined at its attachment to the medial femoral condyle with a cutting diathermy, and the surrounding periosteum is elevated. The centre of the attachment of the medial collateral ligament is pre-drilled with a 3.2 mm drill and tapped in preparation for the fixation screw. Using a fine (2 mm) drill, the attachment is demarcated with multiple drill holes and elevated with a fine flat osteotome (Fig. 7.7), taking great care not to break the bone block. The ligament is turned down distally and dissected down to the joint margins. The base of the defect created in the medial femoral condyle is curetted, lowering the base of the defect by 5–8 mm. The bone plug, with attached ligament, is re-inserted and fixed with a cancellous screw and spiked washer (Fig. 7.8). The ligament insertion is

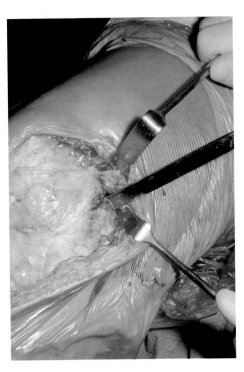

Figure 7.7 – *Elevation of the femoral attachment of the medial collateral ligament.*

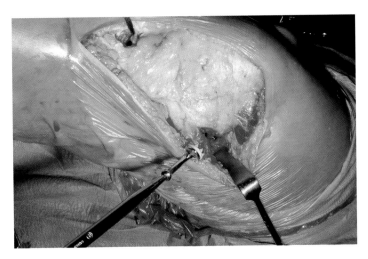

Figure 7.8 – *Recession of the femoral insertion of the medial collateral ligament with a screw and spiked washer.*

recessed by approximately 5 mm and mild to moderate medial ligament laxity will be corrected by this method. Further augmentation of the repair is made by advancing the oblique fibres of the posteromedial capsule anteriorly and slightly superiorly to abolish the redundancy of the capsule.

With more severe laxity of the MCL, where the substance of the ligament is stretched, advancement will not correct the medial instability satisfactorily. Augmentation of the MCL can be effectively performed using the tendon of semitendinosus (Fig. 7.9). The insertion of semitendinosus within the pes anserinus is

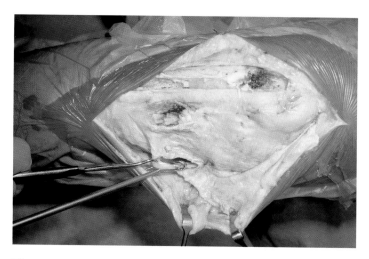

Figure 7.9 – *Isolating semitendinosus and preparing to harvest the tendon with an 'open' tendon stripper, preserving the tibial insertion.*

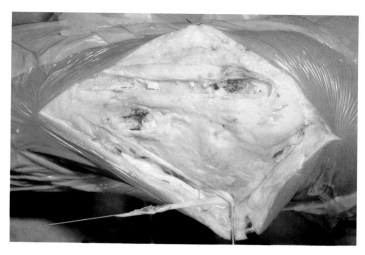

Figure 7.10 – *The tendon is looped over a Steinmann's pin in order to identify the isometric point on the medial femoral condyle.*

identified and the fascial attachment to the medial head of gastrocnemius is incised. The tendon is freed as it passes into the medial compartment of the thigh and an 'open' tendon stripper is used to release the tendon from the muscle belly. The tibial insertion of the medial collateral ligament is identified and the distal part of the semitendinosus tendon is then fixed to the proximal tibia in the centre of the collateral ligament insertion using a cancellous screw with a spiked washer. It is now important to identify the exact point of insertion of the MCL to the femur. This is accomplished by using a Steinmann's pin, which is inserted as closely as possible into the femoral attachment of the MCL (Fig. 7.10). The semitendinosus graft is then looped over the Steinmann's pin and the knee is passed through a full range of flexion and extension, whilst the graft is carefully observed as it passes over the Steinmann's pin. The correct isometric attachment of the graft is identified when the movement of the tendon graft over the pin is less than 2 mm throughout a full range of flexion and extension. This attachment point is then marked out with cutting diathermy. A periosteal elevator is used to expose the bone and a 3.2 mm drill is used to make a drill hole, which is tapped and a cancellous screw with a spiked washer is selected. The graft is looped over the cancellous screw, which is tightened, with the knee in 30° of flexion with the foot in neutral rotation, but with varus force applied to the lower leg, closing the medial joint line (Fig. 7.11). The distal end of the tendon can then be passed down the line of the collateral ligament once again and finally secured beneath the screw at the tibial insertion of the MCL.

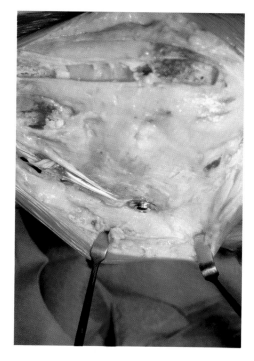

Figure 7.11 – *Tendon graft is fixed to the femoral condyle with a screw and spiked washer and doubled back towards the insertion.*

Having completed the reconstruction of the MCL, the knee is extended with the foot in neutral position and traction is placed on the cruciate ligament graft which is finally secured to the proximal tibia using an interference screw. Regardless of which type of medial ligament reconstruction is performed, it is essential to cycle the knee through a full range of movement to ensure that movement has not been restricted by the reconstruction. Postoperatively, the knee is protected in a knee brace, which allows a full range of knee movement, but the patient is allowed to toe-touch on weight-bearing for the first 6 weeks. After 6 weeks, weight-bearing is increased gradually to achieve full load-bearing without the brace by 10 weeks. Muscle rehabilitation follows the standard programme for isolated ACL reconstructions.

ACL and lateral ligament complex

The lateral ligament complex may be disrupted at the time of the original injury or as a result of repeated episodes of giving way in an ACL-deficient knee. It is important to recognise when the lateral ligament complex is involved. The presence of varus recurvatum and gapping of the lateral joint line on varus stressing when the knee is in extension should alert the surgeon to the possibility of disruption of the lateral ligament complex. However, the most sensitive sign is an increase in tibial external rotation (greater than 10°) when the knee is flexed to 30°. This test is best performed with the patient in the prone position, using the medial side of the foot as a comparison against the uninjured knee. If significant disruption of the lateral ligament complex is detected, then consideration should be given to reconstructing these structures at the same time as performing the ACL reconstruction.

Reconstruction of the ACL may be performed with a patellar tendon or hamstring tendon graft by either an open or arthroscopically assisted method. If an open approach is used, careful planning of the surgical approaches to the knee is needed, as a separate lateral incision will be required to expose the posterolateral complex. At least 130° should separate the incisions if an anteromedial approach is used for the ACL reconstruction.

After the insertion of the ACL graft and femoral fixation (tibial fixation is performed after the lateral ligament reconstruction is completed), the posterolateral aspect of the knee is exposed through a curved lateral incision. The iliotibial band is exposed and the head of the fibula and biceps femoris are identified. The common peroneal nerve runs on the inferior surface of the biceps femoris muscle belly and should be identified. The lateral collateral ligament is located and traced proximally from the tip of the fibula to the lateral epicondyle of the femur. It is convenient to split the fascia lata to identify the insertion of the lateral ligament complex, which can then be seen throughout its course. At this stage, the quality of the tissues is assessed by placing a varus stress on the knee. If the quality of the tissue is satisfactory (usually with less than 10 mm of lateral joint line gapping), an advancement of the posterolateral complex [21] may be considered (Fig. 7.12). Through the split in the fascia lata, the insertions of the lateral collateral ligament, popliteus tendon and arcuate complexes are outlined with cutting diathermy. A curved artery forceps is passed through a hole in the posterolateral capsule and beneath the collateral ligament and popliteus tendon. These structures are elevated on a pre-drilled bone block and advanced proximally in line with the lateral collateral ligament with the knee flexed to 30° and in neutral rotation. The bone block is fixed to the lateral femoral condyle with a four-pronged staple. Care must be taken to ensure that there is no tension on the common peroneal nerve through a full range of knee movement. Judicious release of the nerve may be required if it appears to stretch when the knee is extended. Finally, the knee is placed in extension and the ACL graft is fixed to the tibia.

Frequently, the quality of tissue in the lateral ligament complex is too poor to consider advancement, and consequently augmentation of the lateral collateral ligament and/or the popliteus tendon may be required. An autogenous augmentation of the lateral collateral ligament may be performed using a strip of the biceps femoris tendon, which is left attached to the tip of the fibula and a strip of the tendon is dissected from the muscle belly, tubed and rotated in line with the lateral

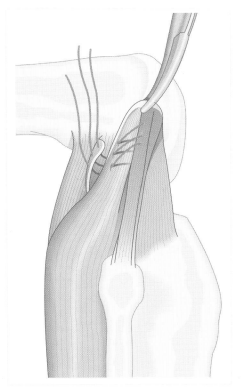

Figure 7.12 – *Advancement of the lateral collateral ligament, popliteus tendon and arcuate ligament to correct laxity of the posterolateral ligament complex. (Reproduced from ref. 21 with permission.)*

collateral ligament [22]. This reconstruction is then attached to the lateral femoral condyle at the epicondyle, producing an anatomically accurate reinforcement of the collateral ligament. Unfortunately, this repair has relatively low tensile strength and is probably only suitable for reconstruction in acute lateral collateral ligament injuries.

The popliteus tendon may also be augmented using a strip of fascia lata, which is tubed, left attached to Gerdy's tubercle and passed through a drill hole in the proximal tibia to the posterior aspect of the lateral tibial condyle. This graft is then passed beneath the lateral collateral ligament in the line of the popliteus tendon and attached anatomically at the point of insertion of the tendon. This reconstruction does not have great tensile strength and is only suitable for reconstructions in the acute situation, rather than in the chronically unstable knee.

Stronger augmentation reconstructions involve using 'free' autogenous grafts, or allograft. Noyes and Barber-Westin [23] have described a 'circle' grafting using either semitendinosus and gracilis autografts or Achilles' tendon allograft to reconstruct the lateral collateral ligament and reinforce the posterolateral corner of the knee (Fig. 7.13). In this reconstruction the head of the fibula is exposed, after identifying and protecting the common peroneal nerve. A 6 mm anteroposterior drill hole is made in the head of the

fibula, which is dilated with a curette to allow passage of the graft. The graft is turned upwards along the line of the lateral collateral ligament, towards the lateral epicondyle. Another 6 mm tunnel is made beneath the epicondyle through which the graft is passed to create a circle of graft material passing on both sides of the lateral collateral ligament. The knee is positioned at 30° and in neutral rotation. The graft is tightened and sutured together. Further reinforcement sutures are criss-crossed between the limbs of the graft and the collateral ligament. The posterolateral capsule can be plicated or advanced antero–superiorly and sutured to the bundle of tissue.

If allograft tissue is available, this may be used to reconstruct the lateral collateral ligament and popliteus tendon. A bone–tendon–bone block of patellar tendon allograft can be implanted into the fibula and lateral femoral condyle to reproduce the collateral ligament. Reconstruction of both the lateral collateral ligament and popliteus tendon can be undertaken using a single Achilles' tendon allograft with an attached bone block. The lateral epicondyle of the femur is identified as the point of attachment of the lateral collateral ligament. A drill hole is made immediately proximal to the attachment of the collateral ligament and the Achilles' tendon bone block is countersunk into this blind tunnel and stabilised with an interference screw. The Achilles' tendon is then split into two strips, producing a so-called 'trouser leg graft' (Fig. 7.14). One leg of the graft is inserted into a vertical drill hole in the fibula and fixed with sutures passed through bone, augmenting the lateral collateral ligament. The other leg of the graft is passed posteriorly beneath the lateral collateral ligament and turned into a drill hole which is made in the proximal tibia (Fig. 7.15). The graft is usually long enough to be pulled into the tunnel and is fixed by

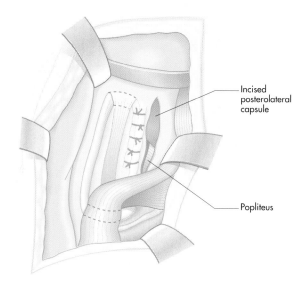

Incised
posterolateral
capsule

Popliteus

Figure 7.13 – *A 'circle graft' reconstruction of the lateral collateral ligament.*

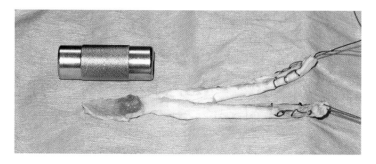

Figure 7.14 – *Achilles' tendon allograft fashioned into a 'trouser-leg' graft for reconstruction of the lateral collateral ligament and popliteus tendon.*

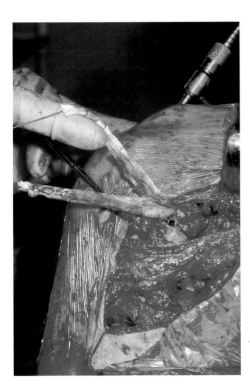

Figure 7.15 – *A trouser-leg graft has been inserted into the drill hole in the lateral femoral condyle and stabilised with an interference screw.*

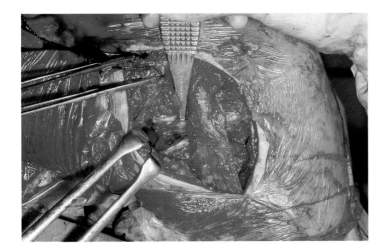

Figure 7.16 – *A trouser-leg graft in place, with one leg augmenting the lateral collateral ligament; the other leg augments the popliteus tendon and is inserted into a drill hole in the posterior aspect of the lateral tibial condyle.*

sutures passed anteriorly and tied over a suture button on the anterior surface of the tibia (Fig. 7.16).

Postoperatively, the reconstruction is protected in a knee brace and touch weight-bearing is allowed for the first 6 weeks, progressing to full weight-bearing by 12 weeks. The patient is recommended to wear a knee brace for a minimum of 6 months.

Reconstruction of the lateral ligament complex is a technically difficult procedure and the results are unpredictable. Several factors may influence the outcome. There is increasing awareness that in a varus knee the tension forces on the reconstruction will cause stretching and may ultimately result in failure of the repair. Noyes and Roberts [24] have described the concept of the primary, double and triple varus knee in relation to ligament deficiency. A primary varus knee refers to the overall tibio-femoral varus alignment, including increased varus due to loss of the medial meniscus and articular cartilage. Mechanical alignment moves over to the medial tibial plateau with increased compressive forces at the joint surface. During weight-bearing, the lateral joint line opens, placing increasing tensile stress on the lateral ligament complex (producing increased lateral 'thrust'), ultimately causing lengthening of the ligaments. This condition is described as double varus of the knee, as the varus alignment is due to medial compression and lateral joint distraction. If this situation continues, other structures are involved, including the ilio-tibial band, biceps femoris, lateral head of gastrocnemius and posterior capsule. This results in a recurvatum deformity, producing hyperextension and tibial external rotation, which increases the apparent varus alignment. In a triple varus knee, individuals may adopt a 'back kneeing gait' in order to compensate for the feeling of instability on weight-bearing. Gait analysis has been used to confirm this abnormal gait pattern [15], which may require gait re-education before reconstructive surgery of the knee can be undertaken.

Only a small proportion of patients with ligament injuries and varus alignment develop a triple varus knee, but detection of this condition before surgery is essential as ligament reconstruction alone will not address the main problems. Consideration must be given to performing a proximal tibial osteotomy to correct the varus alignment before proceeding to ligament reconstruction, usually as a two-stage procedure. Most patients will experience a significant improvement in symptoms after a valgus osteotomy alone, as some of the medial compartment pressure is relieved. It is quite common that patients may improve to an extent that the second stage, the ligament reconstruction procedure, is not required.

In patients with cruciate and lateral complex injuries who have lesser degrees of malalignment, a combined reconstruction of the ACL and lateral ligament complex may be required. The lateral

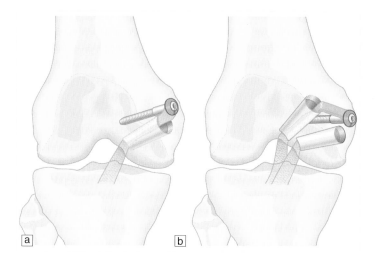

Figure 7.17 – *Reconstruction of the PCL using a combination of graft and prosthetic ligament. The PCL is reconstructed either as a single band (a) or as a bifid reconstruction (b), representing both major bands of the PCL.*

reconstruction, however, will still be subject to tension when the patient commences weight-bearing and there is a significant risk of the repair stretching with time. This problem has been recognised by Jakob [25], who recommends that ligament repairs which will be subjected to tension in the healing period, particularly the PCL and lateral ligament complex, should be 'protected' with a ligament augmentation device (LAD), which is fixed independently of the ligament graft (Fig. 7.17). Theoretically, the LAD will take most of the load placed on the reconstruction during the important phase of revascularisation and remodelling. In the longer term, it is hoped that the graft itself will contribute to the strength of the reconstruction. As failure of prosthetic ligaments by wearing and rupture is a recognised problem in the medium term, it is hoped that the biological graft provides stability in the longer term. The advantage of this method is that early weight-bearing can be commenced and bracing of the knee may not be necessary. There are concerns, however, about the potential for stress protection of the graft which may result in unsatisfactory remodelling during the healing period. At this stage, it is too early to comment on the outcome of this technique for ligament reconstruction, but theoretically the combination of an LAD with a biological graft certainly has appeal in these complex reconstructions.

Combined injuries of PCL and posterolateral or posteromedial complex

The optimum method of treatment for PCL injuries remains controversial. There is a strong body of opinion which feels that PCL injuries have a benign outcome [26,27] with a recovery of knee function without instability. Most orthopaedic surgeons will recall patients under their care who have returned to a high level of sporting activity following definite PCL disruption. There is evidence, however, from longer term reviews [28] that chronic PCL deficiency is associated with a high incidence of degenerative changes, particularly in the patellofemoral and medial compartments of the knee. It is not the remit of this chapter to discuss the advantages and disadvantages of PCL reconstruction; however, it is necessary to recognise that some patients with PCL injuries do develop symptoms of instability in the short term. In general, these patients usually have combination injuries of the PCL and either the lateral or medial ligament complex.

Patients with isolated PCL injuries may have sustained a relatively low energy injury, most commonly involving a blow to the front of the tibia when the knee is flexed at 90°. Higher energy injuries may also be associated with varus, valgus or rotational forces on the knee, which in addition may cause injury to either the medial or lateral ligament complexes. If these injuries remain untreated, patients are more likely to be aware of symptoms of knee instability due to either posterolateral or posteromedial displacement of the tibial plateau, often combined with varus or valgus instability of the knee. This pattern of instability is known as either posteromedial (when the medial collateral ligament and medial capsule is involved) or posterolateral (when the lateral ligament complex is involved) rotatory instability of the knee. Patients commonly complain of a feeling of instability, particularly when descending slopes or stairs and when twisting with weight on the affected knee. Unlike ACL deficiency, however, the patient does not necessarily experience acute giving way of the knee, but rather they experience a feeling of instability and insecurity of the knee, which inhibits activity. Pain within the knee is also a feature of instability associated with PCL tears, which may be due to the increased load within the patellofemoral articulation due to the posterior subluxation of the tibia. In addition, there is also increased load on the medial compartment of the knee, which may result in meniscal tears and premature degeneration of the medial compartment.

Physical examination of the knee reveals a typical posterior tibial sag compared to the uninjured knee. The range of anteroposterior translation of the tibia is increased as the tibia is starting from a subluxated position. It is important that this is not mistaken for an abnormal anterior drawer sign. The posterior translation of the tibia is abnormal, with a soft end-point.

Posterior cruciate ligament injuries associated with a lateral ligament complex disruption will usually be associated with moderate hyperextension of the knee and a positive varus recurvatum sign. Formal testing of the lateral ligament complex will often reveal lateral joint line gapping on varus stressing with the knee in full extension, which increases further when the knee is in 30° of flexion. With disruption of the medial collateral ligament and medial capsule, it is usually possible to demonstrate medial joint line opening on valgus stressing with the knee in full extension, which increases with flexion of the knee.

The commonest combination injury involves the PCL and the lateral ligament complex, which results in PLRI. As mentioned above, in these patients there will be a posterior tibial sag, positive posterior tibial drawer, a positive varus recurvatum sign and increased gapping of the lateral joint line on varus stressing when the knee is in extension and at 30° of flexion. In addition, there will be an increased range of external rotation of the tibia when this test is performed with the knee in 90° of flexion. Finally, the reverse pivot shift test, as described by Jakob [17], may be positive, but it is important to examine the uninjured knee as a positive test is present in 20–30% of the population who have constitutional ligament laxity.

Surgical reconstruction is a more straightforward undertaking in the acutely injured knee when the PCL can be augmented with an autogenous graft, hamstring tendons or patellar tendon, or with an Achilles' tendon allograft. The lateral structures can then be explored and either repaired directly or augmented with a biceps tendon graft or a tubed fascia lata graft for the popliteus tendon. Unfortunately, in the majority of these patients, the severity of the injury is not recognised in the acute phase and they may present months later with established symptoms and signs of posterolateral rotatory instability.

Surgical reconstruction primarily involves reduction of the subluxated position of the tibia and stabilisation by reconstruction of the PCL. Once the tibia has been reduced and stabilised, the collateral ligament structures can be explored and reconstructed using the same techniques described earlier under the sections for combined injuries involving the ACL. The PCL resists forces which displace the tibia posteriorly, mainly the hamstring muscles and the force of gravity. All grafts or prostheses used for reconstruction of the PCL will be subjected to these forces which can result in elongation of the graft or loss of fixation resulting in a recurrence of posterior tibial subluxation. In contrast to an ACL reconstruction, where the only major distracting force arises from quadriceps contraction, the PCL is subject to forces which will result in failure of the graft unless they can be neutralised. Attempts to do this by cross-pinning the joint (olecranonising) or immobilising the knee in extension result in an unacceptably high incidence of complications, mainly due to severe knee stiffness. Alternatively, thicker, stronger grafts may be used, such as Achilles' tendon allografts which can be fashioned to reproduce the dimensions of the natural PCL, but these grafts are also subject to gradual stretching and may be slower to vascularise and remodel than autografts. Prosthetic grafts are an appealing solution, but experience in ACL reconstruction suggests that these may fragment and fail, particularly at the posterior edge of the tibia when used for PCL reconstruction.

A possible solution may be the combination of biological and prosthetic grafts, where the prosthesis acts as an LAD protecting the graft during the healing period from stretching and in maintaining the tibia in a reduced position until the graft remodels and takes over the function of the PCL. Jakob [25] has reported his experience with this technique over a period of 3.5 years, comparing patients who have undergone PCL reconstruction using biological graft alone with those patients who have had a reconstruction with a combination of biological graft and LAD. With the graft alone, tibial subluxation was controlled by 50%, but with the ligament augmentation device tibial subluxation was reduced by a mean of 66%. Although this technique did not control subluxation completely, the use of an LAD allowed more vigorous rehabilitation without bracing, resulting in a more rapid recovery of knee function with fewer complications.

Reconstruction of the PCL can be undertaken either by an arthroscopically assisted technique or by an arthrotomy, usually through a medial parapatellar incision. The intercondylar notch is exposed and the remnant of the PCL is excised, although formal notchplasty is usually not necessary. By pulling forwards on the tibia, the posterior edge of the tibial plateau can be identified and using a combination of curettes and angled rasps the capsular attachments to the posterior edge of the tibia can be freed. The normal attachment of the PCL extends for approximately 1.5 cm down the back of the upper tibia, which is located as accurately as possible with a ligament reconstruction guide system for drilling the tibial tunnel. The guide systems used for PCL reconstruction should consist of a shield which prevents the guide wire from extending beyond the tip of the jig (Fig. 7.18), but as an extra precaution the guide wire can be passed under image intensifier control. When the guide wire is in position, a 12 mm tunnel is made in the tibia using a cannulated drill. Soft tissue is cleared from around the opening of the tunnel in the posterior aspect of the knee to prevent the graft from snagging when it is pulled through. When the femoral tunnel is drilled, the stump of the posterior cruciate ligament is identified and the tip of the guide is inserted into the centre of the stump. A guide wire is passed from the outer surface of the femoral condyle and a 12 mm tunnel is made with a cannulated drill.

The graft is normally pulled through the tibial tunnel into the intercondylar notch before inserting the graft into the femoral tunnel prior to fixation. This can be an extremely difficult and tiresome manoeuvre, as it is difficult to pull the graft around the acute angle at the back of the tibia into the intercondylar notch. Once the graft is in position, however, the knee is positioned in 70° of flexion, the tibial subluxation is corrected and the graft is fixed proximally and then distally.

Initially, this will satisfactorily control the posterior tibial subluxation but, as mentioned above, during the healing period the graft may stretch and tibial

subluxation may recur. If a ligament augmentation device is to be used, the biological graft is inserted inside a prosthetic ligament (Fig. 7.19) and the completed 'parcel' is pulled through the prepared tunnels in the tibia and the femur. The ends of the biological graft are separated from the prosthetic ligament, the knee is reduced with the knee in 70° of flexion and tension is placed on the prosthesis, which is fixed proximally and distally to control the tibial subluxation. The biological graft is then fixed proximally and distally under tension. In doing so, it is hoped that the biological graft will be protected from the stretching forces in the short term by the prosthesis, but in the longer term remodelling of the graft will take place.

After the PCL graft has been inserted and fixed, the tibial subluxation should be corrected and reconstruction of the collateral ligaments can be undertaken, either by advancement or by augmentation, as described previously.

Postoperatively, a full leg hinged knee brace is applied, principally to protect the collateral ligament reconstruction. Initially, touch weight-bearing only is allowed for the first 6 weeks, progressing to full weight-bearing by 3 months. It is important not to allow open chain active knee flexion exercises in the early healing period in order to minimise the forces causing posterior

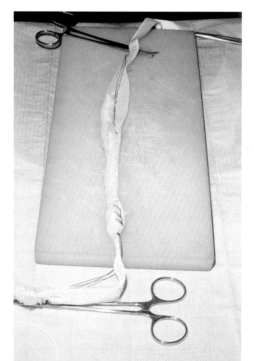

Figure 7.19 – *PCL reconstruction using an Achilles' tendon allograft inside a prosthetic graft. After insertion of the graft, the prosthetic ligament is fixed first to stabilise the tibia, followed by tensioning and fixation of the biological graft.*

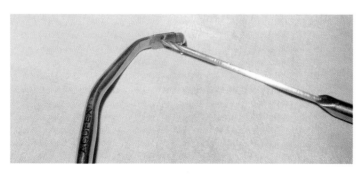

Figure 7.18 – *A drill guide with 'shield' for preparation of the tibial tunnel in a PCL reconstruction.*

tibial subluxation. Knee extension exercises are permitted and, as weight-bearing increases towards 3 months, closed chain kinetic exercises are performed. The knee brace is discarded at 3 months.

Combined injuries to ACL, PCL and collateral ligament

This catastrophic disruption of knee ligaments is almost always due to a knee dislocation, with the associated risk of vascular and nerve injuries. In the acute situation, priority must be given to reducing the dislocation, splinting the knee and arranging for an angiogram. The presence of pedal pulses does not exclude the need for an angiogram, and this should be performed in all cases of knee dislocation. The instance of vascular injury has been reported to be approximately 30% [29]. Whether or not a vascular repair is required, the stability of the knee must be carefully assessed and a decision must be made on the appropriate management of the unstable knee. Conservative treatment in a brace or a split cast is an option and successful results have been reported with this method of treatment [30]; however, most recent reports now favour surgical repair, combined with augmentation of the cruciate ligaments, quoting superior functional results following reconstruction [12–14,31].

Regardless of the method of treatment which has been chosen in the acute situation, a significant proportion of these patients will present later with painful instability of the knee, producing a severe level of disability which impinges on activities of daily living. These individuals frequently become highly reliant on using a knee brace for daily activities, experiencing pain on prolonged standing and walking, difficulty walking over rough ground and with ascending and descending stairs. Assessment of these patients must include a thorough history and detailed physical examination of the knee. It is useful to observe the patient while walking without the support of the knee brace, in order to detect compensatory mechanisms which are often adopted in order to stabilise the knee on weight-bearing. This usually takes the form of hyperextension of the knee, producing a recurvatum of the knee during the stance phase of the gait cycle. It has been suggested that this abnormal pattern of walking should be corrected before undertaking reconstructive knee surgery by teaching the patient to walk with a slightly flexed knee [15]. The adoption of a heel raise may be useful under these circumstances.

Formal examination of the knee ligaments may reveal gross instability to both varus and valgus stressing when the knee is in extension, as well as gross translation of the tibia on the femur when performing anterior and posterior drawer manoeuvres. Although disruption of both collateral and cruciate ligaments can occur, the most common situation is for both cruciate ligaments to be disrupted, combined with either medial or lateral collateral ligaments, depending upon the direction of the force applied to the knee. The capsuler and collateral ligaments on one side may be intact, leaving a soft tissue hinge on this side. If the extent of the soft tissue disruption is difficult to assess on physical examination alone, stress X-rays in varus and valgus, as well as lateral stress views whilst performing a maximum anterior and posterior drawer, can be very helpful. X-rays should also take note of the degree of degenerative changes within the knee joint, as degenerative osteoarthritis may develop rapidly after this injury, particularly if there are fractures of the articular surface. Under these circumstances, knee ligament reconstruction would be fruitless and consideration should be given to alternative methods of treatment, including total knee replacement, when pain and disability is severe.

In the absence of degenerative changes, painful instability is the principal complaint of these patients, the pain probably arising from the abnormal stress placed on the soft tissue structures in the subluxated knee joint. Surgical reconstruction is a formidable undertaking, requiring reduction of the subluxation, stabilisation of the knee by re-establishment of the PCL and reconstruction of the ACL by augmentation grafting and advancement or, more commonly, augmentation of the injured collateral ligament complex. The patient must be aware that the objective of this major surgery is to stabilise the knee to allow activities of daily living, without reliance on a knee brace. The period of recovery will be prolonged and maximum co-operation is required of the patient.

Careful planning of the reconstructive surgery is required before undertaking the operation. The main difficulty is lack of autogenous tissue for augmentation grafts. Consequently, allograft tendons, when available, are invaluable for these reconstructions. At present, the author's preference is to reconstruct the PCL using an Achilles' tendon allograft, combined with a ligament augmentation device. The ACL is reconstructed using a central third patellar tendon autograft, reserving the hamstring tendons to augment the collateral ligament when required.

Under anaesthetic, the knee is carefully examined and when necessary further stress X-rays may be taken to confirm the principal ligament injuries. Preliminary arthroscopy is always performed to inspect the joint surfaces, and particularly the menisci. The knee is then exposed through a medial parapatellar incision, removing the remnants of the ACL and PCL from the intercondylar notch. As the knee is posteriorly subluxated, the first priority is to undertake a reconstruction of the PCL, which is performed by the same technique described on pp. 89–90 – using an Achilles' tendon autograft with a ligament augmentation device. The tibia is reduced on the femoral condyles with the knee in 70° of flexion. The LAD and ligament grafts are fixed proximally and distally. The knee is then passed through a full range of movement, ensuring there is no abnormal tension on the PCL reconstruction. The ACL reconstruction is then performed using the patellar tendon autograft, which is harvested before performing the arthrotomy. A guide system is used to pass guide wires under direct vision into the anatomical sites of attachment of the ACL before drilling the tunnels. A graft is inserted and fixed proximally to the femur with an interference screw, but distal fixation to the tibia is delayed until the collateral ligament reconstruction has been performed.

In most cases the disruption to the collateral ligaments is severe and augmentation with a hamstring tendon graft is required. Medial collateral ligament reconstruction is performed by the technique described previously, having taken care to identify the isometric position on the medial femoral condyle. On the lateral side, disruption of the lateral ligament complex is repaired using the 'loop graft' technique described by Noyes and Barber-Westin [23], passing semitendinosus through a drill hole in the head of the fibula and through a tunnel beneath the lateral collateral ligament attachment to the lateral epicondyle. An incision is made in the posterolateral capsule, which is advanced anteriorly towards the lateral ligament augmentation, which helps to abolish some of the redundancy in the posterolateral capsule. It is important to expose the common peroneal nerve, which is protected during the lateral ligament reconstruction, and care is taken to ensure that there is no undue tension on the nerve when the knee is extended at the completion of the reconstruction.

When the collateral ligament reconstruction has been performed, the knee is placed in 20° of flexion. The ACL

augmentation graft is finally fixed to the proximal tibia with an interference screw, with the tibia in neutral rotation. The tourniquet is released and haemostasis is obtained before closure of the wound and application of a full leg hinged knee brace.

Postoperatively, the patient is mobilised with touch weight-bearing on the affected side. Initially, the brace is locked in extension until straight leg raising is regained, after which the brace is unlocked, allowing free movement of the knee within the brace. At 6 weeks, weight-bearing is progressively increased, achieving full weight-bearing by 10 weeks, at which stage the knee brace is discarded. Muscle bulk is maintained initially for the first 6 weeks by isometric contractions of the quadriceps and hamstring muscles with the knee in extension, progressing to closed chain kinetic exercises commencing at 6 weeks, when increased weight-bearing is allowed.

Patients must be warned that the period of recovery following this type of knee ligament reconstruction surgery is prolonged and priority must be given to maintaining knee movement, if arthrofibrosis is to be prevented. Manipulation under anaesthetic (MUA) is performed if knee flexion is less than 90° at 6 weeks. Knee flexion usually improves after MUA, but if the range deteriorates to less than 90° by 10 weeks, a further MUA, combined with an arthroscopic arthrolysis is performed.

Combined injuries of both cruciate ligaments and collateral ligaments are a rare injury, which can result in severe disability. In most cases, these severe knee injuries should be treated in the acute situation, but when presenting with chronic established instability, careful assessment of the patient's disability is required before undertaking this complex surgery. The surgeon and the patient must be aware that the principal objective of this type of reconstruction is to regain stability of the knee, which will allow activities of daily living without reliance on a knee brace.

Summary

Complex knee instability resulting from combination injuries to the knee ligaments involves a small sub-group of all patients with knee ligament injuries. There is no doubt that early recognition of these injuries, allowing early repair and augmentation in the acute phase, will achieve a better result. Unfortunately, the majority of patients will present with chronic knee instability. It is important to obtain an adequate history and perform a careful systematic examination of the knee ligaments in order to detect these complex patterns of instability. The instability must be defined by the ligaments damaged and the direction and degree of knee instability if an effective reconstruction is to be achieved.

Finally, it is essential that the surgeon has a clear appreciation of the patient's disability and, in turn, the patient understands that reconstructive surgery for this complex condition requires a prolonged period of recovery. Ultimately, it is of paramount importance that the surgeon and the patient have a realistic expectation of what can be achieved by surgery.

Key points

1. Complex instability patterns are difficult to define.
2. The injury mechanism is usually high velocity, e.g. road traffic accident, rather than sport.
3. Most patients present late.
4. There is usually a problem with activities of daily living; sport is impossible.
5. Suspect a missed combined injury if anterior cruciate reconstruction fails.
6. Develop a logical sequence for assessment and examination.
7. Patients should have a realistic expectation of surgery.

CHAPTER 8

Unresolved patellofemoral pain

C. M. Fergusson

Introduction

To the knee specialist, the problem of unresolved anterior knee pain can be one of the most challenging and frustrating to manage. The wealth of symptoms, the dearth of physical signs, the lack of supportive help from investigations and the failure to respond to conservative measures can lead to a very disheartening situation for both patient and doctor. It is hard to resist the temptation to advise empirical surgery, or dismiss the patient as suffering from emotional or psychological problems. Neither approach helps the patient. No surgical procedure will cure anterior knee pain consistently in all patients. Careful patient selection for surgery in this group is more important than in any other because of the potential disappointments, and also because the condition of many patients is actually exacerbated by surgery. A cautious and structured approach to the management of these individuals is critical, especially when they come for a second or third opinion and have had various procedures already performed without success.

As with all controversial subjects, there are no set protocols to follow [1], and each patient must be taken very much on his or her own merits. The goal is to identify those individuals in whom a curative procedure may be possible, and in the others to offer appropriate coping strategies and support, and the advice of other agencies. It is very easy to recommend a surgical approach, and if this fails, to move on to the next procedure. However, this author has seen a patient in whom such an approach had led to an above-knee amputation, with all the attending disabilities, with the pain persisting in an unrelenting fashion. Surgery can too often add a scar to a problem, rather than offering a solution.

Definitions

Right from the outset, one of the initial problems is that there is a great deal of confusion and misuse of terms regarding pain around the front of the knee [2]. Indeed, one of the first questions many frustrated patients ask is: 'What is wrong with me? No one will tell me what is actually going on in my knee.'

Patellofemoral pain, anterior knee pain, anterior knee pain syndrome, chondromalacia patella and patellofemoral dysfunction are all terms one finds in the literature. The term 'patellofemoral pain' has been chosen as the title, as it is the commonest generally descriptive term. The term 'anterior knee pain syndrome' is descriptive but not very helpful in terms of management; chondromalacia patellae dignifies the problem with a Latin name. However, it is a pathological description which may or may not involve pain, and patellofemoral dysfunction, which is possibly most accurate for many individuals, can deny the possibility of true structural causes of pain which may need surgical attention.

Anterior knee pain

This is a useful, descriptive term to describe the aching discomfort many patients complain of. Typically, they hold their whole hand across the front of the joint to describe their pain and it is associated with clicking, crepitus and difficulty going up and especially down stairs. The pain is usually exacerbated by prolonged sitting or driving (cinema knee, clutch knee). Most human beings have suffered from this once or twice in their lives. A direct blow on the patella will give rise to it, and prolonged over-exertion such as descending large hills can lead to it (Sahib's knee). A significant percentage of adolescents suffer from it in a transient way, and in the adult it is often initiated by a change of lifestyle. The best analogy in clinical terms is to liken it to a headache. This describes a recognisable phenomenon which can have a number of causes. It does not indicate any specific treatment immediately, and should not narrow the focus of clinical enquiry into its possible cause or subsequent investigation, but it is a useful handle for clinical record and classification. In loose terms, for example, it separates patients into those presenting with a primarily mechanical pattern of symptoms and those with a more inflammatory pattern of knee symptoms.

Anterior knee pain syndrome

The word syndrome means 'running with' and describes a collection of symptoms and signs which occur in clinical practice, without identifying a single or specific cause. In this category, patients presenting with idiopathic anterior knee pain and with irritable patellofemoral joints, without any other features to suggest a mechanical cause or meniscal pathology, are sometimes described as having anterior knee pain syndrome. There is evidence that if one looks hard enough for structural changes on X-ray and other assessments, one can nearly always identify some form of patellofemoral malalignment or other problem to account for these patients' symptoms. In this case, the syndrome is essentially that of patellofemoral dysfunction. The term 'syndrome', however, implies a degree of clinical defeat in identifying a cause for the condition. Nevertheless, it may be an honest appraisal of a patient's problem, and at least provides, if surgical or simple medical treatment fails to resolve the symptoms, a working term while coping strategies are established. To extend the headache analogy further, one could possibly call this group of patients those with 'migraine' of the knee.

Patellofemoral dysfunction

This term clearly implies that it is the patellofemoral joint which is the source of a patient's symptoms, and that the joint, for whatever reason, is not working correctly. This is probably the most accurate pathological term available, and covers the vast majority of minor patellar malalignment problems, and true chondromalacia, as well as the purely functional pain from imbalance of the vastus lateralis and medialis obliquus muscles. It allows inclusion for pain arising from the patella itself without offering any particular treatment rationale.

Chondromalacia patellae

This term should be restricted to the pathological process of articular surface disruption on the retropatellar surface. It is readily identifiable at arthroscopy and has been classified accurately. Its relationship to pain is not clear, and it is likely that the cause of pain is also the cause of the chondromalacia, rather than one giving rise to the other.

The importance of using these terms correctly is simply to be as honest as possible about the likely causes of pain, so as not to suggest surgical or conservative measures to a patient who does not fully understand the problem. All too often, a patient presents with symptoms which he or she has been told have been caused by roughness of the knee caps, and it is then very difficult to dissuade him or her from the idea that surgical smoothing of this area, or possible removal of the knee-cap, will necessarily solve their problems.

Clinical assessment of unresolved patellofemoral pain

These problems need a significant amount of clinic time, and the first consultation in particular must not be hurried. The initial interview and enquiries of the patient are often confounded with previous doctors' and physiotherapists' opinions, details of minor arthroscopic findings of dubious relevance and complex history of related injuries or sporting activities, all compounded by frustration and indignation, and criticism of previous carers; and the almost universal complaint, 'there must be something wrong because I can't be expected to go on like this'. This common pattern must not dissuade the clinician from gently going back through the history to clarify the clinical details in a logical order.

History

This must be taken carefully to include the age of onset, specifically whether there was any true trauma involved, or whether there was a perceived increase of pain after a certain activity. A common problem in dealing with unremitting anterior knee pain is that what was probably idiopathic patellofemoral dysfunction has been labelled as a sporting injury, and the patient and subsequent carers have expected there to be a mechanical fault. The relevance of any accidental or industrial component to the onset is also important to establish.

Localisation of pain defines the condition, and clearly a finger pointing accurately to a joint line suggests more meniscal pathology, rather than patellofemoral origin. More generalised lower limb pain is common, and probably reflects a generalised dysfunction of the limb, rather than a major psychological overlay in a complaining patient. Popliteal aching is not uncommon. Mechanical symptoms are frequent in patellofemoral pain and often the cause of early misdiagnosis. Giving way is the most obvious symptom, but on careful history this is usually reflex inhibition of the quadriceps with pain before the episode of giving way, rather than the typical pivoting of an unstable knee.

The commonest confusion arises from a history of locking. The clinical term 'locking' implies a knee that will not fully extend. This is not only very rarely described by the patient for any condition, but also when it is, they never describe it in those terms. A sensation of patellofemoral 'locking' is usually an episode of catching, or more commonly seizing when the knee is held bent for a long period. In order to clarify this, it is useful to ask the patient how they 'unlock the knee'. True mechanical unlocking of the joint caused by meniscal or loose body pathology is as distinct an event as the initial jamming, but in seizing from patellofemoral dysfunction, the patient's symptoms subside with time and gentle massage, rather than a single mechanical event.

Swelling is commonly reported in patients with patellofemoral pain, and yet in those individuals who say they have it at the time of presentation there is rarely a palpable effusion. The confusion probably arises from a sense of fullness or indeed slight inflammation of the anterior fat pad, and certainly true swelling of the joint suggests some intra-articular pathology that needs investigation in its own right (see below for clinical examination). Unless the knee swells up dramatically, the patient's history of swelling is rather unreliable. If asked to come back when the knee is swollen, they rarely do.

Bilaterality of symptoms is an integral part of primary patellofemoral dysfunction. That is, there is a constitutional component to patellofemoral pain which would be expected in a symmetrical individual. It can of course also occur in a heavy fall or a road accident where both knees are involved, but a purely unilateral pattern of symptoms suggests another diagnosis.

In gaining a history from a patient with unresolving patellofemoral pain, the value of previous therapeutic attempts must also be established. These are usually freely given, especially if they have been unsuccessful. However, well-managed, supervised physiotherapy to re-balance the quadriceps mechanism properly will almost inevitably improve the patient's symptoms to some extent. A complete lack of response makes one question the diagnosis, the commitment to treatment, or the type of physiotherapy. Arthroscopic surgery often appears to cause an exacerbation, but this may be confounded with disappointment at the lack of a curable lesion, as much as true worsening of the symptoms. The possible complication of haemarthrosis, especially after lateral release, or a true full-blown reflex sympathetic dystrophy pattern, must be established to understand and manage the patient appropriately.

Examination

As with all knee conditions, this starts with an overall assessment of the patient in terms of body weight, fitness and other associated pathology (e.g. psoriasis) which might have a bearing on the knee. Examination of the gait will lead to further benefits, not only in lower limb alignment and foot position, but also possible contribution from proximal pathology in the hip or the spine. Hip examination should be thorough in all cases of knee pathology, especially in patients who have failed to respond to treatment. Careful spinal examination and tension signs will exclude rare L3/4 nerve root compression.

Examination of the knees in question often reveals little in terms of dramatic signs (often to the patient's disappointment). However, careful assessment of patellar height, mobility, tracking, subluxation and points of tenderness, and lower limb alignment, including rear foot posture [3], are important for thorough understanding of the contribution of correctable malalignment in the pathology, in particular tightness of the lateral retinacular structures [4,5]. The patellofemoral joint itself may be irritable, but this is not an uncommon finding in many knee disorders. Provocative tests such as Clark's sign are discouraged by this author because they are almost universally positive. They add little to the understanding of the problem, and certainly can disaffect the patient. The presence of true effusion, locking, joint line tenderness or unilateral muscle wasting, as measured 12 cm above the patella, must make one consider alternative pathology than that from the patellofemoral joint.

Plain X-rays

By the time anterior knee pain has been labelled as unresolved, there will have been at least one set, if not many, of 'normal X-rays', which usually include standard anteroposterior (AP) and lateral views. The latter is useful for establishing patella alta and overt bony pathology which may be contributory, but skyline view at 30° [6] and a tunnel view can be valuable at this stage for the assessment of patellofemoral tilt, dysplasia, joint space loss and loose body formation which may be missed on the standard X-rays. The 30° skyline view is difficult to standardise, and more detailed assessment should be sought if a genuine maltracking component is suspected (see below). Beaconsfield *et al.* have usefully reviewed the radiological measurements [7] (Fig. 8.1).

Summary of initial interview and differential diagnoses

At the end of the formal clinical assessment in unresolved patellofemoral pain, the clinician should be clear as to the pathology being patellofemoral based. It is necessary to exclude proximal hip and lumbar spine problems, arthropathies, patellar tendinitis (jumper's knee) [8], significant degenerative joint disease or mechanical symptoms (not forgetting that bilateral medial meniscal pathology in the posterior horn in middle age is particularly common, and occasionally presents with anterior knee pain). Overt reflex sympathetic dystrophy or other complications of surgical attempts to cure the anterior knee pain, such as

haemarthrosis after lateral release, will also have been quite clearly established and may need specific treatment. Less obvious abnormal pain responses may not be so clear, but allodynia and hyperaesthesia of the knee joint in the clinical assessment may provide clues to this problem (see Chapter 12).

Assuming sufficient time has been allowed for a proper clinical assessment of the patient as above, a proportion of patients will have been identified with a different primary, or indeed a new secondary, problem which requires treatment in its own right. Nevertheless, further specialist investigation is often valuable.

Special investigations

If there is any doubt about an arthropathy, and in the presence of fluid within the joints without an obvious mechanical or degenerative cause, blood should be taken for full blood count, sedimentation rate, C-reactive protein, bone profile, liver function tests, rheumatoid factor and thyroid function tests.

Magnetic resonance imaging

Magnetic resonance imaging (MRI) is hugely valuable in the management of mechanical disorders of the joint and has become an essential tool in the knee clinic, but it does not, of course, replace careful clinical history and examination. Indeed, its use in unresolved patellofemoral pain is mainly to reassure unsuccessfully treated patients that there are no overt meniscal tears, and that reversible pathology has not been overlooked. This can be extremely valuable and may prevent any further

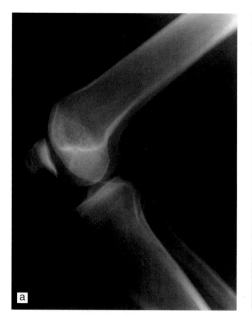 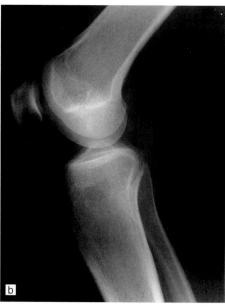

Figure 8.1 – Lateral view of a knee in two differing degrees of flexion. An illusion of patella infera is created. This illustrates the importance of using clear measurements of one of the indices if patella infera or alta is suspected. (a) At about 90° afflexion the patella looks lower than (b). (b) In the same knee at about 30°.

complications from repeat arthroscopy, which could promote further pain. However, although the soft tissues and the patella itself are clearly seen on MRI, it provides little information about the tracking in its static form, and is not particularly useful in the assessment of chondromalacia unless it is fairly far advanced.

In scanning patients over 40 years, it is worth bearing in mind that 5% of asymptomatic individuals in this age group have a torn meniscus, and 20% have minor degenerative change. Surgical treatment to the meniscus in these individuals will not always resolve their anterior knee pain.

Isotope scanning

Technetium-99 bone scanning is a particularly sensitive, but not specific, investigation. It is negative in benign patellofemoral dysfunction, but nearly always strongly positive in reflex sympathetic dystrophy, in significant degenerative joint disease, and in rarities such as osteoid osteoma. In this sense, it is a very useful adjunct in the management of this group of individuals [9]. There is a group of individuals in whom isotope scanning is mildly positive, but there is not the full-blown clinical picture of reflex sympathetic dystrophy. This group may respond better to vascular manipulation such as guanethedine blockade. The value of isotope scanning is that not only does it identify the patella as the source of some pathology, but it also may be the only positive test amongst dozens that the patient will have already had. Even a pathological result can be very reassuring. By the same token, a negative scan can reassure the clinician that there are no missed inflammatory or neoplastic problems (Fig. 8.2).

CT scan

Computerised tomography has been found to be valuable at 30°, 60° and 90° of flexion, in clearly identifying patellar tracking, and conformity of the patella–trochlea position. It is still a static investigation, but in the absence of dynamic tests (see below) it remains the best assessment to establish a true potentially correctable malalignment [10]. It is also particularly good for showing small missed avulsion fragments, suggestive of dislocations in the past (Fig. 8.3).

Dynamic imaging and the future

Patellofemoral dysfunction is a dynamic problem, and all our investigations, other than careful clinical observation, have relied on static imaging. The new

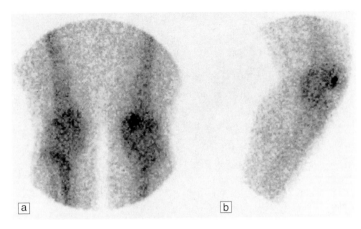

Figure 8.2 – *Isotope scan of a young woman with unresolved patellofemoral pain which shows diffuse uptake. A more extreme scan would be expected in advanced RSD, but a low-grade diffuse pattern is commonly seen, suggesting either a forme fruste of the true syndrome, or another vascularly related phenomenon. Both may respond to guanethedine. (a) AP of both knees showing increased uptake in left knee. (b) Lateral view of left knee showing focal uptake in patella.*

techniques of MRI performed on the moving knee offer some very exciting possibilities, but are not yet widely available. However, this must significantly enhance our understanding of how a patella behaves, given the established knowledge we have of the static situation.

We still cannot image pain, which is the patient's main complaint, and the source of it in patellofemoral dysfunction is still not clear. It may be presumed to be arising from interosseous tension within the patella itself, and a number of facts support this concept. However, we have no way of imaging or measuring this at the present time, although it is the author's belief that this will be the biggest breakthrough in understanding this complex and troublesome condition.

Treatment for unresolved patellofemoral pain

Treatment for the associated pathologies that emerge after assessment and investigation can be conducted in the usual way. Missed meniscal pathology, true degenerative joint disease or an inflammatory arthropathy, for example, will require their own measures. It is very important to identify an abnormal pain response, in reflex sympathetic dystrophy in particular, early on, and refer these sooner rather than later for pain clinic management by a specialist in this field. These problems resolve much faster with earlier

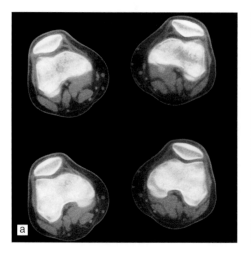

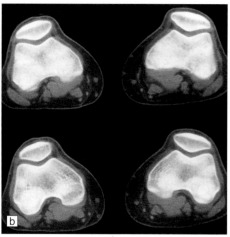

Figure 8.3 – *Serial CT slices of both knees at (a) 0°, (b) 30°, (c) 60° and (d) 90° of flexion. Until the availability of dynamic screening of patellofemoral tracking, this is the best imaging method for assessing the patellofemoral joint throughout its range. The lateral-to-medial movement can be appreciated and a clear comparison made between both sides. This examination was considered symmetrical and within normal limits.*

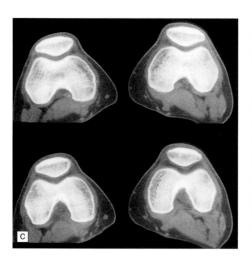

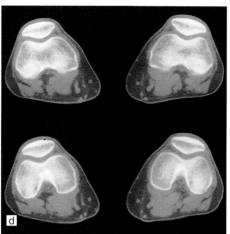

therapy and should not be submitted to the gamut of more conservative options or, in particular, surgical treatment.

Assuming that one is dealing with true persistent patellofemoral pain, initial treatments remain conservative, rather than surgical, even in the face of slight patellar malalignment pathology or a tight retinaculum [11], unless there are overt episodes of patellar dislocation, subluxation or gross abnormality. Just because a minor malalignment problem can be identified does not mean surgical treatment is either advised or likely to be successful.

Physiotherapy

It is a common problem amongst this difficult group of patients that the initial diagnoses and management have been confused and sporadic over a long period of time, and it is essential to re-focus their commitment to a new conservative regime if any success is to be expected [12]. Unfortunately, good evaluation tools [13] are in their

infancy and have usually not been applied. The suggestion of another trip to the physiotherapist early in the interview will often be dismissed, as previous visits have been unsuccessful. Sometimes the term 'physiotherapy' referred to in a general practitioner's letter will have been a single visit to a non-specialist physiotherapist, and will have been of little value. To believe anterior knee pain is caused by patellofemoral dysfunction must be to believe that by re-training patellofemoral function we can relieve the pain. Even in the unresolved cases, this must be re-visited by a dedicated physiotherapy team who will address the imbalance between vastus medialis obliquus and vastus lateralis [14], measurement of this imbalance appears an important primary step in this group [15]. The use of biofeedback therapy to re-train the patient with an exercise programme has been the most useful addition to treatment and management of this disorder for some years. Closed kinetic chain exercises are important [16], and to support this, taping techniques could certainly be tried, as they are non-invasive, safe, functional and often profoundly valuable [17], though not always so [18]. They are very much treater-dependent and not always acceptable to the patient. Bracing, too, has proved effective [19], though it may not be accepted on a long-term basis.

By the same token, correction by simple orthoses of gait problems caused by over-pronation can be very helpful in patellofemoral function. This procedure is non-invasive, reversible and cheap, compared to surgical alternatives.

This whole programme of conservative therapy must be supported by general lifestyle changes, in particular stressing the avoidance of bent-leg activities and the adoption of fitness routines such as free-style swimming and cycling, rather than breast-stroke swimming or running. Encouragement to take part in various activities to try the joints out is useful, as it is important to break the cycle of giving up sporting activities which leads to weakness of the muscle and weight gain. This further aggravates the muscle imbalance of the lower limb and heightens the pain, which in turn reduces the patient's activity. A gym-based physiotherapy programme can help reverse this pattern in all but a few.

Failure to respond to conservative treatment

Even in the presence of suspected tight retinaculum, patellar malalignment and chondromalacia, the conservative options are always re-visited. If no benefit is achieved and nothing emerges from a repeat clinical examination, it is reasonable to proceed to correct overt patellofemoral pathology. This is nearly always at the same time as, or preceded by, arthroscopy. Before making even an arthroscopic surgical approach to a patient, however, it is worth bearing in mind that there is only one study in the literature that claims 100% improvement rate of any patellofemoral disorder, however clear the apparent pathology.

Indications for arthroscopy

Arthoscopy can be valuable in the management of patellofemoral pain [20], but is not essential, and certainly not indicated early on in every case. It can cause complications, some serious, and this must not be overlooked when dealing with an essentially benign disorder, however uncomfortable. The chances of finding a truly reversible lesion which will cure the patient's symptoms are also very small. Nevertheless, there are some indications; these are:

- In association with the alignment procedure, such as lateral release, where there has been a clear clinical and radiological demonstration that this is a primary factor in the pathology (see below).
- To assess patellofemoral tracking if there is some debate, despite the relevant investigations. After thorough assessment, very clear unresolved patellofemoral instability may emerge. This can be rewarding to identify and treat appropriately, as long as there are no other pathological features to the joint, there is no abnormal pain response to previous attempts of treatment, and the patient has a committed approach to rehabilitation. The different assessments and techniques for patellofemoral instability have been covered in a separate chapter of this volume.
- To exclude other pathology such as degenerative joint disease or meniscal change which may have been picked up on the scan and needs pursuing. An examination under anaesthetic is important in this regard, as both anterior and posterior cruciate ligament deficiencies can be associated with patellofemoral pain.
- To identify (and treat?) chondromalacia and plicae.

Chondromalacia patellae

Chondromalacia patellae can, of course, be identified arthroscopically, and indeed debrided manually or with the power tool shaver. However, the value of this is debatable, and only in exceptional cases of established chondromalacia with profound catching and seizing might it be worth pursuing this option. There is very little to support significant abrasion chondroplasty or more extensive techniques compared with simply removing obviously unstable fragments, which can probably be just as well performed with hand tools.

Lateral release in patellofemoral pain

As indicated above, arthroscopic treatment can include arthroscopic lateral release. The author's preferred method is to do this through a mini-open procedure, to remain extra-synovial and to attend to the vessel directly with diathermy in order to reduce the possibility of a haemarthrosis which can complicate lateral release and cause significant deterioration in function and worsening of pain. While either arthroscopic or open technique is relatively straightforward, indication for this procedure is not. Routine lateral release in the absence of tightness should be discouraged [21].

The results are very variable, even in experienced hands. Published reports of satisfactory results for lateral release range from 14 to 100% with both arthroscopic and open techniques employed. Whilst there are no absolute guidelines that can be drawn, evidence of a clear tight lateral retinacular band, as witnessed by reduced patellar glide and tightness on attempts at patella lifting, significant patellar tilt radiologically, and its subsequent correction postoperatively, and few chondromalacic features all favour a more satisfactory outcome. It is important to maintain the vastus medialis pull postoperatively to prevent recurrent lateral tightening. In summary, clear evidence of a tight retinaculum clinically and radiologically without other pathology and unresponsive to conservative treatment, will benefit from a lateral retinacular release in most cases.

Plicae and knee pain

The pathological plica remains a controversial subject in the cause of patellofemoral pain [22]. Plicae are common findings in the knee, and range from minor folds in and around the suprapatellar region to large separated shelves across the medial femoral condyle [23].

In this latter context, they can become thickened and appear to rub along the medial femoral condyle, which is commonly the site of tenderness in anterior knee pain sufferers. Occasionally, a small click can be felt when rubbing them. There is little published evidence to support the plica as a major cause of patellofemoral pain, and yet there are very few arthroscopists who have not removed plicae from time to time, occasionally with good results. However, it is the author's view that they should not be pursued in all cases of patellofemoral dysfunction, and even a suspected plica should be treated conservatively to start with. In unresolved pain with no other pathology in association, it seems reasonable to excise a large and thickened plica.

Patellar subluxation

After thorough assessment a very clear, unresolved patellofemoral instability may emerge. These can be rewarding to identify and treat appropriately [24], as long as there are no other pathological features to the joint, there is no abnormal pain response to previous attempts at treatment, and the patient has a committed approach to rehabilitation. The different assessments and techniques for patellofemoral instability are covered in Chapter 9.

Further surgical procedures for unresolved patellofemoral pain

If all other pathologies have been excluded, lateral retinacular tightness has been relieved, patellofemoral malalignments have been corrected appropriately [25,26], and any intra-articular pathology such as the rare pathological plica has been excised, and the patients' symptoms remain in the patellofemoral region, it is the author's practice to stop operating and re-visit all the conservative avenues and await the passage of a reasonable period of time, supporting the patient if necessary with coping strategies and pain clinic management as indicated (see below).

However, there are a number of other possible surgical options which could be considered.

The bipartite patella

Assuming it is not an un-united fracture, and these are usually readily identifiable on clinical and radiological grounds, bipartite fragment is quite commonly seen, and may be associated with a tight lateral retinacular band which is the cause of both the pain and the bipartite fragment. There is evidence that lateral release alone will effect union in most cases [27]. Surgical treatment directly to unite bipartite fragment has been successful and resulted in pain relief, although the associated lateral release may have been the more valuable component of the procedure. Direct excision of a prominent and directly tender fragment may also be valuable in rare circumstances.

Patellar insertion advancement/medialisation

Macquet described elevation of the tibial tubercle over an extended segment of the upper tibia to reduce the stress across the patellofemoral joint [28]. Bio-mechanical measurements will support the fact that if suitably ventralised, the stress will be reduced, and this has been reported to give benefit [29]. The operation itself is fairly extensive and comes at some cosmetic price, as the shape of the proximal tibia is profoundly altered and not readily accepted by some patients. The results are variable and the risks more considerable and morbidity more significant than measures previously described. Miller and Larochelle described rotation and elevation of the tubercle with encouraging results [30], and the technique developed by Fulkerson *et al.* involves anteromedial displacement of the tubercle. This is a smaller procedure than the Maquet with fewer cosmetic implications, and the results are reported in most cases to be satisfactory [31,32], though they may diminish with time [33].

This technique appears at the present time to be more popular in the US than in the UK.

Patellar osteotomy

In an attempt to normalise patellar tracking, patellar osteotomy through a vertical split and opening has been advocated [34,35], and appears to give satisfactory functional results. Subsequent analysis revealed that pain relief was gained, even at the expense of loss of the apparent correction. This has suggested that it was the decompression of the patella that was effective, although there must have been some profound mechanical changes to the muscle balance at the time of surgery, which may or may not have been involved. Although relatively easy to perform, the author's own experience of this technique has been disappointing and unpredictable. Much clearer indications for it, and more prospective studies, are needed before making it a formal recommendation. The science of patellar dynamics and interosseous pressures may answer these questions in the future, but it does not remain a widespread or recommended technique for unremitting anterior knee pain at the present time.

Surface replacement

Other techniques of articular surface replacement, both with carbon fibre pads in established chondromalacic lesions, and more recently with autografting, have been less successful than the counterparts on the femoral condyle. While the newer techniques have appeared to have great potential, it will be a little while before we can be certain of their long-term value, and they currently have no place in the management of unresolved patellofemoral pain.

Patellectomy

This has been advocated as a measure for patellofemoral pain as 'a last resort'. It still has its advocates, but it should not be used indiscrimately in benign patellofemoral pain [36]. It does not always work, it always decreases knee function by reducing the strength by some 40% [37,38], it effectively reduces the possibility of any future surgical or medical treatment to the patella if developments in medical science provide a more attractive option, and it may promote or accelerate osteoarthritis [39]. Ablative surgery for pain can only be recommended if the surgeon can be absolutely sure that the organ to be excised is the cause of the painful stimulus (Fig. 8.4). In many cases, this may not be the situation.

Pain clinic and other agencies

The involvement of specialists in pain management has been alluded to previously, for clear examples of reflex sympathetic dystrophy (RSD), in which early referral is essential to get good results. Long-term effects of untreated RSD lead to permanent joint stiffness and damage. A good relationship with a pain control specialist can be very valuable in the less clear patterns of patellofemoral pain, when there are no overt malalignment features which should or could be corrected, or there is a component of degenerative joint disease, and yet conservative measures have failed and arthroplasty is not appropriate. There is clear evidence that techniques such as guanethedine blockade can also be useful in anterior knee pain, even in the absence of full-blown RSD, but apart from specialist pain control techniques, the value of teaching coping strategies and a long-term view to this group of patients with this problem cannot be over-estimated.

With the developments of arthroplasty for osteoarthritis of the knee, and the huge success of the arthroscope in soft tissue sports injury management, a patient with a chronically painful joint which is unresolvable by surgical techniques is increasingly frustrated. Coming to terms with an untreatable benign

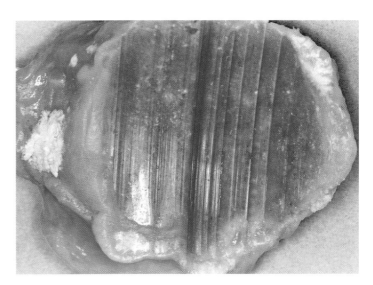

Figure 8.4 – *If a patella has to be removed, ensure there is something wrong with it. This is an advanced case of patellofemoral arthritis in isolation with marked lateral tracking and deep matching scoring of the underlying bone.*

pathology is unfamiliar to the short-suffering population of Britain in the late twentieth century. A team approach in the knee clinic involving physiotherapists, orthotists, anaesthetists and sports therapists, and occasionally clinical psychologists, is far more likely to yield effective results than working one's way through the surgical textbook.

Key points

1. Unresolved anterior knee pain is a complicated problem and requires considerable clinic time.
2. Revisiting the basic clinical details with accurate history and clinical examination is usually more valuable than ordering multiple further investigations.
3. Keep an open mind about rare presentations of common problems, e.g. bilateral torn degenerate medial menisci.
4. Pain from patellofemoral dysfunction is very rarely unilateral. Non-knee causes of pain, such as a high prolapsed intervertebral disc, may present in this way.
5. The use of general descriptive terms is more helpful than specific pathological ones, e.g. chondromalacia patellae, as in the latter case, unless it has actually been proven, it seeds the thought in the patient's mind that a surgical approach to their knee will help, when this is rarely the case.
6. Close co-operation with the physiotherapists is very valuable in establishing protocols of care in chronic patellofemoral dysfunction pain.
7. Involvement of the pain clinic specialists is more successful if considered early, especially in RSD.
8. There is no 100% surgical cure for anterior knee pain.

CHAPTER 9

The unstable patella

D. J. Dandy

Introduction

There are many different types of patellar instability with many different causes. Few textbooks or articles distinguish between the various patterns and most apply a single operation or treatment regime to all, an uncritical approach attended by disappointing results. This article aims to separate the various causes of patellofemoral instability so that the appropriate procedure can be selected. The emphasis is on a selective approach to management rather than one operation used for all unstable patellae regardless of cause.

Dynamics of the patellofemoral joint

Every patella is intrinsically unstable because the tibial tubercle lies lateral to the midline of the knee and the line of action of the quadriceps muscle. When the quadriceps contracts, the patella is subjected to a laterally directed force. This apparent 'design fault' is partially overcome by the median ridge of the patella bearing against the shallow lateral lip of the trochlea during flexion [1]. The lateral side of the trochlea is a gently sloping ramp a few millimetres high, and may be insufficient to resist the pull of the powerful quadriceps even in a normal knee.

In full extension, the patella lies at the upper end of the trochlea, which it enters more deeply as flexion begins. It is essential that the patella is engaged correctly in the trochlea at the start of flexion if it is to remain stable. Once engaged, the patella is held in the trochlear groove by two mechanisms. The first is mechanical

contact between the patella and the lateral edge of the trochlea, which acts as a lateral buffer, and the second is soft tissue tension on the medial side which prevents it slipping laterally.

With the quadriceps relaxed and the knee extended, the patella rests lightly on the femur but moves laterally when the muscle contracts. As flexion begins, the median ridge of the patella in a normal knee lies lateral to the centre of the trochlea during the first 30° of flexion. Between 30 and 60° of flexion, the patella is guided medially to become 'centred' in the trochlea. As flexion proceeds, the patella becomes more deeply engaged in the trochlea and is held firmly by soft tissue tension. When the knee is flexed beyond 90°, the patella tilts so that the medial facet articulates with the medial side of the trochlea.

If the patella is not engaged securely in the trochlea at the start of flexion, it will move laterally and, as flexion continues, will either move completely over the lateral lip of the trochlea and dislocate or move back medially to its correct position.

Factors leading to patellar instability

Poor engagement of the patella in the trochlea
Failure to engage may be due to an abnormally high patella, patellar dysplasia (Fig. 9.1) or a poorly developed trochlea. The consequences of a high patella and a proximally deficient trochlea are the same; the patella is not securely engaged at the start of flexion. Hyperextension of the knee and lax ligaments also contribute to poor engagement by allowing the patella to 'float' off the femur in full extension.

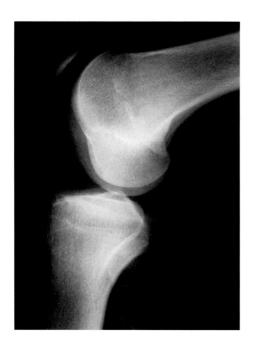

Figure 9.1 – *A lateral X-ray showing a small, high and dysplastic patella with a dysplastic trochlea.*

Causes of poor patellar engagement
- High patella
- Dysplastic patella
- Dysplastic trochlea
- Hyperextension of the knee.

Failure to stay in the trochlea once engaged

Some patellae engage correctly at the start of flexion but sublux or dislocate as flexion continues. This may be due to a trochlea that is defective because it is abnormally shallow, or because the lateral lip is too low at its point of contact with the patella at 30° of flexion.

The tendency to dislocate in flexion is exaggerated if the laterally directed force applied to the patella is increased by excessive genu valgum from trauma, congenital deformity or a very laterally placed tibial tubercle. Poor soft tissue balance around the patella caused by either very tight lateral structures or very lax medial structures may also contribute. The lateral structures may be tight following fibrosis of the vastus lateralis [2] or trauma, but sometimes there may be no obvious cause. Lax medial structures follow trauma to the medial retinaculum, stretching of the tissues from repeated dislocation, severe wasting of the vastus medialis or myopathy.

Causes of failure to stay engaged
- Abnormal trochlea at 30° of flexion
- Tight lateral structures
- Lax medial structures

- Valgus deformity
- Laterally placed tibial tubercle.

Assessment

The purpose of assessment is to identify the factors causing instability so that appropriate treatment can be selected. Assessment follows the usual procedure of a clinical history, clinical examination and investigation.

History

The history will reveal whether the symptoms began with a sudden traumatic event or there was an insidious onset. Normal patellofemoral joints can be dislocated by severe trauma, but if the first dislocation occurred without significant force there is likely to be an underlying anatomical abnormality. The circumstances of the dislocations are also important. Does the patella dislocate with every flexion of the knee or only with twisting movements? Does the patella always dislocate completely or does it sometimes just feel a little unsteady? Can the patient describe a specific movement which causes dislocation?

It is essential to know what effect the symptoms have on the patient's way of life before advising operation. There is little point in advising an extensive operation with prolonged rehabilitation if the dislocations cause only minor inconvenience and are not becoming either more severe or more frequent.

Clinical examination

First, look at the leg as a whole and assess its general appearance. A valgus deformity, lateral scarring and quadriceps wasting are all easily seen. Assess the power of the quadriceps by asking the patient to lift the leg straight, surprisingly difficult for many patients with an unstable patella.

Next, watch the patella while the patient flexes the knee. Does it engage smoothly at the proximal end of the trochlea or more distally than normal? Does it jump suddenly medially as it engages in the trochlea? Does the knee flex fully or is flexion restricted by tight structures?

Next, assess patellar stability by gently holding the patella laterally while flexing the knee. Many patients will be apprehensive when this is done, confirming that the problem is poor patellar engagement. Assess lateral movement by gently moving the patella laterally in full extension; most normal patellae can be made to overhang the lateral edge of the femur by half the patellar diameter, but more than that is usually pathological.

Side-to-side movement of the patella also allows the lateral and medial structures to be assessed and the presence of generalised ligament laxity, hyperextension and abnormally loose patellar retinacula detected.

The Q, for quadriceps, angle is the angle between the long axes of the quadriceps and patellar tendon and it determines the magnitude of the vector pushing the patella laterally when the quadriceps contracts (Fig. 9.2). It is a poor indication of the actual forces on the patella and is difficult to measure. Unstable patellae, particularly if they are abnormally high, lie more laterally than normal in full extension and this reduces the Q angle, while a completely dislocated patella may have a Q angle

of zero or even a negative value (Fig. 9.3). Reducing the Q angle to zero might be expected to eliminate the lateral vector altogether, but patellae still dislocate when this has been done if the trochlea is shallow.

Although the Q angle is a useful dynamic concept, the magnitude of the lateral vector is determined more by the relative positions of the tibial tubercle and the centre of the trochlea in the coronal plane than the axis of the quadriceps. Measurement of this distance is a more useful part of the clinical examination than the Q angle. The distance between the centre of the trochlea and the tibial tubercle (TG–TT) is 10–15 mm in normal patients (Fig. 9.4).

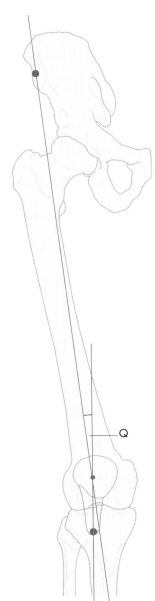

Figure 9.2 – *The Q angle.*

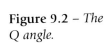

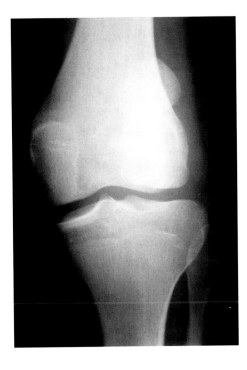

Figure 9.3 – *A small and high patella lying laterally making the Q angle misleadingly low.*

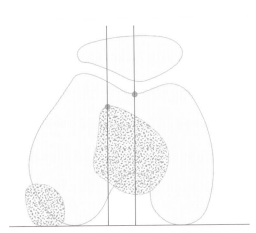

Figure 9.4 – *Transverse section of the lower limb to show the relationship between the femoral trochlea and the tibial tubercle. The tibia and fibula are stippled.*

Goutallier *et al.* [3] have described the TG–TT distance by radiological measurements, but a rough estimate of this relationship can be made by examining the knee in 90°, of flexion. The centre of the trochlea usually lies in the midline of the lower end of the femur, i.e. at the mid-epicondylar point. With the knee flexed to 90°, the tibial tubercle should be less than 20 mm lateral to the midline of the femur at the level of the epicondyles. More than 20 mm indicates a tubercle that is abnormally far lateral and an increased lateral force on the patella.

Patellar height can only be measured accurately on X-rays but, again, a rough estimate can be made clinically. The patella is usually a little shorter than the patellar tendon and an abnormally high patella is quite easily detected by comparing the lengths of the patella and patellar tendon.

Radiological examination

Plain X-rays show the position and shape of the patella and may also show small ossicles on the medial side of the patella. These ossicles, first described by Coleman [4], are sometimes called 'Coleman's fractures', even though they are more likely to be the result of ossification within a haematoma rather than a true fracture.

Radiological measurements of patellar height

Patella alta is the Latin for 'high patella' (Fig. 9.5). American surgeons, particularly those from California, have recently begun to refer to an abnormally low patella as 'patella baja'. While it is true that alta and baja are the Spanish for high and low, the Spanish for patella is 'rotula'. Mixing ancient Latin with modern Spanish has little to recommend it, particularly when those who do not speak Spanish write, phonetically, of 'patella baha'. Patella infera is Latin for 'low patella' but it is hard to know why we need another language to express this simple concept. English will be used in this chapter.

Many methods exist for measuring the height of the patella on radiographs. The Insall–Salvati index [5] (Fig. 9.6a), which compares the length of the patella with the length of the patellar tendon (men 0.9–1.1, women 0.94–1.18) is often used, but has a number of practical disadvantages. The point of attachment of the patellar tendon to the tibia is indistinct and measurement after tibial tubercle transposition is very difficult. Further, the total length of the patella is not always an indication of the length of the articular surface of the patella in contact with the femur. Long pointed patellae can produce misleading measurements.

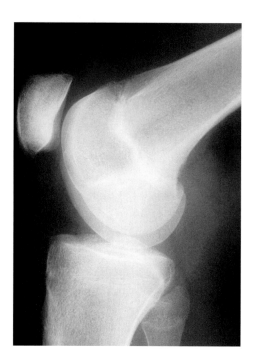

Figure 9.5 – *A high patella. There is also a positive crossing sign.*

The Blackburne and Peel index [6] (Fig. 9.6b) relates the length of the articular surface of the patella to its distance above the tibial plateau (men 0.85–1.09, women 0.79–1.09) and provides a more useful measure of the relationship of the patella with the trochlea than the Insall–Salvati index. The measurements are influenced by the angle of flexion but errors caused by variations in flexion are probably less than the errors of measurement.

Perhaps the easiest and most useful method is that of Caton [7] which compares the length of the articular surface of the patella with the distance between the lower end of the articular surface and the nearest point on the tibia, its antero-superior angle (Fig. 9.6c). The ratio of these two measurements in the normal knee is close to 1 (men 0.96 ± 0.134, women 0.99 ± 0.129). The Caton index is simple, is not dependent on the angle of flexion and is not affected by long patellae or abnormal tibial tubercles.

Observations on a true lateral radiograph

Dejour *et al.* [8] have described how a true lateral X-ray can provide much information about the anatomy of the femoral trochlea. Detailed examination of the lateral X-ray has received little attention in the English literature, apart from measurements of patellar height, but the shape and depth of the trochlea can be measured with great precision provided the radiograph is a true lateral view in which the posterior margins of the condyles are superimposed.

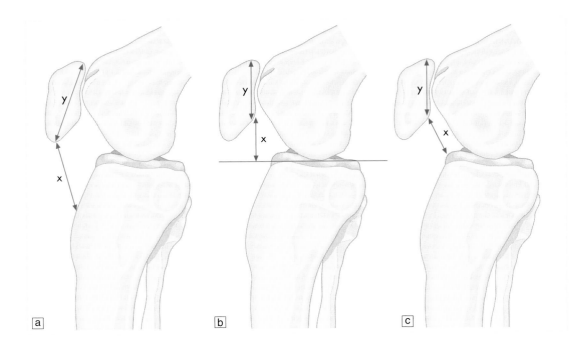

Figure 9.6 – *Methods of measuring patellar height. (a) Insall–Salvati index; (b) Blackburne and Peel index; (c) Caton's index.*

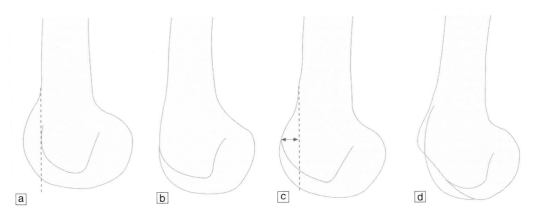

Figure 9.7 – *Appearances of the femoral trochlea on the true lateral X-ray. (a) Normal appearance; (b) crossing sign; (c) the 'bump' sign; (d) dysplastic trochlea.*

The floor of the trochlea can be seen as a radio-dense line linking the anterior cortex of the femur with the roof of the intercondylar notch (Blumensaat's line [9]). In the normal knee, the floor of the trochlea is a direct continuation of the anterior cortex of the femur (Figs 9.7a, 9.8). Examining a real femur, perhaps during joint replacement or arthrotomy for other reasons, makes it easier to appreciate this relationship. Several abnormal variants of this arrangement are seen.

The 'crossing sign'

If the line indicating the floor of the trochlea intersects or crosses the lateral lip of the trochlea (Figs 9.7b, 9.9) the trochlea must be deficient proximally and the patella will not engage correctly. The proximal third of the trochlea has no lateral lip in these patients and secure engagement at the start of flexion is impossible.

The 'bump' sign

The 'bump' sign indicates a more serious abnormality than the crossing sign (Figs 9.7c, 9.10). If the radio-dense line linking the anterior cortex of the femur and the floor of the trochlea presents an anterior convexity, or bump, the proximal third of the trochlea is convex instead of concave and patellar engagement will be mechanically impossible because there is no groove to hold the patella. A slight anterior convexity is not unusual, but a bump of more than 3 mm is pathological [8].

Dysplastic condyles

Trochleae with grossly dysplastic condyles often show a small beak or spike at the proximal end of the trochlea resembling a small osteophyte (Figs 9.7d, 9.11) and in very severe examples the two lips of the trochlea are asymmetrical. Such trochleae cannot engage the patella correctly.

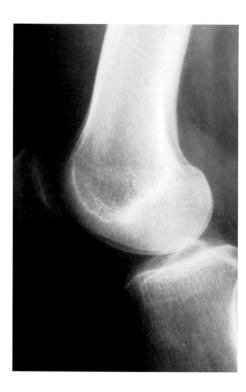

Figure 9.8 –
*Lateral X-ray
showing a normal
trochlea.*

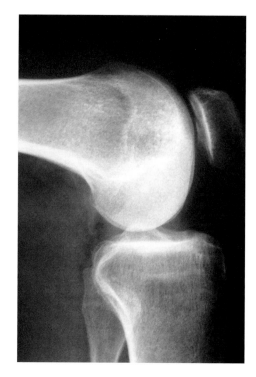

Figure 9.10 –
*A lateral X-ray
showing the 'bump'
sign.*

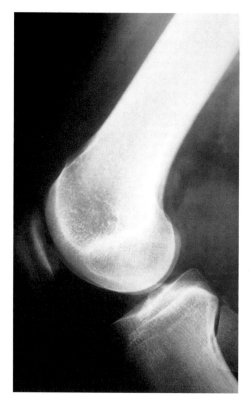

Figure 9.9 –
*The crossing sign
in the presence
of a slightly high
patella.*

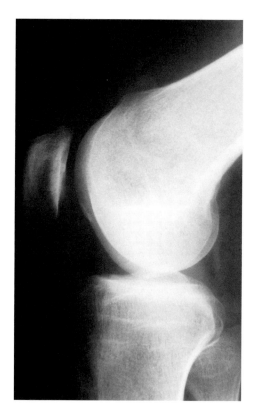

Figure 9.11 –
*A dysplastic and
asymmetrical
trochlea with a
proximal spike.*

Trochlear depth
The line indicating the floor of the trochlea lies posterior to the anterior margins of the condyles and the distance between the two indicates the depth of the trochlea (Figs 9.12, 9.13). The normal trochlea has a depth of

7–8 mm [8]. A shallow trochlea may be insufficient to prevent the patella dislocating laterally, even it engages correctly in the trochlea at the start of flexion.

It is not unusual to find more than one of these radiological abnormalities in the same knee. High

Figure 9.12 – *Measurement of the trochlear depth on a lateral X-ray.*

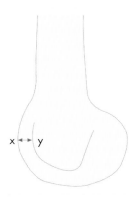

Figure 9.13 – *A shallow trochlea. The patient also has a high patella and a shallow bump.*

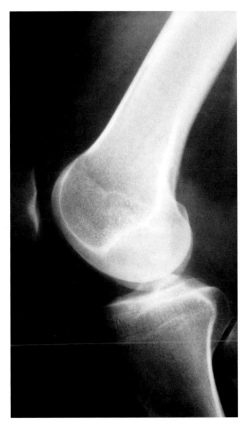

patellae than in normal patients, while if measured from the centre of the trochlea it is greater in patients with unstable patellae. This information is not surprising and does not help greatly with the management of individual patients. CT is a time-consuming and expensive technique for measuring something of little importance.

Relationship of tibial tubercle and trochlea (TG–TT)

The TG–TT distance is more useful than the Q angle. The distance can be estimated clinically and measurements can be made on X-rays, but precise measurement requires the superimposition of transverse CT images. Clinical examination is usually sufficient to determine how far the tubercle should be moved at operation.

Patellar angle

MRI or CT scans also give information about the condition of the trochlea, the shape of the patella and the angle at which it lies in the trochlea. Tangential X-rays of the patella [10] have been widely used in the past, but obtaining good X-rays consistently in the first 30° of flexion is extremely difficult. Basing management on these angles was seldom practical and they are now largely obsolete. One does not need an X-ray to know that the patella is subluxed or tilted, but if accurate measurements are needed they can be obtained with CT or MRI.

Abnormal angles may indicate a deficient trochlea or sulcus, a dysplastic patella, shallow trochlear lip or tight lateral structures. Similar information can be obtained from clinical examination or a true lateral X-ray as already described.

Arthroscopy

Although not needed to diagnose patellar instability, arthroscopy is a valuable preliminary to surgical stabilisation. The patella can be seen engaging in the trochlea from the anterolateral or lateral suprapatellar approaches. A normal patella centres between 30 and 60° of flexion and failure to centre is easily seen. The contour of the trochlea and the shape of the patella can be seen directly and related to the appearance of the lateral X-ray. A dysplastic or flattened trochlea, for example, can be seen clearly and the technical problems of achieving stability assesssed. The medial retinaculum can also be examined. Abnormally loose tissues may be an indication for medial plication.

A useful view of the patella can be obtained by placing the telescope in the lateral gutter from the

patellae and shallow trochleae are often seen together [7].

Q angle

For the reasons already described, measurement of the Q angle based on the position of the patella is much less useful in practice than in theory, but it may be more valuable if the centre of the trochlea is used for measurement instead of the centre of the patella. With the help of computerised tomography (CT) it can be confirmed that the Q angle measured from the centre of the patella is actually less in patients with unstable anterolateral approach and looking upwards (anteriorly). The normal patella usually overhangs the femur by one-third of its width and pushing the patella laterally may bring the whole of the lateral half into view. Unstable patellae may sublux completely.

Finally, the joint surfaces can be examined. Vertical fissures resembling the side of a clinker-built boat [11,12] are almost diagnostic of patellar instability. If the patella is pushed laterally and allowed to reduce the cartilage, ridges may been seen catching on the edge of the lateral condyle, suggesting that they are probably caused as the patella reduces after dislocation. Osteochondral separations of both the patellar and trochlear surfaces may also be present. Articular surface lesions, which may lead to progressive osteoarthritis and indicate a poor prognosis, should be recorded.

Selecting the operation

Broadly speaking, stabilising operations can be classed as distal realignments to transpose the tibial tubercle, proximal realignments or releases to alter the tension of tissues attached to the patella, or operations to deepen the trochlea.

It is essential when selecting an operation to choose the procedure which will correct the underlying problem in the individual patient. It is incorrect to use the same procedure for operation on all patients regardless of the underlying cause.

Distal realignment

Distal transposition of the tibial tubercle is required if the patella is abnormally high and the trochlea normal. The tubercle should be transposed far enough distally to allow the patella to engage correctly in the trochlea and bring the indices of patellar height to the lower end of the normal range (Fig. 9.14). The amount of transposition required is variable, but can be measured on the lateral X-ray and is commonly between 10 and 20 mm.

Hauser [13] described a technique for distal and medial transposition which fell into undeserved disrepute because it was often applied uncritically to all patients with unstable patellae, regardless of patellar height. Distal transposition, whether by the Hauser technique or another, is only appropriate if the patella is abnormally high and produces serious problems if it produces a very low patella.

Although distal transposition is not indicated if the patella is already at the correct height and the problem lies

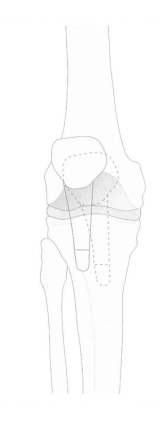

Figure 9.14 – *Correction of a high and lateral patella by distal and medial tibial tubercle transfer.*

in the trochlea, distal transposition may be appropriate if the trochlea is only slightly deficient at its upper end, even though this may bring the index of patellar height a little below the lower limit of its normal range.

Techniques exist for lifting the tibial tubercle anteriorly at the time of transposition. Such procedures are based on the work of Maquet [14] in patients with patellofemoral osteoarthritis, but are not applicable to patellofemoral instability. Moving the tibial tubercle anteriorly can only reduce patellar stability.

Medial transposition

Medial transposition of the tubercle is indicated if it lies too far laterally, but is commonly done as an adjunct to distal transposition (Fig. 9.15). Care should be taken not to move the tubercle medial more than 10 mm medial to the midline of the trochlea, thus producing a negative Q angle or negative TG–TT distance, because this may lead to recurrent medial dislocation.

Medial transposition alone may also be appropriate when the trochlea is dysplastic and a patella of normal size and height engages poorly in the trochlea, but only if a trial at the time of operation confirms that the patella is stable. Testing the effect of simple medial transposition is easily achieved by holding the patellar tendon medially with a bone awl driven into the tibia.

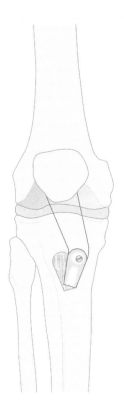

Figure 9.15 – *Medial transposition using the Elmslie–Trillat technique.*

Medial transposition alone is not adequate for a high patella or gross ligament laxity.

Adjustment of tissue tension
The tension of the soft tissues around the patella can be altered by releasing lateral structures or tightening medial structures.

Lateral release
Both tibial tubercle transposition and medial plication are usually accompanied by lateral release. In the early days of arthroscopic surgery, it seemed reasonable to perform arthroscopic lateral release before tibial tubercle transposition on the grounds that the morbidity was lower, rehabilitation faster, and that a more extensive procedure could always be performed later if the result was unsatisfactory. The results showed that lateral release alone is a surprisingly reliable procedure for recurrent dislocation, provided the patella is not abnormally high and the ligaments are not abnormally loose [15].

One might have expected lateral release to produce good results only in patients with tight lateral structures, but it has proved to be effective for many other patients. The overall results [15] are better than tibial tubercle transfer or medial plication, although it is not clear why this should be. The release perhaps alters the balance between vastus medialis and vastus lateralis or the tilt of the patella at the moment of engagement, but it can have no effect on bony anatomy.

Apart from the unexpectedly good results, the operation also has the advantage of fewer complications and a shorter rehabilitation period than open realignment. An unsuccessful lateral release has less serious consequences than a failed tubercle transposition and is easier to revise. The present position of lateral release in the author's practice is that it is the treatment of choice unless there is patella alta, generalised ligament laxity, subluxation of the patella on extension or a shallow trochlea.

Medial tightening
The medial structures may be plicated or tightened using a number of techniques involving fascia, tendon, imbrication or advancement of the vastus medialis. All of these procedures increase the Q angle, illustrating the shortcomings of this measurement. Advancing the insertion of the most distal fibres of vastus medialis, sometimes called vastus medialis obliquus (VMO), is commonly performed. The VMO is a powerful muscle and secure fixation to the patella may not be achieved. The procedure has the additional effects of tilting the lateral edge of the patella anteriorly and pulling it proximally.

Medial tightening alone will only correct the underlying problem if there is abnormal laxity of the medial structures, a rare problem. In other situations, medial plication is an adjunct to the main corrective procedure.

Improving the trochlea
The trochlea may be deepened by elevating the lateral condyle or removing bone from its centre. Both approaches damage the articular surface of the trochlea and may be expected to predispose to late osteoarthritis. There are no satisfactory long-term results of any of these procedures.

Elevation of the lateral condyle
Techniques are described [16] to increase the height of a dysplastic lateral trochlear margin (Fig. 9.16). These procedures are easy to describe on a two-dimensional page but transferring the technique to the complex three-dimensional geometry of the trochlea may not be so easy. The dissection required for total knee replacement provides an opportunity to examine the practical problems of this procedure.

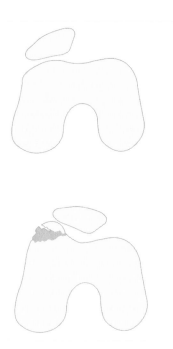

Figure 9.16 – *Elevation of a dysplastic lateral condyle.*

The indications for increasing the height of the lateral margin of the trochlea are comparatively rare and reported results are hard to find. In the absence of good published results, there must be a strong suspicion that the results are poor.

Deepening the trochlea

The trochlea can be deepened by removing bone from beneath its articular surface or covering the excavated area with osteochondral flaps. Although an attractive solution to the problem of a defective femoral trochlea, damage to the articular surface is inevitable and long-term results are elusive.

The technique is appropriate for knees with a defective trochlea, particularly if there is a marked bump or crossing sign.

Operative techniques

There is no space in this chapter to describe all the many procedures for stabilising the patella, but illustrations of each type will be given. Hundreds of operative techniques have been described for both proximal and distal realignment of the patella and most surgeons develop their own variation of an established technique. None is entirely satisfactory and it is more important to select the right type of operation than adopt a specific technique as the answer to every problem.

Tibial tubercle transfer

It is essential to plan the operation before the leg is draped. Accurate measurements should be made on the lateral X-ray and the required amount of medial and distal transposition clearly established. Precise measurement is difficult when a saw blade removes a millimetre of bone, but it is possible to decide within 2–3 mm how much movement is required to bring the various indices within the normal range.

Sound fixation of the transposed tibial tubercle is difficult and separation of the transposed bone block is a complication of all techniques of tibial tubercle transfer. The quadriceps is a powerful muscle with a small insertion and the forces imposed on the fixation are very great. Immobilisation in extension reduces, but does not eliminate, the risk of separation at the expense of postoperative stiffness.

The comments that follow are based on personal experience of many attempts to produce fixation sound enough to permit early motion without immobilisation.

Fixation with an ASIF screw through the centre of the tubercle creates a stress raiser, particularly if the screw is countersunk, and the transposed tubercle may split on either side of the screw. Such a screw is not secure unless its tip passes through the posterior cortex and this can place the posterior structures at risk. The drill must be advanced slowly and with great caution.

Staple fixation is inherently insecure because the legs of the staple only provide fixation where they pass through the cortex and they cannot be attached to the posterior cortex. Staples also create stress raisers if they pass through the tubercle itself, but if a large staple is used to straddle the tubercle the fragment can slip from beneath it. Staples do not provide sound fixation.

The Goldthwait operation [17], in which the lateral half of the patellar tendon is passed behind the medial and stitched to the periosteum of the tibia, may be followed by rupture of the remaining half (Fig. 9.17). This technique has the additional disadvantage that the amount of medial transposition of the insertion is dictated by the anatomy of the tendon itself and cannot be more than half the width of the patellar tendon. No distal transposition is possible and moving the lateral slip medially tilts the lateral edge of the patella posteriorly.

Fixation by re-implanting the fragment beneath the cortex without internal fixation requires accurate bone cuts and places great strain on the proximal cortical lip of the mobilised bone block. The cortex in this area is

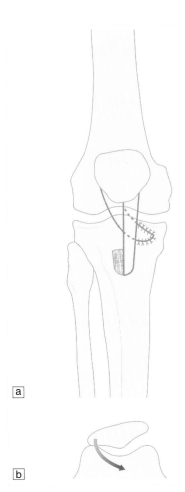

Figure 9.17 – *The Goldthwait procedure. (a) The lateral slip of patellar tendon is passed beneath the medial slip; (b) the lateral edge of the patella is tilted downwards by the transposition.*

laterally. The end result is a medial transposition which may be sufficient to obtain stability and reattachment may not be required. The separated fragment of bone may need later excision.

If the patella remains unstable it can be secured at a second operation with a screw and washer in most cases, but the fragment is sometimes too small or too soft to take a screw. If sound reattachment cannot be secured by staple or screw fixation, a figure-of-eight tension band wire passed through patella and tibia is effective, but the wire must be removed between 8 and 12 weeks after operation if damage to the patellar tendon and tendon contracture are to be avoided.

The third dimension

The upper end of the tibia is triangular in cross-section at the level of the tibial tubercle but this cannot be seen on a two-dimensional page or screen and two-dimensional descriptions of three-dimensional operations can be very misleading. A simple illustration of medial tibial tubercle transposition shows movement in one plane only; it does not show how the patella rotates about its long axis as it moves from one side of the triangular tibia to another, or how it is moved posteriorly by transposition (Fig. 9.18).

Anterior transposition

Moving the tibial tubercle anteriorly was originally proposed by Maquet [14] as a salvage procedure for gross patellofemoral osteoarthritis on the basis that lifting the patella away from the femur and lengthening the lever arm acting on the knee would unload the joint surface. Maquet lifted the tubercle a full 2 cm and had many problems with wound healing. Maquet's operation is a major procedure and was not devised for patellar instability.

Although it has been said that anterior transposition unloads the patellofemoral joint, the detailed mechanics

comparatively thin and easily fractured if the patient flexes the knee unexpectedly.

Retained screws, staples or sutures around the tibial tubercle may cause persistent pain and make kneeling difficult or impossible. The pain and tenderness may settle after two years but seldom disappear completely. The problem can only be avoided by omitting all internal fixation devices.

The author's current preference is to re-implant the tibial tubercle using a cortical ASIF screw and washer. The precise amount of transposition required is measured on the lateral X-ray, a lateral release performed to a point about 4 cm above the upper pole of the patella and the tibial tubercle raised with a block of bone approximately 15 mm wide. A window is cut in the tibia at the desired point of attachment and the block of bone placed into the cavity of the tibia where it is held with a screw and washer.

Management of the detached fragment

When the fragment becomes detached from the tibia, it moves proximally to its original level but seldom

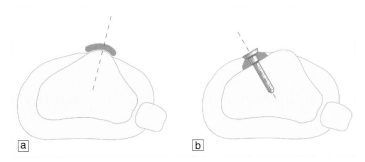

Figure 9.18 – *The effect of medial transposition on rotation of the patella. (a) The tibial tubercle normally faces anterolaterally but (b) after transposition it faces anteromedially.*

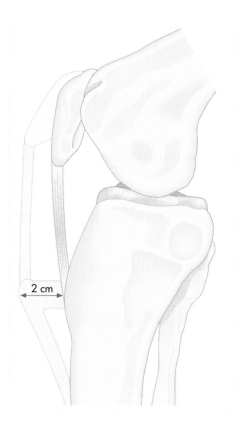

Figure 9.19 – *Anterior transposition of the tibial tubercle lifts the patella out of the trochlea and makes it less stable.*

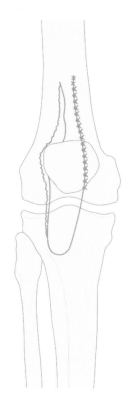

Figure 9.20 – *Lateral release and medial plication of the patellar mechanism.*

of this are not universally agreed [18]. Even if it does unload the patellofemoral joint, it is difficult to see how lifting the patella off the femur in full extension can do anything but make it more unstable (Fig. 9.19). Anterior transposition would appear to be theoretically unsound in patients with patellar instability.

The theoretical advantage of anterior transposition has been extended to suggest that posterior transposition has a similar theoretical disadvantage and Fulkerson has described a technique to avoid this movement [19]. A long strip of the anterior cortex of the tibia is lifted, in a similar manner to that described by Maquet, and swung medially so that the tubercle is not moved posteriorly. Although theoretically attractive, the operation is more extensive than a simple transposition and the cosmetic appearance may be unsightly. There is little evidence that the theoretical advantages are reflected in the results.

Medial plication

Medial plication alone increases the Q angle and has no effect on either patellar height or the anatomy of the trochlea. The indications for performing this procedure in isolation are rare. The operation is usually accompanied by a lateral release and this may be the only reason the operation is effective (Fig. 9.20).

The procedure is straightforward and consists of a lateral release of the patellar tendon from its insertion distally to vastus lateralis proximally. Vastus lateralis may also need to be divided in order to bring the patella medially. The medial retinaculum and capsule are then divided and repaired so that the patella is drawn medially. It is preferable to use absorbable sutures to avoid tender and unsightly subcutaneous knots.

If vastus medialis is to be advanced, it is first raised from the patella and medial retinaculum and moved distally and laterally to be held with absorbable sutures (Fig. 9.21). A lateral release is necessary.

Both procedures may require cast immobilisation for 6 weeks.

Lateral release

Lateral release (Fig. 9.22) is often followed by a large haematoma. The lateral superior geniculate artery is divided during the procedure and is difficult to control if the operation is performed arthroscopically. There is much to be said for releasing the patella through a short incision at the upper end of the patella so that the artery can be identified and coagulated.

Many techniques for lateral release have been described. The author's present technique is to inject

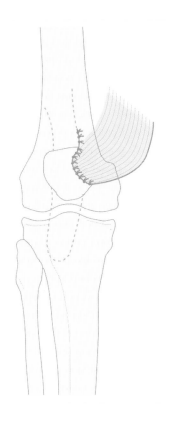

Figure 9.21 –
Distal and lateral transposition of the vastus medialis.

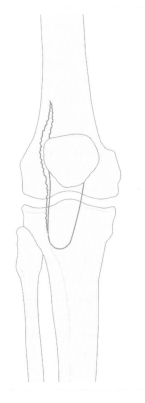

Figure 9.22 –
The site of lateral release of the extensor mechanism.

laparoscopy. The joint is then examined with an arthroscope in the usual manner, noting the extent of damage on the patella and the congruity of the patellofemoral joint. The capsule is next divided with a Smillie knife introduced at the anterolateral portal and pushed proximally to at least 4 cm above the upper pole of the patella [20]. The release is not complete until the lateral edge of the patella can be lifted so that the patella lies vertically.

The edges of the capsule are then coagulated with a diathermy ball electrode from the suprapatellar approach and the tourniquet released. Any remaining bleeding points are coagulated, a suction drain placed in the wound and a pressure dressing applied along the line of incision. The drain is removed the following day and mobilisation begun. The operation is not done as a day case.

Patterns of dislocation

Acute versus chronic dislocation

Many reports of the management of patellar instability fail to distinguish between acute and recurrent dislocation. This is a serious shortcoming because the prognosis for anatomically normal knees is far better than for those with, for example, an absent trochlea. Anatomically normal patellofemoral joints dislocated by acute trauma may suffer no further dislocations and can be effectively treated by conservative means, but those which continue to dislocate frequently have abnormal anatomy and present a much greater challenge. No conclusion can be drawn from a series which fails to differentiate between acute and chronic dislocations.

Even papers reporting the results of managing a patella with no history of previous dislocation are unsatisfactory. It is obvious that all recurrently dislocating patellae must at some stage have suffered a first dislocation, even those which have a much worse prognosis because of abnormal anatomy, and it is possible that operative treatment may be appropriate for such patellae after the first dislocation. A study relating the anatomical features and clinical outcome of acute patellar dislocation is long overdue and could be very instructive.

Some confusion exists over the terminology applied to recurrent patellofemoral instability.

Recurrent dislocation is generally taken to mean repeated occasional dislocation and is the commonest pattern of dislocation. Dislocations may occur at intervals of weeks or months.

Marcain with added adrenaline along the proposed line of capsular incision and to distend the knee with CO_2 from an abdominal insufflator normally used for

Recurrent subluxation implies a less drastic event than a dislocation but the distinction between subluxation and dislocation is often unclear, particularly in patients with very lax joints. Luxation and dislocation are synonymous and a subluxation is a 'subdislocation'. A feeling of unsteadiness accompanied by abnormal movement is usually interpreted as subluxation.

The terminology has been confused by some authors who misunderstood the word and applied it to patellae that were laterally placed but entirely stable. This led to the lateral pressure syndrome of Ficat being described as lateral subluxation of the patella [21], and much of the literature on subluxation is bedevilled by this error.

Habitual dislocation was probably first used to describe voluntary dislocation of the patella by children with lax ligaments. The same patients may dislocate the temporo-mandibular joints, shoulders, and first carpometacarpal joints as a party trick. These patients should be encouraged not to dislocate their patellae but some cannot control the dislocation and require both tibial tubercle transposition and medial plication to achieve stability.

The term is also applied to those patellae which dislocate with every flexion of the knee and cannot be held in the reduced position during the full range of flexion. The description 'inevitable dislocation' is sometimes applied to such patellae even though it is very different. Common causes for this phenomenon are a deficient or shallow trochlea combined with tight lateral structures and it is a separate condition from habitual dislocation due to lax ligaments.

The 'inevitable' type of 'habitual' dislocation requires an extensive soft tissue release, often extending far up the thigh, combined with a tibial transfer and medial plication. Flexion may be reduced because of quadriceps contracture and some authors have added a proximal release of the straight head of rectus femoris to overcome this problem.

Permanent dislocation

Permanently dislocated patellae lie on the lateral side of the femur and cannot be reduced (Fig. 9.23). Active extension by the quadriceps is negligible and the knee is often held in valgus because the quadriceps has been acting as an abductor of the knee. The trochlea is also abnormal because the patella has not articulated with the front of the femur and stability is then very difficult to achieve [7].

Congenital dislocations

Some permanently dislocated patellae may be present at birth but others arise from congenital deformities or

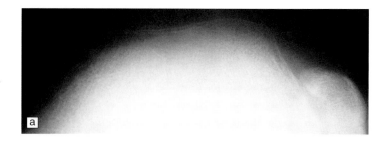

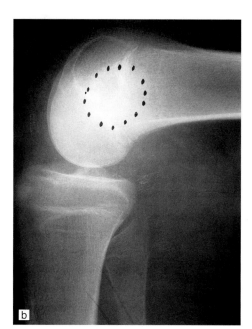

Figure 9.23 – *Permanent congenital dislocation of the patella. (a) Axial X-ray showing laterally placed patella and absent trochlea; (b) lateral X-ray with the patella indicated by dots.*

contractures of the vastus lateralis [22]. Contractures of the quadriceps muscle may also occur following intramuscular injections in the neonatal period [23].

Permanently and congenitally dislocated patellae require an extensive soft tissue release, tibial tubercle transfer and medial plication. The patellofemoral joint is not congruent and the articular cartilage is usually deficient. The prognosis is poor.

Replacement of the patella on the front of the femur may restore extension in these patients, but flexion is usually severely restricted. Release of the rectus femoris from its attachment to the pelvis may be required, but the author has no personal experience of this.

Special situations

There are a few special situations which require a different approach from those outlined above.

Dislocation in the immature skeleton

It is not possible to perform a distal realignment involving the tibial tubercle until growth is complete

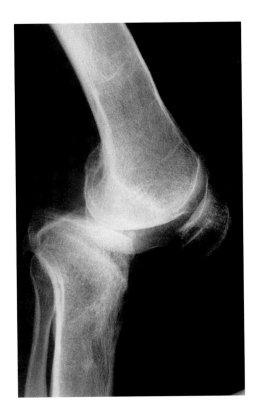

Figure 9.24 – *The late effects of premature growth arrest at the upper end of the tibia following tibial tubercle transposition before skeletal maturity.*

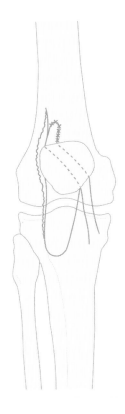

Figure 9.25 – *Semitendinosus tenodesis combined with lateral release.*

because of the risk of producing premature fusion at the front of the tibia and a genu recurvatum deformity [24,25] (Fig. 9.24). Stabilising procedures in children must use soft tissue only. Many of these will fail and can be considered as the first of a two-stage procedure, the second performed when growth is complete.

Stabilisation is important in children for two reasons. First, it is important to replace the patella in the trochlea to encourage normal development and moulding of the patellofemoral joint. Secondly, articular surface lesions in children lead to osteoarthritis of the patellofemoral joint in early adult life.

Of the many soft tissue procedures described, medial plication combined with lateral release is probably the treatment of choice. If this does not control the stability, a semitendinosus tenodesis [26] (Fig. 9.25) is effective. The tenodesis is performed by detaching the tendon proximally, passing it subcutaneously to reach the inferomedial corner of the patella in a straight line from its tibial insertion and then passing it through a 6 mm drill hole running from the inferomedial to the superolateral corners of the patella in the coronal plane.

The tenodesis may need to be dismantled when growth is complete in order to avoid osteoarthritis of the medial facet.

Pathological ligament laxity

Ligament laxity at the knee may be part of generalised joint laxity [27] or, less commonly, be confined to the knee. Patellae can be very difficult to stabilise in the presence of abnormal laxity because the soft tissues neither guide the patella into the trochlea at the start of flexion nor hold it there once engaged. Lateral release alone is ineffective and must be combined with medial tightening and tibial tubercle transposition. Care must be taken not to produce a medial dislocation of the patella in these knees. Precise soft tissue balance is essential.

Subluxation on extension

Some patellae sublux laterally on full extension and reduce on flexion as the patella engages in the trochlea [28,29]. The underlying pathology in these patients is extreme and usually includes a high patella, ligament laxity and often a deficient lateral condyle. The trochlea may be deficient, perhaps because it has not been moulded by the patella during growth. Many patients have another congenital anomaly such as talipes or congenital dislocation of the hip in the same limb.

Lateral release alone is never sufficient to stabilise these patellae. An extensive procedure erring on the side of excessive stabilisation is required.

Dislocation after patellectomy

Patellectomy enjoyed a brief period of popularity for patellofemoral instability, but is ineffective as a stabilising procedure. The ensuing dislocation of the patellar tendon may be more difficult to stabilise than the patella itself because it lacks a median keel. Dislocation may also follow patellectomy for trauma.

Stabilisation requires a wide lateral release combined with tibial tubercle transposition. Medial transposition alone may be adequate, but distal transposition is helpful if there is an extensor lag. These procedures are insufficient in themselves because the undersurface of the tendon becomes concave to conform with the convexity of the lateral edge of the trochlea. This concavity does not sit easily in the trochlea and must be converted to a convexity by a series of transverse cuts along the lateral edge of the tendon which can then be everted so that the tendon lies comfortably in the trochlea (Figs 9.26, 9.27).

A convenient technique is to split the lateral half of the tendon in the coronal plane and make the transverse cuts in such a way that they coincide with an intact leaf of tendon above and below (Fig. 9.15). For additional

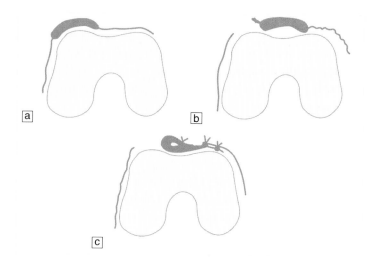

Figure 9.27 – *Stabilisation of patellar tendon following patellectomy. (a) The laterally placed patellar tendon becomes convex to conform with the lateral condyle; (b) the convexity of the tendon is retained after lateral release; (c) the position of the tendon can be maintained by rolling the lengthened lateral margin of the tendon to make it convex and plicating the medial capsule.*

security, the flap can be rolled anteriorly and stitched to the medial half of the tendon.

Instability in the presence of patellofemoral osteoarthritis

Severe osteoarthritis combined with patellar instability presents a difficult problem because stabilisation may aggravate the osteoarthritis and patellectomy does not stabilise the patella. Careful explanation is important so that the patient understands the complexity of the problem. Both patellectomy and stabilisation may be required, either combined or as staged procedures. Many of these knees also have a valgus deformity with osteoarthritis of the lateral compartment, and it is often wiser to wait until a total knee replacement is indicated.

Complications

Patellofemoral osteoarthritis is common in the presence of patellar instability, whether treated or untreated. Inappropriate transfer of the tubercle is said to aggravate the condition by exposing the patellar surface to severe loads but there is no evidence that judicious transposition to correct a high patella carries the same risk. There is no evidence either to show that anterior advancement of the tibial tubercle at the time of transposition reduces the incidence of later osteoarthritis.

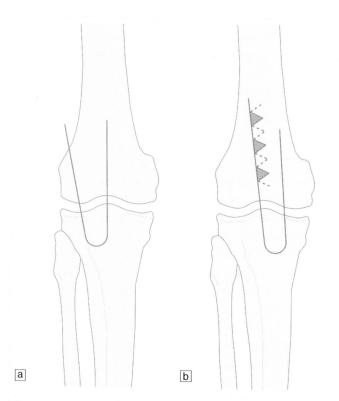

Figure 9.26 – *Patellar tendon stabilisation following patellectomy. (a) The patellar tendon comes to lie over the lateral condyle; (b) staggered transverse cuts lengthen the lateral edge of the tendon and allow it to lie in the trochlea.*

Medial dislocation of the patella may follow excessive medial transposition of the tubercle, particularly in the presence of abnormal ligament laxity, a defective trochlea and excessive medial plication.

The tubercle should never be moved more than 10 mm medial to the centre of the trochlea and the movement of the patella along the trochlea should be observed at the end of operation to exclude medial subluxation.

Loss of flexion may follow distal transposition or relocation of a permanently dislocated patella. Persistent gentle physiotherapy will eventually restore flexion but may take as long as a year. Release of the rectus femoris from the pelvis is said to relieve this problem [8].

Recurrence of dislocation following stabilisation. The management of a failed stabilisation is no different from that of a patella which has not undergone previous surgery. Thorough assessment to discover the cause of failure is essential. Corrective surgery is usually effective, but some patellae continue to dislocate even when all underlying causes appear to have been removed.

Detachment of the transposed tibial tubercle. This complication has already been described in the section on operative techniques.

Assessment of results

There is no general agreement on the best way to assess the outcome of surgery for chronic patellar instability. The score of Crosby and Insall [30] is widely used, but the good and excellent grades are generous and may include patients with a recurrence of dislocation.

The situation is complicated because some patients experience an occasional dislocation in the immediate postoperative period before the tissues have matured and the quadriceps has regained power. These patients may still go on to achieve an excellent result. The symptoms of osteoarthritis may also interfere with the assessment of stability if a simple subjective grading such as the Crosby and Insall score is used.

Finally, few scoring systems take account of the complaint of many patients that although their patella has never dislocated, it feels as though it might. The subjective grading of:

■ 'feels completely stable'
■ 'feels occasionally unstable but never dislocates'
■ 'continues to dislocate'

is simple to apply and may yield more information than complicated knee scores.

Key points

1. The patella is intrinsically unstable.
2. There are many different types and many different causes of instability.
3. The patella will be unstable because of either failure to engage or failure to stay in the trochlea.
4. The factors causing instability must be assessed clinically and radiologically so that appropriate treatment can be selected.
5. The true plain lateral X-ray gives much useful information about the trochlea.
6. Operations fall into three broad groups, distal realignment, proximal realignment or release, and deepening of the trochlea.
7. The operation selected must correct the underlying problem.

CHAPTER 10

Treatment of meniscal injuries in the young adult

N. A. K. Flynn and N. P. Thomas

Introduction

Knee injuries are the most common sporting injury and of these, injury to the meniscus abounds, with sports injuries being responsible for over 30% of the total number of lesions [1]. Treatment will determine the long-term outcome for the involved knee, because the menisci play an important biomechanical role in the function of the normal knee joint. Total meniscectomy is clearly implicated as a major factor in the premature development of osteoarthritis of the knee joint [2]. Our understanding of the anatomy and function of the meniscus is paramount in determining the correct treatment for its injury. This chapter will concentrate on the adolescent/young adult meniscus before the advent of degenerative change in the knee joint.

Historical perspective

Treatment of the injured meniscus has evolved over many years as our understanding of its function has improved and the aftermath of total meniscectomy has been recognised. The first published treatment was by Annandale (1883), who performed an open meniscal repair (Figs 10.1, 10.2) [3]. This technique was not popularised and for years arthrotomy and total meniscectomy was felt to give the best results [4]. Smillie influenced a generation by suggesting that regeneration of the meniscus occurred and that any injury should be treated with a total meniscectomy. He felt that any retained portions of a meniscus would actually accelerate degeneration [5]. The 'regenerate' is scar tissue with no functional capability. Follow-up studies have all shown progressive deterioration both clinically and

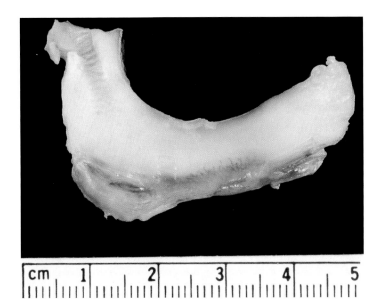

Figure 10.1 – *Meniscus removed via an open procedure with a healing peripheral tear.*

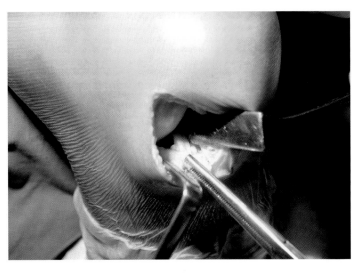

Figure 10.2 – *Open meniscectomy.*

123

radiologically following meniscectomy [6–8]. Medlar *et al.* found a direct correlation between the extent of radiographic changes and the degree of clinical symptoms [9]. The incidence of concomitant anterior cruciate ligament (ACL) tears is high, although in the past these were not recognised and many patients had normal menisci removed for the symptom of giving way. The effect of a meniscectomy on an unstable knee is to increase instability and thus accelerate the degenerative process.

Developmental/functional anatomy

Menisci develop from the mesenchyme of the proximal tibia and are clearly formed at 8 weeks of gestation [10]. Their shape is configured early in their development, but at this prenatal stage they are very cellular and fully vascularised. After birth, the changes are gradual with decreasing vascularity from the centre towards the periphery, growth of the menisci in parallel with the femur and tibia, and the collagen fibre arrangement changing progressively in response to biomechanical function [10,11].

Anatomy

The menisci are biconcave fibrocartilaginous discs that are triangular in cross-section. They cover approximately two-thirds of the articular surface of the tibia. The medial meniscus is semicircular, broader at its posterior horn than the anterior. The lateral meniscus is more circular, with a uniform size throughout. Both menisci are loosely attached at their peripheries to the tibial plateau by the coronary ligament, although the medial is attached to the deep elements of the medial collateral ligament. The lateral meniscus is more mobile than the medial, moving up to 1 cm. This is due to its more circular shape, the attachments to the ligaments of Humphry and Wrisberg posteriorly and the lack of attachment to its collateral ligament. This may explain the propensity for medial meniscal injuries in comparison with lateral meniscal injuries.

The blood supply of the meniscus is via terminal branches of the medial and lateral geniculate arteries (superior and inferior), which form a 'circum-meniscal anastomosis' [12]. At birth 50% of the meniscus is vascularised and by skeletal maturity this has fallen to

20–30%, as shown by Arnoczky and Warren and also Danzig *et al.* (Fig. 10.3) [13,14]. In the young patient the posterior horns are very vascular [15]. The peripheral vascular meniscus, as opposed to the central avascular portion, is a factor in the decision-making process in the treatment of injury. The periphery has a synovial reflection that extends for some 3 mm over both sides. It does not contribute to the vascularity but has been shown to be a valuable source of vascular ingrowth during healing after injury [13,16].

The meniscus is a soft, hydrated fibrocartilaginous structure [18]. It is composed of 75% collagen, of which 98% is type I. There are also small quantities of types II,

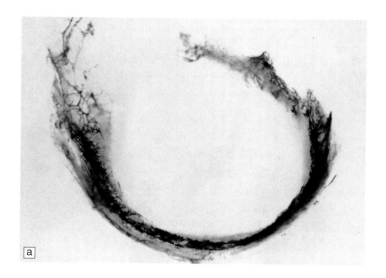

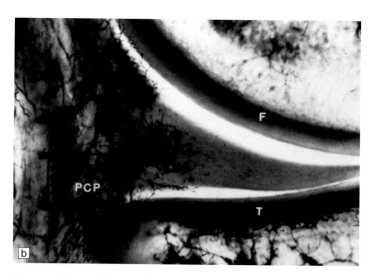

Figure 10.3 – *(a) Round view of peripheral vasculature of meniscus. (b) Transverse section showing peripheral vasculature of meniscus. F = femur, T = tibia, PCP = pericapsular plexus. Peripheral vasculature demonstrated with injection techniques (Reproduced from ref. 13 with permission).*

III, V, and VI. The content of collagen increases until the third decade and remains fairly constant until the eighth decade, whereupon it decreases [19]. Bullough *et al.* [20] have shown that the collagen fibres mainly have a circumferential orientation which gives the meniscus its tensile strength (Fig. 10.4). There are some radially orientated fibres which provide shear strength; these are mainly situated in the superficial layers of the meniscus [11].

The ground substance has a mechanical property for resisting compressive forces [19]. Fibrochondroblasts are present in the visceral portion of the meniscus and have a role to play in formation of fibrocartilage which may be a factor in repair of the avascular area [18].

The functional role of the meniscus is shown in Table 10.1 [21]. The arrangement of the collagen bundles circumferentially from anterior to posterior horns allows for absorption and translation of vertical compressive forces into circumferential forces which have been termed 'hoop stresses' by Bullough *et al.* [20]. This

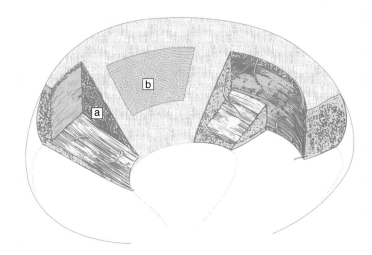

Figure 10.4 – *Diagram of the collagen arrangement within the meniscus showing (a) circumferential fibres and (b) radial fibres in the superficial layers of the meniscus. (Reproduced from ref. 20 with permission).*

Table 10.1 – Functions of the meniscus

- Shock absorption
- Joint stabilisation
- Nutrition of the articular cartilage
- Lubrication of the knee joint

protects the underlying articular cartilage from focal concentrations of stress and their viscoelasticity attenuates shock waves generated by impulse loading [22]. The menisci transmit 45–50% of an applied load across the knee in extension, which increases to 85% in flexion [23]. The medial compartment takes 90% of any load transmitted through the knee joint and this is shared evenly between the meniscus and the articular cartilage. Of the 10% through the lateral joint, the lateral meniscus takes 70% [24]. Consequently, disruption of the menisci, whether by meniscectomy or a large tear, will lead to higher peak stresses, greater stress concentration, and decreased shock-absorbing capabilities [21]. The lateral meniscus plays such an important role in shock absorption that lateral meniscectomy leads to increased degenerative changes in comparison with medial meniscectomy [25].

The meniscus has a role as a secondary stabiliser of the knee in the anteroposterior plane. This is particularly important in the ACL-deficient knee. Levy *et al.* showed that the posterior horn of the medial meniscus provided the greatest contribution in this respect [26].

With this knowledge of the function of the meniscus, attempts at salvage and preservation should be undertaken to prevent early degenerative change occurring. This was first noted by Fairbank, who concluded that the joint space narrowing, osteophyte formation and flattening of the femoral condyles that was seen after meniscectomy occurred because of the failure of the shock-absorbing effect [7].

Causes of traumatic injury

The meniscus is injured when the shear stress exceeds the tissue strength. In the young patient this is due to abnormal forces taking place on a normal meniscus. These form either vertical longitudinal or radial tears. If the menisci were degenerate, then the tear would be horizontal in character. When the knee is flexed, the menisci are displaced posteriorly. In this position the medial meniscus is prone to injury, with external rotation of the tibia, and the lateral meniscus with internal rotation. Medial meniscal injuries are seen five times more commonly than lateral meniscal injuries. The reason for this is the attachment of the periphery to the deep fibres of the medial collateral ligament and the propensity for valgus injury from side-on tackles in sport [27].

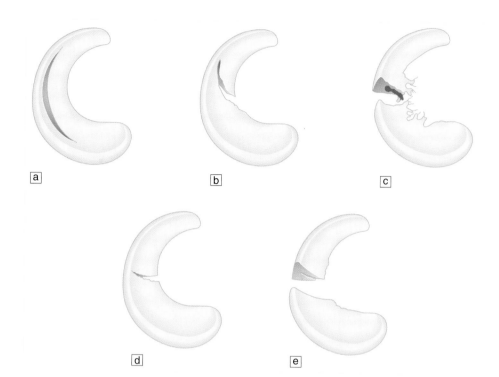

Figure 10.5 – *Types of meniscal tear: (a) vertical longitudinal; (b) oblique; (c) degenerative; (d) transverse (radial); (e) horizontal.*

Types of tears

Figure 10.5 shows the various types of meniscal tears [28].

Clinical presentation

In order to effect treatment at the optimum time, early diagnosis is very important. The majority of injuries in the young will be from sporting activities. Many will present to accident and emergency departments with a swollen knee with or without locking. With a true haemarthrosis, in the absence of a fracture, there is a 75–80% chance of a tear of the ACL and a 50% chance of a peripheral tear of the meniscus [29]. A careful history and examination are the most important factors in making a diagnosis. Table 10.2 covers the major points to be elicited. Plain X-rays must be taken to exclude fracture or other pathology such as osteochondritis dissecans. Magnetic resonance imaging (MRI) can be of value if the findings on examination are not definite and the patient fails to settle. Accuracy rates of 77%, 91% and 96% for medial meniscus, lateral meniscus and ACL lesions, respectively, have been reported [30]. Mackenzie *et al.* found that MRI did allow correct assessment of the knee for both ACL and menisci, but other structural pathologies were not as well diagnosed [31], although in patella dislocations that

Table 10.2 – Clinical pointers in initial assessment of the injured knee

History	■ Time of injury
	■ Mechanism of injury
	■ contact
	■ non-contact
	■ Duration of symptoms
	■ Pain
	■ Swelling
	■ Locking
	■ Instability
Examination	■ Range of movement
	■ Swelling
	■ Joint line tenderness
	■ Tibial rotation tests
	■ Quadriceps wasting
	■ Laxity
Investigations	■ Plain X-rays
	■ MRI

present with swelling, the soft tissue damage to structures such as the media patellofemoral ligament can be readily delineated [32].

Treatment

Precise knowledge of the meniscal tear is important. A decision must be made as to whether the tear is to be treated surgically or conservatively (Table 10.3). Not all meniscal tears produce clinical symptoms, and a torn meniscus can function biomechanically if the peripheral fibres remain intact [33]. Partial thickness tears and short full-thickness tears that are stable to probing arthroscopically can be left alone.

Usually the tears that are found in these categories are associated with other pathology in the knee, such as an ACL rupture. If they are the only pathology in the symptomatic knee, then clinical judgement must be used as to whether the tear requires treatment. Peripheral stable tears appear to heal without the need for repair [34].

Partial meniscectomy

Meniscal tears that are not suitable for repair because there is extensive damage or they are in the avascular central zone are treated by partial meniscectomy [33]. The aim of partial meniscectomy is to preserve as much of the functioning rim of the meniscus as possible. Metcalf put this most eloquently when he said that partial meniscectomy entails the removal of a portion of the meniscus necessary to leave a well contoured, stable, balanced rim [35]. In the canine model, the amount of degenerative change in the knee is directly proportional to the amount of meniscus removed [36]. The tibio-femoral contact stresses increase in proportion to the amount of meniscus excised, but even a damaged

meniscus can transmit loads as long as the rim remains intact. A significant proportion of the load is taken by the intact periphery, with no increase in the load at the cut edge [37–39]. Partial meniscectomy has been shown to have better functional results than total meniscectomy [40–43]. The long-term results of Schimmer *et al.* give figures of 78.1% good or excellent results at 12 years, although they point out that the outcome is affected by concomitant chondral damage at the time of meniscectomy. Isolated meniscal injuries had a 94.8% good or excellent rating, in comparison with only 62% in knees with cartilage damage and meniscectomy combined [44].

Repair

'Healing is a matter of time, but is also sometimes also a matter of opportunity.' Hippocrates

The function of the meniscus has been shown to be of importance in preventing degenerative change within the knee joint. Annandale was a lone pioneer in 1883 [3] and it was only after work by King in 1936 that it became evident that the meniscus could heal in its periphery [45]. The microvascular environment in the periphery is paramount for healing of the collagen fibres [46]. There are three zones within the meniscus, based on its blood supply and thus the potential for healing. The 'red–red' zone occurs within the peripheral vascular area approximately 3 mm from the meniscocapsular junction. There is a blood supply to both sides of this tear, which therefore has an excellent healing potential. The 'red–white' zone occurs at the junction of the vascular and avascular areas. It is approximately 3–5 mm from the meniscocapsular junction. The vascularity is only in the peripheral side of the tear; thus there is a reasonable potential for healing but less than the 'red–red' tears. The 'white–white' zone occurs in the avascular region centrally. These tears are over 5 mm from the periphery. Their potential for healing is poor [32,47].

Tears that are suitable for repair are ideally acute, traumatic tears in young patients within the 'red–red' zone, greater than 7 mm long, unstable to probing and without major structural damage (Table 10.4). Tears of dubious vascularity and with damage to the body of the meniscus provide a difficult clinical decision. Large radial tears that encroach on the periphery will have damaged the circumferential collagen fibres (Fig. 10.6). The repaired meniscus may therefore not function normally. In the young patient, the consequence of a

Table 10.3 – Decision-making factors in the treatment of meniscal injuries

Conservative	Surgical
Peripheral	Any tears
Stable	Unstable
Partial thickness	Full or partial thickness
<7 mm	>7 mm

Table 10.4 – Steps in meniscus repair

Arthroscopic evaluation	■ Site
	■ Length
	■ Stability
	■ Structural damage
Rim preparation	■ Rasp
Repair	■ Open, 'outside-in', 'inside-out', or 'inside-in'
	■ Suture type
	■ Orientation of suture
Concomitant surgery	■ ACL reconstruction
	■ Chondral surgery
Rehabilitation	

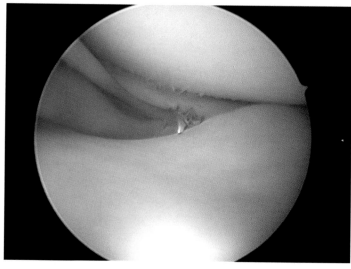

Figure 10.7 –*Meniscal rasp roughening in the edges of a white–white tear prior to suture.*

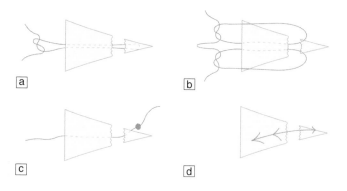

Figure 10.6 – *Schematic representation of meniscal repair techniques: (a) horizontal mattress; (b) vertical mattress; (c) 'mulberry' knot; (d) meniscal arrows.*

virtually total meniscectomy is early degenerative change and thus repair of these lesions is necessary. However, the patient will need to be counselled as to the possible need for further surgery. Chronicity does not appear to be a problem, as DeHaven has reported successful repairs some 8 years after the index injury and he has stated that re-tears following repair do not require excision, but repeat repair [33]. Chronic tears can undergo 'plastic' deformation; thus there is structural deformity that precludes repair and partial meniscectomy will be required.

Preparation of the tear site by rasping (Fig. 10.7) is an essential step in meniscal repair. This can be undertaken with a proprietary arthroscopic rasp.

The aims are to remove any avascular scar tissue that may have formed and to stimulate vascular in-growth that will aid healing. The use of a mechanical shaver is not recommended, as it may remove too much tissue.

Repair can be undertaken by a variety of techniques: 'open', 'outside-in', 'inside-out', and 'inside-in'. The latter three are arthroscopically assisted. The type of repair is dependent on the surgeon's own preference and expertise.

'Open' repair

This type of repair is suitable for peripheral tears only. It requires a longitudinal incision posteromedially or posterolaterally with an oblique capsular incision. Vertical sutures can then be placed across the tear after rim preparation. Long-term results are excellent, with 79% remaining successful at 10.9 years. This technique is used almost exclusively for 'red–red' tears as the other types cannot be visualised satisfactorily [48].

'Outside-in' repair

Multiple small incisions are made along the joint line and the soft tissue is bluntly dissected down to the capsule. A spinal needle is passed across the tear and is visualised within the knee by the arthroscope. Rim preparation is undertaken and then a suture is passed down the needle, grasped within the knee and withdrawn through the anteromedial portal. A 'mulberry' knot is tied and the suture pulled back into the knee to abut up against the meniscus. Adjacent sutures are tied to one another over the capsule. This repair is very difficult to accomplish in posterior horn tears. It is more applicable to the anterior portion of the meniscus.

'Inside-out' repair

This is the authors' preferred method of meniscal repair and is the most popular technique in use at the present time [49]. It combines an incision on the joint line with placement of sutures from the inside of the knee under arthroscopic control, capture of the sutures through the skin incision and tying the sutures onto the capsule of the knee joint.

For medial meniscal tears a posteromedial incision is made longitudinally in line with the neurovascular structures. Transillumination can assist in identifying the saphenous vein and thus the nerve that accompanies it. Blunt dissection can then be made down to the joint line and peripheral meniscus after incision of the superficial fascia and pes anserinus.

Lateral meniscal repairs require an oblique incision posterolaterally. The important anatomical landmark is the tendon of biceps femoris because the lateral popliteal nerve runs posterior to it. Provided that the dissection is kept anterior to biceps, injury to the nerve should not occur. The interval between the lateral collateral ligament and the biceps tendon is then developed, giving access to the joint line and the peripheral meniscus.

The tear is prepared with a rasp on both sides of the meniscus. Cannulae are used to place sutures into the meniscal tear. Various types of cannula are available, from double lumen (Fig. 10.8) to single lumen (Fig. 10.9). The authors' choice is a single lumen 'zone-specific' cannula (Fig. 10.10) placed through the contralateral portal whilst viewing through the ipsilateral portal. These cannulae are so designed that the sutures are 'kicked-out', thus aiding repair of even the most posterior of tears, especially tears that are medial to the popliteus tendon in the lateral meniscus.

A variety of suture techniques can be used, but vertical mattress sutures (Fig. 10.11) are superior mechanically in pull-out studies when compared with horizontal or knot-end techniques and are thus the preferred option.

Braided non-absorbable suture is preferable, as it allows for a longer and more stable fixation which enhances maturation of meniscal healing [50–52]. This technique requires an assistant to retrieve the sutures under direct vision (Fig. 10.12), whilst retracting the soft tissues and thus protecting the neurovascular structures.

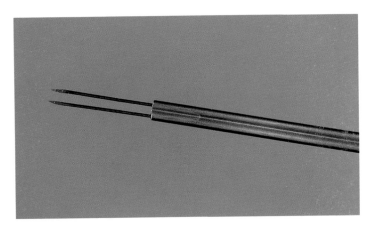

Figure 10.8 – *Double lumen cannula.*

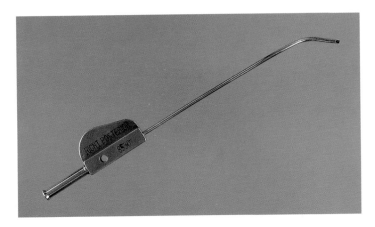

Figure 10.9 – *Single lumen 'zone specific' cannula.*

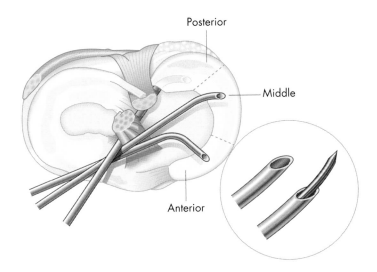

Figure 10.10 – *'Zone-specific' cannula crossing from the contralateral portal to various positions on the meniscus showing the way the suture is 'kicked' out to ease retrieval of the suture and to prevent any damage to the popliteal structures.*

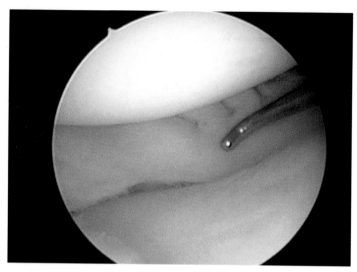

Figure 10.11 – *Stacked vertical sutures holding a peripheral lateral meniscal tear.*

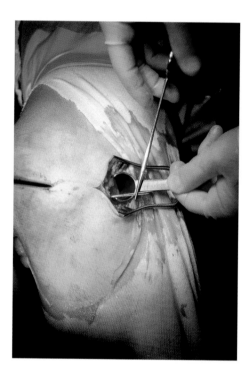

Figure 10.12 – *Retrieval of the suture in an 'inside-out' repair with protection of the neurovascular structures.*

'Inside-in' repair

Morgan has described a technique for an arthroscopic 'all-inside' approach to meniscal repair. It is technically demanding and can only be used for peripheral tears in the posterior horns [53].

Recent developments have tried to simplify the 'inside-in' approach. The 'T-fix' is a non-absorbable suture on a T-shaped anchor. The anchor is driven through the meniscus to hold the suture. The latter are tied outside the knee and snugged down onto the meniscus. There are no long-term evaluation studies for this system as yet, but the technique is demanding and time-consuming compared with other methods [54].

Biodegradable meniscal staples and arrows have been developed (Fig. 10.13). They are easier to place than previous 'inside-in' techniques and the pull-out strengths are comparable to 'inside-out' sutures [55–58].

The young patient with a white–white tear can be helped by meniscal repair if it is accompanied by fibrin clot insertion into the tear prior to tying of the sutures (Fig. 10.14). Arnoczky *et al.* [59] first showed that repair of canine meniscal tears in the avascular zone using fibrin clot was possible and Henning *et al.* [60] showed increased healing of repairs in the avascular portion of the meniscus. This has been confirmed by Rudman *et al.* [61], although their re-operation rate was higher than repair in the periphery. The fibrin clot technique is not easy to perform in the knee. A quantity of blood is drawn from the patient in an aseptic manner and using a glass rod in a sterile bowl, the

The sutures are clipped and held on a 'kilt' pin in order to facilitate tying over the capsule after all the sutures have been placed. Gentle traction on the sutures before tying can allow probing to ensure that a stable repair has been performed. A combination of vertical and horizontal sutures may be required to allow the meniscus to 'sit' in its anatomical position, as if horizontal sutures are used alone, the meniscus can evert after repair. Stacked vertical sutures give the best result, but can be difficult to place in the tight knee.

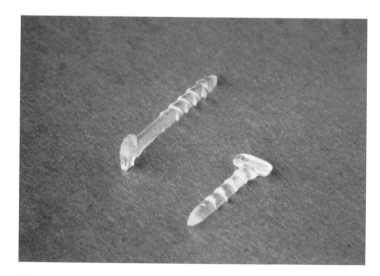

Figure 10.13 – *Biodegradeable meniscal arrows. (Transparency with the compliments of Atlantech Harrowgate Yorkshire, UK.)*

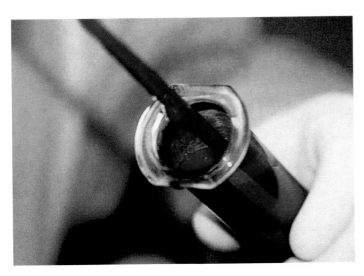

Figure 10.14 – *Fibrin clot being prepared. (Reproduced from ref. 77 with permission.)*

Table 10.5 – Author's rehabilitation regime	
Immediately	■ Early movement – CPM 0–90°
	■ Weight-bearing
	■ Avoidance of twisting
First 4 weeks	0–90°
4–6 weeks	0–120°
6 weeks	> 120°

blood is stirred until a clot forms on the rod. The clot is then placed within the edges of the tear and the sutures tightened to effect the repair. There is an excellent explanation of this technique in an article by Swenson and Harner [23].

The incidence of meniscal tears associated with ACL injuries is high: 65% in acute ACL injuries, rising to 98% in chronic ACL disruptions [62,63]. The results of repairs in ACL-deficient knees are very poor, with high failure rates [64,65]. The reason for this is that the meniscal repair will be subjected to increased shear stresses and thus fail. Reconstructing the ACL at the same time as meniscal repair or as a staged procedure is the preferred option, as the stability of the knee is enhanced. If the two procedures are performed concomitantly, then the haemarthrosis that occurs after the surgery acts like a fibrin clot and enhances the healing of the tear. A meniscus should not be repaired in isolation in an ACL-deficient knee.

Rehabilitation

Protocols for rehabilitation following meniscal repair are many and varied (Table 10.5). Long-term immobilisation of the knee joint causes adverse effects within the articular cartilage and the meniscus itself; thus early controlled exercise is advocated [66,67]. If the ACL has been reconstructed at the same time as a meniscal repair, there is felt to be no restriction to the normal ACL rehabilitation [68].

The future

It has been stated that the goal of meniscal surgery is to preserve as much functioning meniscus as possible to prevent long-term degenerative disease. In some cases the damage to the structure of the meniscus will be such that preservation will be impossible. This may be due to the complex nature of the tear or the long history and thus deformed nature of the meniscal remnant.

Meniscal allograft

Meniscal allograft techniques are in their infancy but there are some promising early results. The functional capabilities of allografts are maintained if they are kept in tissue culture media rather than frozen, gamma sterilised or lyophilised [22]. The grafts usually require an open procedure to insert them, although some centres perform the surgery arthroscopically which is technically very demanding [69]. It appears that the functional characteristics of the allograft are preserved if the anterior and posterior horns are attached by bone blocks [70,71]. Only one paper has indicated possible early rejection and this was in a cryopreserved allograft [72]. The meniscal allograft appears to be repopulated by fibrochondrocytes that migrate from the synovial rim [73] and the grafts appear to protect the underlying articular cartilage [74]. Short-term studies have shown possible benefits, but longer follow-up is required at the present time [22].

Collagen scaffold

This has also been evaluated and it has been found to permit regeneration of meniscal cartilage, acting as a reabsorbable regeneration template for the regrowth of new menisci. *In vivo* experiments in a canine model have been encouraging: the results in human knees are awaited [75,76].

Summary

The prompt diagnosis and correct treatment of meniscal injuries in the young is mandatory if we are to minimise degenerative disease within the knee joint. Recognition of the role of the meniscus is relatively recent so that once the injury pattern and extent of the lesion is recognised emphasis is placed on preserving as much functioning meniscal tissue as possible as well as preventing further injury. The choice between conservative treatment, partial resection or meniscal repair will depend on the type and position of the lesion, the overall complexity of the injury, the experience of the surgeon and the patient's wishes, e.g. a professional footballer may choose to have a partial meniscectomy rather than a meniscal repair which would mean that he would miss a shorter part of the playing season.

Newer developments with inside-in techniques may make meniscal repair technically easier and faster and thus more attractive to the non-specialist surgeon. We must be vigorous in our protection of the meniscus. The treatment of white–white tears should not be 'reflex' partial meniscectomy; if the rim is 5 mm or less and the meniscal body is undamaged then the surgeon should ask himself, 'Why am I removing this?'

Meniscal repair has an overall success rate of 60–85% and patients should be aware that further surgery may be required. It is hoped that with the advent of the newer techniques and a more respectful approach to the meniscus the presentation of middle-aged patients with degenerative arthritis secondary to meniscal lesion will decrease over the next 20–30 years. However, it must also be recognised that other factors, i.e. genetic, primary articular cartilage damage and lifestyle, also play their part in the aetiology of joint degeneration.

Key points

1. Meniscectomy leads to progressive clinical and radiological deterioration.
2. Early, precise diagnosis is important.
3. A torn meniscus can function biomechanically if the peripheral fibres remain intact.
4. Partial thickness tears and short full-thickness tears that are stable can be left alone.
5. Using an 'inside-out' technique for meniscal repair, the lateral popliteal nerve is protected by dissecting anterior to the biceps tendon and retrieving the sutures under direct vision with a retractor protecting the soft tissues posteriorly.
6. Meniscal repair in the ACL-deficient knee will almost certainly fail and if repair is to be undertaken the knee should be stabilised.
7. Allografts hold promise for the future.

CHAPTER 11

Osteochondritis dissecans of the knee

P. Aichroth

Introduction

Osteochondritis dissecans is the process whereby a segment of cartilage, together with subchondral bone, separates from an articular surface. It may be found in many joints, but it is most common in the knee. The lesion is commonly unilateral, but bilateral and symmetrical lesions are not unusual.

Osteochondritis dissecans is the most common cause of a loose body in the knee joint in a young person. The fragment may stay in its crater, remaining silent, or alternatively producing symptoms of pain, giving way, swelling and occasionally locking. The cause of the separation of the fragment has been the subject of much discussion and many theories over the past century. There have been two main schools, one supporting injury and the other supporting vascular insufficiency leading to bone infarction.

Loose bodies in joints were first recognised by Ambroise Paré in the 16th century, who must be credited not only with the first recognition of the disease but also with the first reported case of surgical removal of a loose body from the knee. In a soldier, he isolated the loose body clinically. He fixed it with a spike, he cut down onto it and extracted it with a toothed instrument, and he stated that the patient lived!

In Sir James Paget's classic description of the disease in 1870 [1], he mentioned in the first case a girl who had a habit of breaking thick pieces of wood across her thigh. The second case was of an athletic schoolboy from Harrow, who sustained many blows and strains of the knee. He felt that the condition was traumatic. König [2] in Münster in 1887 was the first to name the disease osteochondritis dissecans. This was an unfortunate name, for there is nothing inflammatory about it, but he did believe the cause of this 'dissection' was traumatic.

Fairbank [3] in the 1930s endorsed the suggestion that osteochondritis dissecans might be caused by an un-united subchondral fracture. He envisaged such a lesion as being frequently sustained in sports in the 'heat of the game'.

Ian Smillie [4] in the 1960s believed there were many types of osteochondritis dissecans. He thought that osteochondritis dissecans in a patient aged 10 years was an anomaly of ossification. He thought the juvenile type was due to local ischaemia with subsequent trauma, and the adult type was due to trauma producing the ischaemia.

Many authors in the last three decades have shown that in the immature skeleton joint surface damage produces an osteochondral fracture but, in the adult, the lesion is more frequently localised to a chondral fracture.

Clinical features

Osteochondritis dissecans commonly occurs in children and young adults between 10 and 20 years of age. The condition is more prevalent in boys than in girls, with a sex incidence of 2 to 1. In the author's series [5], there were unilateral lesions in 74% and bilateral in 26%. In those in whom there was bilateral disease, the lesions were surprisingly symmetrical. In the author's series of 200, the medial femoral condyle was affected in 85% and the lateral in 15%. The classic site on the lateral aspect of the medial femoral condyle was present in 69% (Fig. 11.1). Those on the lateral side were most frequently associated with patellar dislocation. The lesion can also affect the trochlea of the femur, and

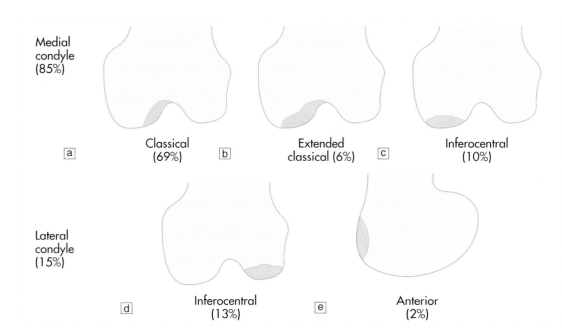

Medial condyle (85%)

[a] Classical (69%)

[b] Extended classical (6%)

[c] Inferocentral (10%)

Lateral condyle (15%)

[d] Inferocentral (13%)

[e] Anterior (2%)

Figure 11.1 – *The sites of osteochondritis dissecans at the knee. A review of 200 cases.*

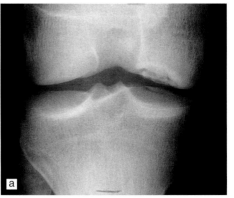

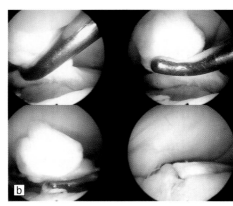

Figure 11.2 – *(a) An X-ray of osteochondritis dissecans of the medial femoral condyle. There is an unhealed fragment* in situ, *with a sclerotic base to the crater. (b) The arthroscopic appearance of a fragment in the crater. The fragment is being hinged from the crater with a probe.*

although this is an unusual site, it is being seen more commonly; it now constitutes 4% of the total seen in the author's unit.

The symptoms of osteochondritis dissecans of the knee are often vague and intermittent. The patient presents with low grade pain, recurrent swelling, joint irritability and giving way or locking. The clinical signs may be inconclusive. Examination findings include localised tenderness over the affected area, effusion, quadriceps atrophy, crepitus, restriction of knee movement and sometimes a positive Wilson's [6] sign (pain with extension of the knee and internal rotation of the tibia). On some occasions, a detached loose body may be palpated in the knee.

Plain X-rays usually show a well circumscribed fragment of subchondral bone, which is demarcated from the surrounding femoral condyle by a radiolucent crescentic shaped line (Fig. 11.2). The affected bone may appear denser than the surrounding parent bone. As the

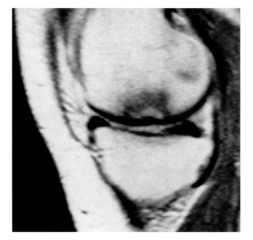

Figure 11.3 – *The magnetic resonance image of an osteochondritis dissecans – sagittal section.*

fragment gradually separates, a crater or depression is seen. Radioisotope bone scan, tomography, computed tomography (CT) and magnetic resonance imaging (MRI) are useful for the evaluation of this lesion (Fig. 11.3).

Osteochondral fractures of the knee

Osteochondral fractures of any part of the articular surface of the knee may occur in traumatic incidents. Direct blows, ligament ruptures and patellar dislocations are frequently responsible. Indirect violence and especially pivoting on an extending knee produces shearing forces severe enough to avulse a segment of articular cartilage and subchondral bone. The lateral femoral condyle is especially involved with an osteochondral fracture after this type of sports injury [7].

Kennedy *et al.* [8] found clinical examples where fractures of most areas of both condyles were present with separation of a fragment, and he produced experimental work in the cadaveric knee, in which strong axial compression and rotary forces were applied. Osteochondral fractures of the weight-bearing surfaces could be produced by this method. It has been pointed out by Landells [9] that adult articular cartilage tears at the junction between the calcified and the uncalcified zones. The immature adolescent cartilage does not have this calcified zone. Hence, the shearing forces are transmitted to the subchondral bone and it is here that osteochondral fractures occur. O'Donoghue believed that there was no real difference between an osteochondral fracture and osteochondritis dissecans, and this is certainly the author's feeling.

Aetiology of osteochondritis dissecans

A significant injury was sustained in 46% in the author's series; approximately half had an injury of substance, but the other half reported no specific knee injury. Nevertheless, the teenage males who made up most of the cases of osteochondritis dissecans were excellent or good at their sports. Ten percent were national or county players, and another 40% were league or school first players. Fifty percent can therefore be considered excellent or good at sports, and most were involved in contact field games.

Some 15% had associated meniscal or cruciate ligament injuries and it is interesting that in my series of discoid menisci, some 10% had an associated osteochondritis dissecans. Presumably, this was some mechanical problem affecting the joint surface. Those who had symmetrical bilateral disease frequently had an epiphyseal dysplasia, Blount's disease or some metabolic

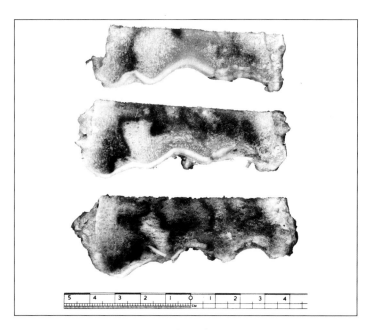

Figure 11.4 – *Osteonecrosis of the femoral condyle in steroid arthropathy. The peripheral segments of the large necrotic area are separating. This is in contradistinction to osteochondritis dissecans where the fragment crater consists of normal vascularised bone.*

abnormality. It is probable that some anatomical variation was a causative factor at the joint surface.

Osteochondritis dissecans is certainly *not* a primary osteonecrosis. Avascular necrosis occurs in steroid therapy, renal transplantation, haemoglobinopathies and Caisson's disease. In systemic disease the area involved is very large and in Caisson's disease a substantial area of avascularity may be seen. In transplantation arthropathy, the steroid necrosis again is substantial and the fragment separation is purely from the periphery of a large avascular zone (Fig. 11.4). The so-called idiopathic avascularity of a small area of the femoral condyle is again quite different from osteochondritis dissecans. The area of avascularity affecting the condyle is large. In an osteochondritis dissecans, the crater is covered with a fibrocartilagenous zone. Once this is removed, bleeding bone is exposed. In an avascular necrosis, the crater remains avascular and this is quite different to osteochondritis dissecans.

Experimental osteochondral fractures in animals

The author has studied the natural history of experimental osteochondral fractures of various types in an attempt to relate these fractures to the clinical disease [10]. Sixty adult

	31 Fragments			29 Fractures	
Group 1	Group 2	Group 3	Group 4	Group 5
Shifting	Stable	Pinned	Bridged	Unstable bridge
Animals 8	13	10	12	17
United 1	8	10	12	8
Not united 7	5	0	0	9

Figure 11.5 – *Experimental osteochondral fractures in the rabbit (60 animals studied). The cuts of various types healed when stable but remained unhealed when unstable, and these resembled osteochondritis dissecans.*

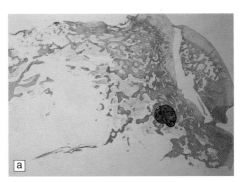
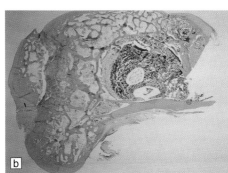

Figure 11.6 – *Both sections (a) and (b) are experimental un-united osteochondral fractures in rabbits, showing the fragment consisting of living hyaline cartilage, together with avascular bone. The crater is lined with fibrous and fibrocartilaginous tissue.*

New Zealand white rabbits were used. A knee arthrotomy was undertaken under general anaesthetic and various osteochondral cuts were made into the medial femoral condyle. The fragments were cut in different ways, so that they remained unstable and would shift on joint movement. Others were internally fixed (Fig. 11.5).

Osteochondral fractures which were cut in such a way that shift occurred progressed to a non-union state. Those adequately fixed did unite. Non-union of an osteochondral fragment was characterised by a necrotic osseous portion with viable cartilage. The junction or zone between the crater and the fragment contained much fibrous tissue and fibrocartilaginous material. The appearance of the un-united osteochondral fragment was similar to that in osteochondritis dissecans in the human (Fig. 11.6). Cadaver studies were also undertaken, showing that the medial patellar facet articulates with the medial femoral condyle in increasing flexion along the line of the classical site of osteochondritis dissecans. The classic site may be injured by falls onto the flexed knee with the patella damaging the condylar surface (Fig. 11.7).

Treatment

Removal of the loose body is essential if repeated episodes of pain, swelling and locking have occurred. Arthroscopic removal of the loose fragment depends upon observation and isolation of the fragment, its fixation with a needle or some other restraining method, its entrapment by means of a rongeur or some type of grabbing instrument and its final removal, which sometimes requires an extension of the portal if its size is large.

In a child, a stable lesion will frequently heal. The author reviewed 31 knees in 28 patients with arthroscopically confirmed osteochondritis dissecans of the femoral condyle treated at the Westminster Children's Hospital. The stability of the fragment was assessed arthroscopically by the use of a hook and the stable fragments were left *in situ*. Of these 28 patients, there were 14 males and 14 females with a mean age of 12 years. The mean interval between arthroscopy and review was 7.5 years. Of the 31 lesions, 21 were considered stable at arthroscopy and were left *in situ*. At

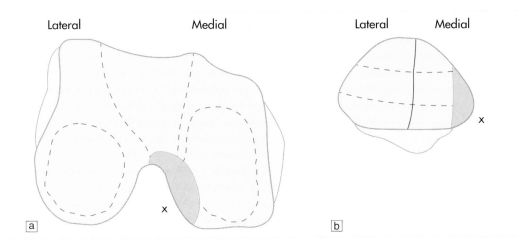

Lateral　　　Medial　　　　　Lateral　　Medial

a　　　　　　　　　　b

Figure 11.7 – *The medial patellar facet articulates with the medial femoral intercondylar region in increasing flexion, and this is the site of osteochondritis dissecans. Contact zone between medial patella and femoral condyle in increasing flexion indicated by x.*

review, 13 of the 21 stable lesions had healed and the distribution is as shown in Figure 11.8.

Further analysis showed that of the 10 lesions in the classic position on the medial femoral condyle, only three had healed, whereas elsewhere in the knee they had all healed, with only one exception. There was no correlation between healing and the size of the lesions, the age of onset or sex of the patient.

Some surgeons feel that symptomatic stable fragments should be drilled in an effort to increase the vascularity of the non-union. There has been no controlled trial of drilling, but Bradley and Dandy [11] showed in 10 children that the lesions in the classic site had healed within 12 months. The drilling can be undertaken arthroscopically. In the author's series there seemed to be no improvement with drilling.

Replacement fixation of a loose fragment is accurate and frequently successful in an acute osteochondral fracture. The re-attachment of chronic osteochondritis dissecans loose bodies is a different matter, as the osseous fragment is always covered by fibrous tissue or by hyperplastic hyaline cartilage. When the fibrous or cartilaginous tissue is removed, the bone apposition is less accurate and the fragment may fit poorly into its crater. The fit can be improved by curettage of the crater to remove all the fibrocartilaginous material present, and bone graft may be added. The fixation device was initially pins as advocated by Smillie. Compression screws may be used and the screws may be of different types, including Herbert screws. However, they must be removed at a moderately early stage and a period of immobilisation and non-weight-bearing is advocated in this type of fixation.

The ideal fixation material has not yet been found, and the author has used biodegradable Orthosorb pins,

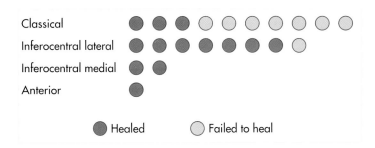

Classical
Inferocentral lateral
Inferocentral medial
Anterior

● Healed　　○ Failed to heal

Figure 11.8 – *Healing of stable osteochondritis dissecans lesions in the child.*

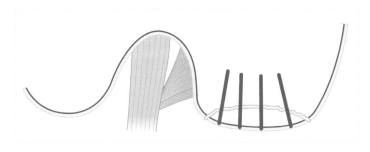

Figure 11.9 – *Pins of poly-L-lactide are used to fix an osteochondral fragment in the medial femoral condyle, which fits well in its crater.*

made of poly-P-dioxanone, successfully undertaking 10 fixations with multiple pins spread out on the fragment. Pins made of poly-L-lactide are now probably better (Fig. 11.9).

The author has recently reported the treatment of seven patients where six showed radiographic evidence of full incorporation at $2^{1}/_{2}$ years [12]. There is no need to retrieve the fixation device, and no specific erosions or other untoward radiological or clinical signs were found postoperatively (Fig. 11.10).

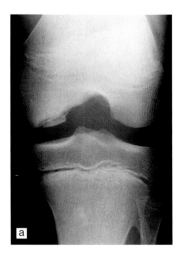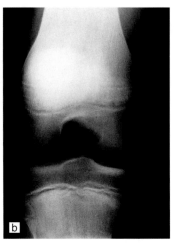

Figure 11.10 – *(a) A medial condyle osteochondritis dissecans was fixed with absorbable pins. (b) A well healed and united fragment after absorbable pin fixation. No reaction around the pins.*

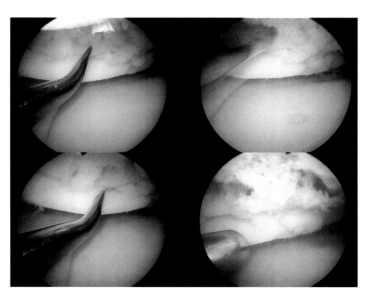

Figure 11.11 – *Arthroscopic appearance of the crater. Bone surface microfractured with a pick. The surface bleeding is seen after release of tourniquet.*

Excision of the unstable fragment is suggested if the lesion is small, if it is impossible to fix the fragment internally due to its mechanical characteristics, or if the defect contains multiple small broken fragments. The crater should be curetted down to bleeding subchondral bone with an arthroscopic curette and rongeurs, burr and picks are used for microfracture (Fig. 11.11) into the vascularised bone. The edges of the crater should be cut cleanly to make absolutely certain there are no loose osteochondral fragments at this site. There is no doubt that the reparative *fibrocartilage* resurfacing is often satisfactory, but the the quality and quantity is variable. Homminga [13] from the Netherlands has added an autogenous strip of costal perichondrium with improvement. The Japanese have used periosteum with improvement.

If after preparing the crater and so-called 'microfracture' of the bone surface, the lesion is very deep, I have added fluffy cancellous upper tibial graft by pressing this into the defect. If carefully pressed in, it sticks adequately and has tended in my hands to decrease the depth of the crater, producing again a fibrocartilaginous surface layer. Kevin Stone [14], however, has had the idea of adding a mush of hyaline cartilage to this cancellous mass as a paste (Fig. 11.12) and has shown the improvement in the surface and the production of a hyaline surface. This is an important advance.

Hangody *et al.* [15] and Bobic [16] have produced novel methods of osteochondral autografts, using plugs of bone and cartilage to fill osteochondral defects in the femoral condyles (Fig. 11.13). Their results are exciting

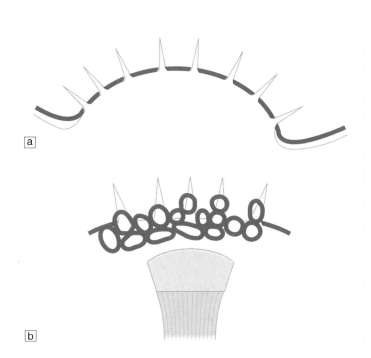

Figure 11.12 – *(a,b) The bone of the crater is microfractured and morselised osteochondral graft taken from the intercondylar notch is pushed into the crater interstices and punched home.*

and encouraging. Aston and Bentley have shown that chondrocyte grafting is a possibility and their work in animals [17] indicates that a supporting matrix base is required to maintain the chondrocyte position and to allow hyaline cartilage development.

Brittberg *et al.* [18] have recently described their method of autologous chondrocyte transplantation. The patient's chondrocytes are harvested from articular hyaline cartilage at arthroscopy. Culture of the chondrocytes occurs and they are then transplanted back to the chondral defect, which is covered with a strip of periosteum sutured in position and producing a water-tight seal. The chondrocytes are injected beneath this periosteal layer. In 2- to 9-year follow-ups, good and excellent results were obtained in 88%.

Massive and large shell osteochondral allografts have been undertaken in experimental studies [19]. This is difficult and non-routine work with multiple problems of tissue transplant and harvesting. Osteotomies are frequently required and the work is only being undertaken in specific experimental centres.

Human chondrocytes may be cultured and grown on a bioabsorbable mesh framework in a nutrient-rich environment. The cells are attached to this scaffold and excrete extracellular matrix. Plaques are then designed and may be permanently implanted on this surface. This experimental work undertaken in animals will soon be extended to the human [20].

We are on the verge of great progress in the filling of these defects in joint surfaces. The traumatic defect, such

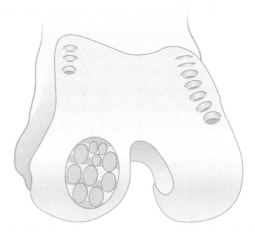

Figure 11.13 – *Mosaicplasty. Cylinders of osteochondral grafts are carefully harvested from the notch region and from the periphery of the trochlear surface. These cylinders are then pushed into exactly fitting holes drilled in the bone defect. Fibrocartilaginous tissue fills the spaces between the areas of transplanted hyaline cartilage.*

as osteochondritis dissecans, will soon be well filled with hyaline cartilage by these various means.

Degenerative changes and defects in joint surfaces will take much longer to solve and to resurface.

We are on the edge of an era of *biological* engineering.

Summary

Osteochondritis dissecans treatment plan

In young children:

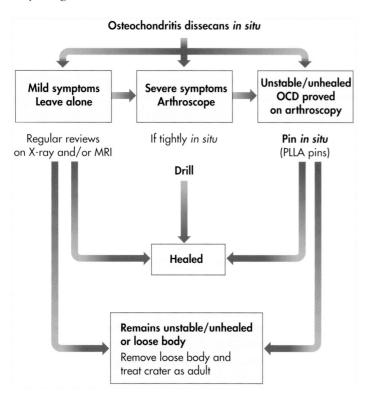

In adolescents and young adults:

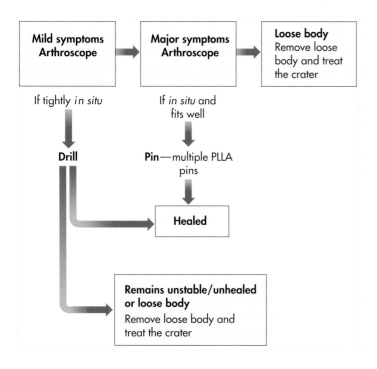

For the crater or defect:

**Small lesion
(less than 1×1 cm)**
Microfracture

**Medium sized lesion
(2×2 cm)**
Consider mosaicplasty or
Peterson technique or
morselised osteoarticular
graft

**Large lesion
(4×4 cm)**
Peterson technique
or morselised
osteochondral graft

Whole condyle with collapse
Consider osteochondral shell
allograft with osteotomy

Key points

1. There are two main theories of aetiology: injury and infarction. Osteochondritis dissecans is an unhealed osteochondral or subchondral fracture.
2. Significant injury is common (46%) and the condition is different from primary osteonecrosis.
3. The condition is commoner in boys, with a sex ratio of 2:1.
4. The condition is approximately 25% bilateral.
5. Symptoms and signs may be vague.
6. Advances in articular cartilage replacement hold promise for the future.

CHAPTER 12

Complex regional pain syndromes of the knee

R. L. Allum and R. H. Fell

Introduction

The International Association for the Study of Pain (IASP) [1] has agreed in the course of the last decade to rename the reflex sympathetic dystrophies (RSD) which include causalgia, Sudek's dystrophy, shoulder/hand syndrome and 'kangaroo's paw'. The new nomenclature applies equally to the knee.

Complex regional pain syndrome (CRPS) type I is the new name for post-traumatic reflex sympathetic dystrophy, whilst CRPS type II (causalgia) includes all the features of type I but, in addition, includes a peripheral nerve lesion [1]. The object of the change in the nomenclature was to introduce a descriptive diagnosis as opposed to one based on the questionable assumptions that the syndrome was always first, post-traumatic, second, reflex in nature, third, mediated through the sympathetic nervous system, and fourth, displayed dystrophy.

The new definition expresses the complexity and infinite variety of clinical presentations of the condition and the regional distribution of the characteristics presented, whilst pain is considered to be a constant feature. In addition, the new name for the condition allows a third group of presentations which may present regionally but in an unusual way and are classified by Stanton–Hicks et al. as 'not otherwise specified' (NOS) [2]. These authors also stress that any other known pathology in a region would preclude a diagnosis of either type of CRPS. Inevitably in a change-over period, the terms RSD and causalgia will continue to be used.

CRPS of the knee displays a great variety of symptoms and signs which are characterised particularly by a disproportionate amount of pain, loss of function and a number of features which appear at first sight to be difficult to evaluate. Some of these features are so random, bizarre and unconfined to dermatomes that it is tempting to regard the patient as mentally disturbed; however, most features are sufficiently constant to demand further questioning and investigation.

In making a diagnosis when a patient presents with a painful knee, it is clearly essential to carry out appropriate investigations first in order to exclude a mechanical or inflammatory disorder. It is when these have been eliminated that features which would support a diagnosis of CRPS should be sought. This search is simplified if the patient's symptoms and signs are matched to the definitions of well-known conditions described below. If there is no such match, it is then worth enquiring into the factors which predispose to complex regional pain syndrome, including such conditions as Raynaud's disease and migraine outlined in subsequent paragraphs.

Definitions

Reflex sympathetic dystrophy

As stated above, this syndrome follows minor or major trauma and is characterised by regional pain, non-dermatomal sensory changes, thermal and sudomotor changes and alterations in the turgor and colour of the skin. The word 'dystrophy' indicates malformation and malfunction, from the Greek words meaning 'poorly nourished'. The modern definition is CRPS type I.

Causalgia

Shumacker has reported that after an accident or after major surgery, a limb may become extremely painful, swollen, discoloured and lose its function [3]. In the absence of evidence of thrombosis and when a nerve injury can be demonstrated, this group of symptoms would be ascribed to causalgia, now CRPS type II. For the present, the IASP has retained the term causalgia to help communication and for historical reasons. The term RSD is also retained for CRPS type I [2].

Sudek's dystrophy
A limb or part of a limb may respond to trauma or surgery by becoming blue, painful and swollen and losing function, but in this case the X-ray of the region affected will display patchy osteoporosis in the bones particularly above and below a joint. The striking similarity between this condition and causalgia indicates that it is another example of CRPS but, in the absence of nerve injury, is classified as type I.

Sympathetically mediated pain (SMP = CRPS type I)
This expression is self-explanatory, since the pain responds to sympathetic blockade.

Shoulder/hand syndrome
This is a well-known combined syndrome in which the shoulder is held in adduction and in which the wrist is flexed and often supported by the opposite hand with both elbows held in flexion. In addition, Rosen and Graham have described changes in autonomic function [4].

Kangaroo's paw
When CRPS affects the wrist, the joint displays flexion associated with extension of the fingers and thumb in a characteristic position which resembles that of an Australian plant called kangaroo's paw. The affected wrist is often supported by the other hand.

Neuropathic pains in the knee
A number of patients present to orthopaedic surgeons with pains in the knee which are disproportionate to the physical signs and whose degree exceeds that which arthroscopic or magnetic resonance imaging (MRI) findings would support. Careful questioning of these patients should reveal whether the pain is a feature of an underlying neurological disorder such as diabetic, alcoholic, idiopathic or other peripheral neuropathy; if not, it is reasonable provisionally to diagnose CRPS.

Central
Apart from the sympathetic dystrophies, there may be a thalamic component to a peripheral neuropathic pain and it may also follow cerebral infarction or tumour.

Pathogenesis
Predisposition
One of the features of patients with CPRS is that they often display a history of an overactive sympathetic nervous system. It is not surprising that those suffering from Raynaud's syndrome, migraine, and carcinoid would be more likely to develop reflex dystrophy in response to trauma than those who have a 'normal' autonomic balance. In anorexia nervosa, the hypoglycaemic tendency triggers adrenaline secretion which in turn maintains blood sugar levels but increases the risk of CRPS. We encountered a patient with anorexia whose hands and feet were constantly cyanosed. After a fracture of the wrist she developed classical CRPS which responded to stellate ganglion block, and in the absence of response to guanethidine to transthoracic ganglionectomy.

Medication may predispose to CRPS particularly in asthmatics who regularly take beta-agonist adrenergic drugs. Conversely, patients stopping treatment with antihypertensives develop an adrenergic bias, as do those whose treatment for depression or epilepsy is being withdrawn when autonomic neurotransmission may be re-enhanced.

Distress of any kind will augment the tendency to CRPS and examples of this would include the death of a close relative, moving house, divorce or the actual or perceived loss of employment. Anticipation of surgery and suffering a road accident are also typical examples of factors inducing stress.

Clearly, the greater the number of predisposing factors associated with trauma, the more likely this excessive autonomic response will be.

Environmental factors which predispose to dystrophic reactions to injury include exposure to repetitive trauma or cold as in the use of jack-hammers or horse riding, particularly if two or more of these predisposing factors are combined.

Females appear to be at considerably greater risk from developing CRPS than males. This is a consistent finding in all the reported series. This syndrome can occur at any age and indeed occurs both in children and the elderly, but the peak incidence is in the third and fourth decades. In the knee, the patellofemoral joint seems to be particularly vulnerable and the majority of series in the literature report a relatively high incidence of problems associated with patellofemoral joint injury, disease or surgery. Injury to cutaneous nerves may also precipitate an exaggerated autonomic response and the saphenous nerve and its branches appear to be particularly vulnerable [5,6].

Katz and Hungerford [5] reported on 36 patients with RSD, 69% of whom were female. The mean age was 39.6 years with a range from 13 to 70 years. Sixty-four percent of these patients had had either an injury or an operation involving the patellofemoral joint. Forty-one percent had had previous surgery and 47% had had trauma to the front of the knee. The average number of operations prior to diagnosis was 1.2 and in 17% there was evidence of nerve injury. The mean delay in diagnosis was 29 months, with a range from 3 weeks to 11 years. One patient had been submitted to an arthroscopy, three manipulations, another arthroscopy, an arthrotomy and patellar realignment, a posterior cruciate ligament reconstruction and a further manipulation followed by a total knee replacement without resolution of symptoms! In a review of 19 patients, Ogilvie-Harris and Roscoe [6] reported 13 females and six males with an average age of 40 years, range 15–49. Sixteen had sustained injuries and three had undergone surgery, two menisectomies and one Maquet procedure. Poehling *et al.* [7] found that 100% of 35 patients with RSD had evidence of damage to the infrapatellar branch of the saphenous nerve, either by trauma or by surgery. The mean age in their series was 42 years, with a range from 19 to 80, and 73% were women. Cooper *et al.* [8], reviewing the results of epidural anaesthesia in RSD in 14 patients, had a rather younger age group with a mean of 29 years, range 21–39, eight women and six men. Eleven of the 14 patients had had surgery to the patella. Fulkerson and Hungerford [9] also highlight the vulnerability of the patellofemoral joint due to the superficial subcutaneous position of the patella. In their experience, the most common type of trauma is a direct blow to the patella, such as occurs in a dashboard injury or a fall onto the front of the knee. Indirect injuries such as twisting injuries or patellar dislocation are considered to be less likely to lead to RSD.

In a large series of 60 patients from the Hospital for Special Surgery, New York, O'Brien *et al.* [10] reported a similar age distribution with a mean age of 37.5 years and a range from 15 to 70. Forty-one of the 60 patients were female. Two thirds of the patients had had previous knee surgery and 13 of the remaining 20 patients had pain arising from the patellofemoral joint.

It would seem, therefore, that the typical CRPS victim is a woman in her late 30s or early 40s with a history of vasospasm or Raynaud's phenomenon who either sustains an injury to the patellofemoral joint by some form of direct trauma or who has surgery to the patellofemoral joint, possibly with an injury to a superficial cutaneous nerve.

An accomplished equestrian lady who competed in cross-country events found that her knees had become so painful that she was unable to walk across the field from her house to the stables and had given up all thoughts of a longed-for visit to Antarctica. She had none of the bony changes of reflex dystrophy but did have patchy hair growth over the outside of one leg and extremely cold toes on the other. A series of three guanethidine blocks, first at a fortnight's interval and then after a month, led to such complete recovery that she found it possible to ride horses even in cold weather and to carry out her trip across the winds and currents of Cape Horn to visit the elephant seal breeding grounds in Antarctica.

Mechanism

Prior to the conversion of nomenclature from RSD and causalgia to CRPS types I and II, it was considered that a sympathetic response to trauma is a normal component of the overall response, so that if there is a range of responses varying from 'normal' to causalgia, it is reasonable to suppose that CRPS of any severity can develop after trauma, depending on the circumstances in which the damage was sustained.

The theories proposed to explain the mechanism whereby a single or repeated skeletal stimulus can bring about chronic autonomic overactivity are many, and were selectively reviewed by Lindenfield *et al.* [11]. They reported the work of Barasi and Lynn [12] and others indicating that peripheral nocioceptors and mechanoreceptors could be sensitised by sympathetic stimulation. Scadding, together with Devor and Janig, has suggested that coupling of sympathetic to afferent fibres could be effected through alpha-adrenergic receptors, perhaps sensitised by trauma, whilst excess adrenaline is known to stimulate the afferent nerves of the spinothalamic tract [13,14]. Another very attractive theory by Janig [15] suggests the development of post-traumatic synapses (ephapses) which shunt information from efferent to afferent fibres in the same way that demyelinating disease leads to a shunt of information. Cross-stimulation between injured sensory fibres and sympathetic efferent fibres thus proposed would explain the localised nature of the autonomic response.

Sunderland has shown that chronic irritation of a peripheral sensory nerve may evoke a reflex arc through normal sympathetic connections at spinal level or at interjunctional neurone centres, either by recruitment or after discharge in the efferent loop of the reflex [16]. The only certainty is that the adrenergic mechanisms become overactive in many cases of CRPS. However, it is clear to clinicians that well-motivated patients overcome this sympathetic overdrive much more readily than those of a depressive nature, indicating that this reflex reaches a very high level of central nervous function. The systemic effect is demonstrated by the fact that in our pain relief unit, we have encountered several patients with unquestionable CRPS who have alterations in the growth of the hair in their head, recognised by their hairdressers.

It has certainly been observed that excitement and emotional upset already mentioned, unconnected stimuli from the eyes or ears or vibration sense, or even laughter can bring about an exacerbation of the dystrophic response in a sufferer. What has certainly not been explained is why only a few aspects of sympathetic activity should be displayed rather than a whole gamut of physical signs. Furthermore, the tendency of a particular patient to develop the same rather than a variety of dystrophic responses to different physical insults in different areas cannot be explained.

Negative observations seem to be every bit as important as positive objective findings in considering the pathogenesis of CRPS, as syringomyelia, poliomyelitis and prolonged unconsciousness have not been associated with this group of syndromes.

Wall and Devor [17] have demonstrated that the activation of inhibitor nerves by stimulation of the skin or by activity can suppress pain at the spinal level, but conversely, inactivity and protecting skin which is sensitive to touch can bring about an enhancement, particularly of sympathetically mediated pain. It is interesting that one of the earliest treatments of CRPS in amputee sailors was the use of hammers to stimulate the stumps and thus overcome 'negative input'. These were found in the medical stores when HMS *Mary Rose*, King Henry VIII's flagship, was raised from the Solent.

Clinical features

The certainties about this syndrome are unpredictability and variability. The spectrum of severity ranges from mild transient symptoms to a severe disabling long-term problem. The causative injury, if any, is also variable, ranging from a minor knock or bruise to major trauma, fracture or surgery. The autonomic nervous system will react to any trauma, no matter how minor, and an abnormal or exaggerated response could therefore be expected to occur after any injury. Over the years, the majority of reports in the literature have concentrated on the upper limb and the syndrome has not been well recognised in the lower limb. The author's group has found that looking at problems in the knee from an autonomic point of view can elucidate many confusing clinical presentations.

Pain

This is of course the main symptom which causes the patient to seek medical advice. The prime feature of this syndrome is pain which is out of proportion to the precipitating injury or operation. The onset is variable, and Fulkerson and Hungerford [9] have described three different modes of onset. Firstly, the pain begins immediately following the precipitating trauma and from the outset is out of proportion to the degree of injury. Secondly, the initial pain is of expected intensity but it does not settle as expected and persists or increases. In the third pattern of onset, the patient initially makes satisfactory progress with resolution of symptoms but the pain then reappears, possibly in response to manipulation or over-vigorous attempts at rehabilitation. The pain is described as being different to the pain of the injury. It is more intense, often described as burning and is persistent and unremitting. Night pain may be particularly troublesome. Autonomic pain does not follow an anatomical distribution, that is it does not specifically follow the distribution of a single peripheral sensory nerve [11]. The knee is diffusely tender and hyperaesthetic and there may be trigger points which cause excruciating pain. Hyperpathia and allodynia can both occur. Hyperpathia or hyperalgesia is overreaction to a painful stimulus. Allodynia is pain produced by what is normally a non-noxious stimulus. Light touch such as the brushing of clothes or a bed sheet over the skin may cause extreme irritation. The pain may also be made worse by changes in temperature, loud unexpected noises or changes in the emotional state of the patient.

Other symptoms and signs

The other clinical features of this syndrome relate to the vasomotor instability. Pain and intolerance to cold is often the first sign of a problem. The initial response is one of vasodilatation and the skin becomes pink, warm and dry. Changes in sweating are termed sudomotor changes. There is oedema. The combination of swelling and inactivity due to the constant pain soon leads to joint stiffness. The clinical picture then changes and after a variable period of time vasoconstriction occurs. The knee becomes blue and cold and the skin shiny or shrivelled. Hair growth is affected in a variety of ways. Tufts of extra growth are commonest, but bare patches or marked thinning may be present. Delicate questioning is required in women who shave their legs regularly. In some hand and foot problems, ipsilateral nail growth is also affected; occasionally the same applies when the knee is involved. Later the knee becomes atrophic with thinning of the skin and loss of subcutaneous fat. Pigmentation changes may also occur, leading to dark or pale patches of melanin redistribution. One patient was accused of smoking by his daughter because his nails became brown. A businessman who had patchy translucency in X-rays of the condyles of the femur and in the patella and had an extremely painful knee, responded to a series of three guanethidine blocks. His case was particularly interesting in that on visiting Spain after a successful outcome, he went sunbathing and returned with three brown limbs and one which resembled a lobster! This supports the concept that melanophore activity is under autonomic control and the observation that is mentioned above, that changes in melanin concentration in the affected limb may be a physical sign of CRPS. Travellers should therefore be advised to take the highest level of sun block creams and use them liberally after sympathetic block.

Most authors have described three phases in the vasomotor changes in CRPS:
- Phase 1. The early vasomotor response with swelling, vasodilatation where the knee is hot, pink and dry. This usually occurs within 3 months of the precipitating episode.
- Phase 2. The dystrophic phase with predominant vasoconstriction, continuing oedema and cold thin skin together with increasing stiffness developing between 3 and 12 months after the onset.
- Phase 3. The atrophic phase with increasing skin, muscle and soft tissue atrophy with fibrosis and contractures. Diffuse bony changes also occur and these later changes may well be irreversible and cause a permanent disability. This phase occurs at a variable time but usually after at least 12 months.

Atkins [18], on the other hand, has described a more practical classification. The critical issue is the onset of late atrophic changes and the disease is therefore divided into two stages.
- Stage 1. Early RSD with vasomotor instability, either dilatation or constriction. As atrophy and fixed contractures have not yet occurred, in theory this stage is reversible.
- Stage 2. Late RSD. Established atrophy and contracture have now occurred and some of these changes are irreversible.

The timescale is variable, but stage 2 normally occurs 6–12 months after the onset of the condition, although it may take longer.

Investigations and diagnosis

Awareness is one of the key factors in the diagnosis of this condition which should be considered in any patient who fails to make satisfactory progress following knee injury or surgery, however limited. The difference between the normal autonomic response to the injury and the abnormal lies in the rate of progress. It is important to make the diagnosis at as early a stage as possible for a number of reasons. The symptoms are always distressing and will inevitably lead to a reaction with a degree of depression. This will affect the individual patient's ability to cope with the disorder, often causing a vicious circle of pain, depression and more pain. The sooner treatment is started, the better the chance of breaking the cycle.

Initially, the pathological changes are reversible but as time goes by, irreversible changes occur which will obviously lead to a degree of permanent disability. Continuing uncertainty regarding diagnosis will almost certainly cause problems with the doctor/patient relationship. Both parties will become increasingly frustrated and possibly angry with the failure to progress after what is often a trivial injury or a relatively minor surgical procedure, with high expectations on the part of the patient (and doctor) of a prompt return to full activity.

The incidence of RSD varies in reported series but it may occur in up to 30% of patients following a distal radial fracture [18]. The diagnosis, as in the majority of medical conditions, is essentially a clinical one.

If a patient's pain and symptoms cannot be readily explained by local pathology in the knee, it is also important to rule out referred pain. Examination and investigation of the hip and lumbar spine may be appropriate. The possibility of an underlying neurological disorder should also be borne in mind as a source of pain, and investigations such as MRI scanning of the lumbar spine may need to be considered.

The clinical features are as stated above, with a wide range of severity. O'Brien *et al.* [10] report that few patients with RSD of the knee have an effusion and vasomotor symptoms were not present in approximately one-third of the patients in their series. The radiological changes are not universally present and may be absent in up to one third of patients.

Other causes of unresolved pain are infection, inflammatory joint disease and circulatory disturbances including venous thrombosis. The patient with CRPS will be well with no systemic signs and the appropriate haematological investigations including full blood count, erythrocyte sedimentation rate, C-reactive protein, rheumatoid factor, uric acid and serum biochemistry will be normal. The radiological signs will be confined to the bone and the joint space will be normal, or at least unchanged from previous X-rays. A venogram is advisable if deep venous thrombosis is clinically suspected.

Radiological changes

The X-ray changes normally appear between 2 and 8 weeks after the onset of symptoms. The essential change is one of demineralisation. The osteoporosis is commonly patchy with a band-like distribution, predominantly affecting the subchondral bone, epiphysis and metaphyseal regions. Both cortical and cancellous bone are involved. The changes are different from the generalised ground-glass appearance of disuse atrophy. The joint space is normal and there is no evidence of inflammatory arthropathy such as erosions. Comparison with the opposite knee is helpful. In patellofemoral problems, the osteoporosis may be confined to the ipsilateral patella or to the patella and trochlea only (Figs 12.1, 12.2). Soft tissue swelling may also be visible. The severity of the radiological changes is very variable, as is the clinical syndrome, and in a small proportion of patients the X-rays may be normal. The osteoporosis resolves after clinical recovery, but some of the radiological changes may be irreversible.

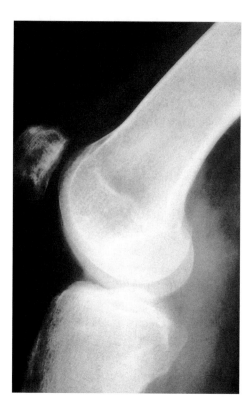

Figure 12.1 – *Selective osteoporosis of the patella, lateral view.*

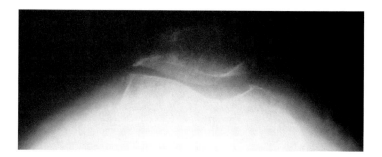

Figure 12.2 – *Selective osteoporosis of the patella, skyline view.*

Bone scanning

This is a very useful investigation and is certainly sensitive, although not specific. Typically, the technetium-99 scan will show increased uptake in the early stages of the disease (Fig. 12.3). The bone scan is abnormal before the X-ray changes appear. There is increased uptake in the whole area affected by the disease. Both the blood pool phase and the delayed image show increased activity. The changes can be widespread with increased activity in the other joints of the affected limb; the whole limb itself may be involved and there may also be changes in the contralateral limb. The exception to this is in children, where the bone scan may not change. Later the scan returns to normal. Ogilvie-Harris and Roscoe [6] reported that in patients presenting early, all had positive scans,

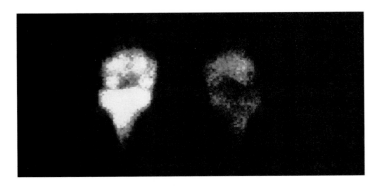

Figure 12.3 – *Increased uptake in CRPS on technetium-99 scan.*

whereas in the group presenting later, only six of eight scans were positive. In the large series reported by O'Brien *et al.* [10], all 19 patients who had bone scans demonstrated some asymmetry of uptake and two patients with good results from treatment had repeat scans which showed decreasing activity. Bone scanning is therefore a reliable indicator of CRPS and, if the bone scan is normal in an adult, particularly in the early stages, then the diagnosis must be thrown into considerable doubt.

Magnetic resonance imaging

MRI has not been found to be particularly useful in the diagnosis, being insensitive and non-specific. There are no consistent bone or soft tissue abnormalities.

Computerised tomography

Computerised tomography (CT) shows patchy osteoporosis in the cancellous bone with cortical thinning and soft tissue swelling. It has not been demonstrated to have any specific advantage over the plain X-ray.

Thermography

Thermography can be useful, giving an objective assessment of temperature changes around the knee and later measuring the response to treatment, but it is not widely or readily available in the routine clinical setting. In the early stages, the affected area shows an increase in temperature and later the painful area becomes cooler than normal. In the series reported by Katz and Hungerford [5], eight patients had thermography with an average temperature decrease of $1.6\,°C$ (range $1-2.5\,°C$).

Densitometry

The extent of the osteoporosis may be quantified using densitometry, but this is really a research rather than a clinical tool.

Pathology

There is little information in the literature on the histological findings, as biopsy has rarely been recommended or carried out, particularly because of concern that an invasive procedure will cause a deterioration in the condition. The soft tissues and synovial membrane may initially show an inflammatory response and oedema which later progresses to fibrosis.

Ogilvie-Harris and Roscoe [6] however, reported in the early cases non-specific subsynovial fibrosis with synovial proliferation but without inflammatory changes. In cases presenting later, the degree of fibrosis appeared to be greater. They concluded that the synovial changes take some months to develop and are therefore not always present in the early cases.

Arlet has described bone lesions which are more specific [19] and can be diagnostic. There are essentially three lesions: stasis and oedema of the bone marrow, osteoclastic erosion of the trabeculae and subchondral plate and marked osteogenic and osteoblastic activity.

Sympathetic blockade

The role of sympathetic blockade as a diagnostic agent is somewhat controversial. Some authors believe [9,11] that by definition sympathetically mediated pain must be abolished by sympathetic blockade and, if the symptoms are not relieved, the diagnosis is most unlikely. However, this syndrome is not entirely clear cut and there are certainly cases of clinical CRPS where other conditions have been excluded which do not respond to a sympathetic block or respond only partially.

In the full-blown case the diagnosis is easy, but this is such a variable condition that awareness and a high level of suspicion may well be the keys to diagnosis. Bone scanning is probably the single most reliable investigation, but the diagnosis can prove to be exceedingly difficult.

Treatment

The prime objective of the clinician when the diagnosis of CRPS is made is to get rid of the pain as a prelude to rehabilitation [2].

The mainstays of treatment of CRPS are the use of analgesics, including non-steroidal anti-inflammatory drugs (NSAIDs), neurotransmitter blockers, physiotherapy, and regional blocks. The transcutaneous nerve stimulator (TENS) is also said to be effective if any of the above modalities, singly or together, fail to achieve progress. Melzak and Wall have recommended that interventional regional blockade is instituted when stimulation of the afferent loop of reflex arcs is associated with pain [20].

The neurostransmitter blockers include the tricyclic antidepressants amitriptyline and nortriptyline in particular, the anticonvulsants and the centrally acting anti-hypertensives, particularly clonidine. In resistant cases, it becomes necessary to use a combination of two or even three of these substances, with or without the use of nerve blocks of the skeletal sensory and/or autonomic nervous systems.

It is noticeable that those determined to recover will take treatment more readily and to a higher dosage than those who are more concerned about the many side effects of these agents. It is up to the clinician to try and push each patient as far as possible towards the maximum tolerable dose. It is also important to use these agents immediately the diagnosis is suspected, whilst arrangements are made for regional autonomic blockade to be carried out. Physiotherapy has often been used before the diagnosis is considered and should continue in the manner recommended by the algorithms of Stanton–Hicks *et al.* [2] if possible and TENS can be used at any time. Again, it is the most motivated patients who will be moved to use all therapeutic techniques available to them.

Analgesics

Until recently, each pain control group has adopted a hit-or-miss approach to the use of analgesic agents in CRPS; the use of opioids and mixtures of simple and more powerful agents is debatable. On the one hand, Arner and Meyerson [21] regard opioids as ineffective in neuropathic pain, but Portenoy *et al.* [22] and Rowbotham *et al.* [23] groups claim good results with post-herpetic neuralgia. Suffice it to say that a trial of therapy is well worthwhile very early in the treatment plan to see if the prime objective, analgesia, can be achieved by this means. Children and addicts should not receive these drugs.

Non-steroidal anti-inflammatory drugs (NSAIDs)

These agents should be tried for the same reason as analgesics, but the response is unpredictable.

Amitriptyline and congeners

Amitriptyline and clomipramine are without doubt the best of the tricyclic neurotransmitter blockers in the treatment of CRPS. The dose required is between 75 mg and 150 mg, well below the antidepressant dose. However, it is vital to explain the four common side effects to the patient so that non-compliance can be avoided. These are dry mouth, constipation, drowsiness and increase in weight. The drowsiness is combated by starting at a very low dose, such as 10 mg at night, and gradually advancing up to 50 mg at night and then offering doses of 10 or 20 mg twice a day in addition. Further increases are possible in motivated patients and may go up to a total of 150 mg per day. Constipation can be overcome by the use of lactulose or danthron derivatives at an effective dosage, whilst dryness of the mouth can be overcome by taking more liquids. The patient can be reassured that weight gain due to these agents will reverse when treatment becomes unnecessary. It is also essential to point out to the patient that the benefit may not be noticed until a month into treatment.

If the side effects of amitriptyline are intolerable to the patient, then nortriptyline or clomipramine and other tricyclic antidepressants should be tried. The serotonin re-uptake inhibitors are not nearly as effective as the tricyclics, but they do elevate the mood and could be used in combination if necessary, particularly in chronic cases [2]. Above all, the essential message is not to give up unless the side effects are intolerable.

Anticonvulsants

Probably the most popular agent in this group is carbamazepine, which may be used in doses up to 600 mg a day with gradual progression from a dose of 100 mg at night to 200 mg three times a day. If amitriptyline is unacceptable to the patient at high dosage, it may be used in a lower dose at night with the above dosage of carbamazepine added gradually. If 600 mg carbamazepine per day does not affect the liver and symptoms are still present, this dosage can be raised to 900 mg a day with 6-weekly liver function tests to ensure safety.

The second most popular anticonvulsant is sodium valproate, which can be given in the same dosage and with the same precautions regarding the liver. This often has a better side-effect profile than carbamazepine, but may not be quite as effective. It has a particular advantage when the patient complains of shooting pain. Gabapentin is also useful [24].

Alternatively, clonazepam may be used at night in dosages up to 2 mg if side effects are experienced in the use of the other two agents. It is important to recognise that any of these neurotransmitter blockers needs to be withdrawn slowly to avoid symptoms of deep hallucination with or without depersonalisation.

Finally, an oral congener of lignocaine, mexiletine, which is also capable of membrane stabilisation, is helpful in neuropathies [23] and may be so in CRPS.

Anti-adrenergic drugs

Clonidine is usually administered in CRPS following a period of admission to a specialist unit for epidural block using a very weak solution of this agent. It can, however, be used by mouth in a dose of 200 μg first daily and then twice a day and finally three times a day if the patient is not subject to postural syncope. Davies *et al.* have shown that patches applied dermally may work in discretely painful areas [25].

Alpha-blockers often used for the treatment of Raynaud's disease have a poor therapeutic to side-effect ratio, but can be used if an intravenous phentolamine trial has been effective. Topical capsaicin may be similarly effective.

Additional therapies

At the same time as management using drugs, it is essential that the patient is instructed to use the affected limb as much as possible, to try to avoid limping and to carry out specific exercises recommended by the physiotherapist. In addition to the above, the use of alternating hot and cold packs on the affected area may give at least psychological support and may be very beneficial in its own right.

TENS devices may be attached as recommended by the manufacturers on either side of the painful area and the stimulating current adjusted so that it can just be perceived by the patient. Again, this form of treatment may take 2 or 3 weeks to have an effect and should be persisted with even if initial results are disappointing.

Regional anaesthetic techniques

When pharmacological treatment has proved inadequate to control the pain of CRPS, it is essential to provide sufficient local analgesia early to allow mobilisation of the affected part and to enable the patient to return to a more normal 'bilaterally active' life. Great psychological benefits accrue from this. In addition, sympathetic blockade may accompany the analgesic effect of a peripheral block [2].

The nerve blocks in any part of the body may be prolonged for up to 6 weeks by the insertion of a catheter connected to an infusion pump containing low concentrations of local anaesthetics. Raj and Denson have added opioids [26] and Rauck *et al.* used clonidine [27] to enhance their efficiency. The risks of infection and displacement of the catheter and the minor loss of motor power and control which accompany their use are a small price to pay for the likely benefit of re-mobilisation. Prolonged nerve blocks may be followed by surgically implanted neuromodulators in the peri-spinal tissues, spinal cord stimulation (SCS) or peripheral nerve stimulation (PNS) as described by Barolet *et al.* [28]. These implants have proved effective over months and even years in controlling the pain and disability caused by CRPS.

Techniques for sympathetic block

Blockade of the sympathetic outflow to the upper limb may be carried out by stellate ganglion block perhaps followed by ganglionectomy, brachial plexus perfusion or guanethidine block. In the lower limb, the two groups of techniques for achieving sympathetic blockade are lumbar sympathetic block, paravertebral block, chemical or even surgical sympathectomy in resistant cases, and guanethidine block under tourniquet originally described by Hannington Kiff [29]. Repeated paravertebral blocks have been carried out in the US in order to reduce the outflow of sympathetic impulses without using techniques which can interfere with potency [11]. The disadvantages of repetitive paravertebral blocks are that the patient is considerably inconvenienced and the resources required are not generally available in the UK. The choice of sympathetic block depends on the highest point to which symptoms travel. If pain in the knee is associated with pain in the thigh and buttock, a chemical sympathetic block (Figs 12.4, 12.5) followed, if necessary, by a surgical sympathectomy is the best way to proceed. If the pain is distal to the mid thigh, then a guanethidine block is carried out with appropriate precautions using 30 mg guanethidine under tourniquet for 20 min on three occasions preferably at fortnightly intervals (Fig. 12.6). However, the value of this technique has been questioned by Jadad *et al.* [30]. In the most severe and resistant cases, who have responded transiently to sympathetic blockade or guanethidine blocks, a surgical sympathectomy may be carried out traditionally. Darzi and Fell are investigating a micro-surgical approach employing minimally invasive techniques [31].

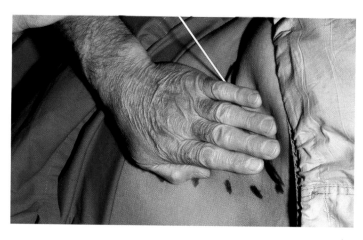

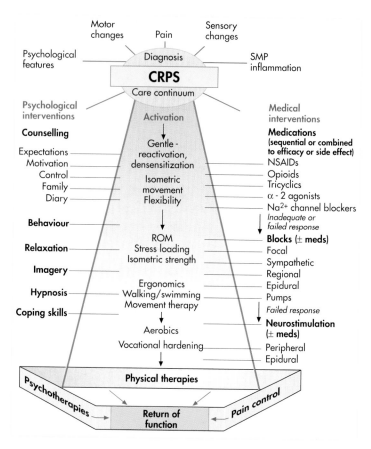

Figure 12.4 – *Technique of chemical sympathectomy (Kappis technique). The needle is introduced at 45° to the horizontal at the apex of the renal triangle one hand's breadth lateral to the lumbar spine with the patient in the lateral position.*

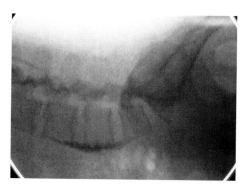

Figure 12.5 – *X-ray control of needle introduction in chemical sympathectomy. Contrast medium (2 ml) is seen between the lumbar spine and the psoas muscle.*

Figure 12.7 – *Algorithm for management of CRPS. (Reproduced from ref. 2 with permission .)*

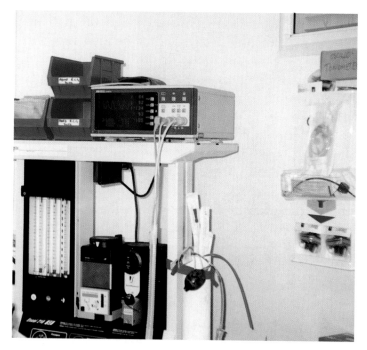

Figure 12.6 – *Monitoring and resuscitation equipment available for guanethidine block.*

Algorithm

A summary of the management of CRPS is displayed in Figure 12.7. This includes the psychotherapeutic and complementary medical techniques used in this condition.

Outcome

Most workers agree that early diagnosis is a key factor in a good outcome. There is no shame in treating CRPS when it does not exist; the true diagnosis may still emerge. In general, the outcome of treatment of CRPS is as varied and as random as the pain itself. Sometimes a single injection of bupivacaine into the space between the psoas muscle and the lumbar spine can bring about a dramatic improvement which is sustained by medical treatment; conversely, recovery may either never occur or be slow or followed by recurrence of symptoms. The majority of outcomes fall between these two extremes.

It is noticeable that the psychological makeup of the patient has a major effect on the outcome where depression and the stress factors already mentioned exist, and the possible presence of litigation may have a deleterious effect. A series of three guanethidine blocks is frequently successful in the author's experience when supported by psychotherapy, a rigorous programme of physiotherapy and neurotransmitter blockade. Chemical sympathectomy may be successful after the first, second or third visit but surgical sympathectomy is often more effective in the long term. Patients who decline invasive techniques will often respond eventually to neurotransmitter blockade alone or in combination with physiotherapy techniques.

This variety of responses is best illustrated by case histories of patients encountered by the authors.

A lady who had intensely tender and hypersensitive scars at the sites of previous knee surgery underwent guanethidine blocks at regular intervals for almost 2 years, but gradually the need for guanethidine blocks diminished and has now become an annual requirement. This lady had additional psychological problems which manifested themselves in an hysterical response to TENS and the need for nortriptyline in high dosage for depression. Nine years on, she still finds the need to smoke and still displays some inappropriate physical signs in addition to the extreme tenderness mentioned.

A young man of 18 years of age displayed patchy tufts of hair with bare patches between on a very painful knee which he claimed not to be able to flex at all. He could not tolerate a guanethidine block without a general anaesthetic and during this it was noted that the stiff knee could be flexed almost to a right angle. After the first guanethidine block he displayed an ability to flex the knee to 45° but, after subsequent blocks, resolutely refused to bend the knee even though during anaesthesia it had been possible to achieve flexion. It subsequently emerged that the changes in hair growth had been fabricated by shaving and the final indicator of hysteria was that the patient had been seen manoeuvring himself from a car to his front door backwards over gravel using his heels to push himself along on his buttocks with good knee flexion!

A young 23-year-old female athlete developed an intensely tender spot adjacent to the insertion of the patellar tendon which responded well for approximately a fortnight each time she received guanethidine blockade. Subsequently she responded to TENS treatment alone which she maintained for a number of years.

Identical twins presented with knee pains and were managed in different units with and without sympathetic blockade with markedly different results, the twin receiving sympathetic blockade having a much better result.

Conclusion

There is no doubt that CRPS is now more readily recognised by clinicians who are puzzled when there is a disparity between symptoms, particularly pain, and physical, imaging and arthroscopic findings in the knee joint. The authors believe that this syndrome is much commoner than many surgeons think and that the symptoms and disabilities suffered by patients are augmented by sympathetic restriction of blood supply and nutrition to the joint and surrounding structures. Severe vasoconstriction, if sustained, may lead in itself to intra-articular and peri-articular damage.

Key points

1. Reflex sympathetic dystrophy and associated conditions have been renamed as the complex regional pain syndromes.
2. Females are more commonly affected than males.
3. The patellofemoral joint is particularly vulnerable.
4. Clinical features are variable and it is important to bear the condition in mind in a patient who fails to make satisfactory progress following injury or surgery.
5. The bone scan is the single most reliable investigation.
6. The main aim of treatment is to rid the patient of pain so that they can progress with their rehabilitation.

CHAPTER 13

Biology, injury and healing of articular cartilage

V. Bobic

Introduction

In 1743, Hunter stated: 'From Hippocrates to the present age it is universally allowed that ulcerated cartilage is a troublesome thing and that once destroyed, it is not repaired' [1]. The inability of cartilage to repair itself after traumatic injuries and the incapacity of the treatment to stop further degenerative process, leading to osteoarthrosis, has been described repeatedly for at least 250 years.

It is well known that the capacity of articular cartilage for repair is limited. Partial-thickness defects in the articular cartilage do not heal spontaneously. Injuries of the articular cartilage that do not penetrate the subchondral bone do not heal and usually progress to the degeneration of the articular surface [2]. A short-lived tissue response fails to provide sufficient cells and matrix to repair even small defects. Injuries that penetrate the subchondral bone undergo repair through the formation of fibrocartilage. Although fibrocartilage fills and covers the defect, this tissue is suboptimal from the biomechanical standpoint. Fibrocartilage is made to resist tension forces, while hyaline cartilage is made to resist compression forces, to enable smooth articulation, and to withstand long-term variable cyclic load and shearing forces.

Normal hyaline articular cartilage

Hyaline articular cartilage has a glossy, bluish-white, opalescent, homogeneous appearance, firm consistency and some elasticity. Articular cartilage serves as the load-bearing material of joints which has excellent friction, lubrication and wear characteristics. Articular cartilage is a complex structure, which is self-renewing and responds to alterations in use. It provides smooth articulation under variable loads and impaction for very long periods of time. It varies in thickness, cell density, matrix composition, and mechanical properties within the same joint, among joints, and among species. However, in all synovial joints it consists of the same components, has the same general structure, and performs the same functions (Fig. 13.1). Although it is at most only a few millimetres thick, it has surprising stiffness to compression, resilience and an exceptional ability to distribute variable loads. The cartilage thickness varies significantly across articular surfaces of the same joint. Stiffer cartilage tends to be thinner than softer cartilage. Cartilage subject to higher prevalent stress tends to be thinner than cartilage subject to lower prevalent stress. There are significant directional, topographical and zonal variations in the fatigue properties of cartilage [3,4]. Macroscopically and histologically, adult articular cartilage has an unimpressive appearance and seems to be a simple inert tissue. When it is examined macroscopically, normal articular cartilage has a smooth, shiny and firm surface that resists deformation. Microscopic examination shows that it consists primarily of extracellular matrix, with only one type of cell, the chondrocyte, and that it lacks blood and lymphatic vessels and nerves [2,5–7].

Cartilage is often described as totally avascular, which is not entirely correct. Cartilage contains an anti-angiogenic factor that inhibits vascular invasion, and inhibitors to many chondrolytic proteinases.

Chondrocytes surround themselves with their extracellular matrix and do not form cell-to-cell contacts

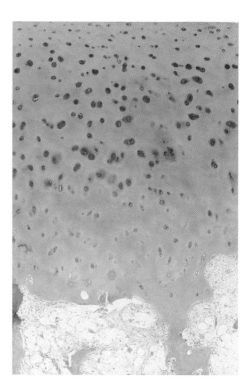

Figure 13.1 – *Histology of normal hyaline cartilage.*

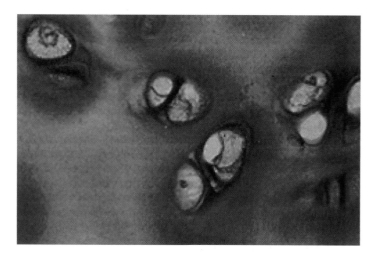

Figure 13.2 – *Clusters of chondrocytes, surrounded by proteoglycan clouds.*

(Fig. 13.2). Chondrocytes seem to be observers rather than participants in the function of mature articular cartilage as a joint surface. They appear to remain unchanged in location, appearance and activity for decades. Chondrocytes derive their nutrition from nutrients in the synovial fluid, which, to reach the cell, must pass through two diffusion barriers: the synovial tissue and synovial fluid, and the cartilage matrix, which is a restrictive barrier. The nature of this system leaves chondrocytes with a low concentration of oxygen relative to most other tissues, and therefore they depend

primarily on anaerobic metabolism. Individual chondrocytes are surprisingly active metabolically, but the total metabolic activity of the tissue is low because of the low cell density. Although the cartilage has a low level of metabolic activity, it is a highly ordered structure where a variety of complex interactions between the chondrocytes and the matrix actively maintain the tissue. The articular cartilage derives its form and mechanical properties from its matrix. The cells contribute little to the volume of the tissue, about 1% in adult human articular cartilage. In other species, especially small animals such as rabbits, which have thin articular cartilage, the cell density is many times greater than in humans. Cytokines and growth factors can have profound effects on chondrocytes. It is apparent that, as well as regulating normal matrix synthesis, they are also involved in cartilage destruction during disease. Growth factors such as transforming growth factor-beta (TGF-β) and insulin-like growth factor-I (IGF-I) are present in high amounts in cartilage, bound to various components of the extracellular matrix. Both have a protective effect on cartilage by stimulating matrix synthesis and blocking the effects of pro-inflammatory cytokines.

The extracellular matrix of the articular cartilage consists of two components: the tissue fluid and the framework of structural macromolecules that give the tissue its form and stability. The interaction of the tissue fluid with the macromolecular framework gives the tissue its mechanical properties of stiffness and resilience. Water contributes as much as 80% of the wet weight of articular cartilage.

The structural macromolecules of the cartilage, collagens, proteoglycans and non-collagenous proteins, contribute 20–40% of the wet weight of the tissue. Collagens (types II, VI, IX, X, and XI) contribute about 60% of the dry weight of cartilage. The principal collagen, type II, accounts for 90–95% of the collagen in articular cartilage. Proteoglycans account for 25–35%, and non-collagenous proteins and glycoproteins, 15–20%. Collagens are distributed relatively uniformly throughout the depth of the cartilage, except for the collagen-rich superficial zone. The collagen fibrillar meshwork gives cartilage its form and tensile strength. Proteoglycans and non-collagenous proteins bind to the collagenous meshwork or become mechanically entrapped within it, and water fills this molecular framework.

Proteoglycans consist of a protein core and one or more glycosaminoglycan chains. Articular cartilage contains two major classes of proteoglycans: large aggregating proteoglycan monomers or aggrecans, and small proteoglycans including decorin, biglycan and fibromodulin. It has been suggested that the proteoglycans may act as minute compressed springs, storing energy when further compacted, then releasing it on recoil, and so conferring elastic properties on the matrix. Glycosaminoglycans (GAGs) include chondroitin 4-sulphate, chondroitin 6-sulphate, dermatan sulphate and keratin sulphate. Groups of GAGs are bound to a filament of protein. Several such proteoglycan assemblies are bound along the length of a relatively huge hyaluronic acid molecule to form highly complex filamentous aggregates [2,5–7].

Structure of hyaline articular cartilage

To form articular cartilage, chondrocytes organise the collagens, proteoglycans and non-collagenous proteins into a unique, highly ordered structure. The composition, organisation and mechanical properties of the matrix, cell morphology and cell function vary according to the depth from the articular surface.

There are four layers: a superficial zone, a transitional zone, a middle or deep zone and a zone of calcified cartilage. Although each zone has different morphological features, the boundaries between the zones cannot be sharply defined, but the zonal organisation has functional importance (Fig. 13.3).

The superficial zone has specialised mechanical and biological properties. This zone consists of two layers: a sheet of fine fibrils with little polysaccharide and no cells covers the joint surface, and corresponds to the clear film often identified as the *lamina splendens*. Deep to this layer, flattened ellipsoid-shaped chondrocytes arrange themselves so that their major axes are parallel to the articular surface.

The chondrocytes synthesise a matrix that has a high concentration of collagen and a low concentration of proteoglycan relative to the other cartilage zones. The dense matrix of collagen fibrils lying parallel to the joint surface in the superficial zone helps to determine the mechanical properties of the tissue and affects the movement of molecules in and out of the cartilage. These fibrils give this zone greater tensile stiffness and strength than the deeper zones, and they may resist shear forces generated during use of the joint. The superficial zone also makes an important contribution to the compressive behaviour of articular cartilage. Removal of this zone increases the permeability of the tissue and probably increases loading of the macromolecular framework during compression. Disruption or remodelling of the dense collagenous matrix of the superficial zone is one of the first detectable structural changes in experimentally induced degeneration of articular cartilage, suggesting that alterations in this zone may contribute to the development of osteoarthrosis by changing the mechanical behaviour of the tissue. The morphology and the matrix composition of the *transitional zone* are intermediate between the superficial zone and the middle zone. The transitional zone usually has several times the volume of the superficial zone. Cells in the transitional zone assume a spheroidal shape and synthesise a matrix that has larger-diameter collagen fibrils, a higher concentration of proteoglycan and lower concentrations of water and collagen than does the

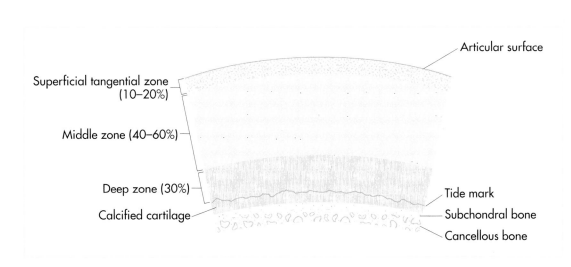

Superficial tangential zone (10–20%)

Middle zone (40–60%)

Deep zone (30%)

Calcified cartilage

Articular surface

Tide mark

Subchondral bone

Cancellous bone

Figure 13.3 – *Zonal structure of articular cartilage.*

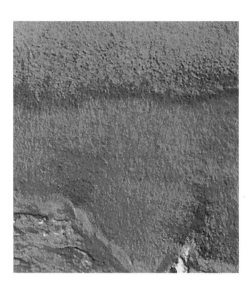

Figure 13.4 – *The tidemark (junction of non-calcified and calcified cartilage).*

matrix of the superficial zone. The chondrocytes in the *middle zone* are spheroidal in shape and tend to align themselves in columns perpendicular to the joint surface. This zone contains the largest-diameter collagen fibrils, the highest concentration of proteoglycans and the lowest concentration of water. A thin zone of *calcified cartilage* separates the middle zone (uncalcified cartilage) from the subchondral bone. The cells of the zone of calcified cartilage have a smaller volume than the cells of the radial zone. In some regions, these cells appear to be surrounded completely by calcified cartilage; they appear to be buried in individual 'calcific sepulchres', suggesting that the cells have an extremely low level of metabolic activity. However, recent work suggests that they may have a role in the development and progression of osteoarthrosis.

The collagen fibres pass into the *tidemark*, a thin basophilic line that roughly corresponds to the boundary between calcified and uncalcified cartilage. The nature of the tidemark remains uncertain. The collagen fibres of the cartilage are not anchored into the bone, but the cartilage tissue is keyed into the irregular surface of the bone, like a jigsaw puzzle (Fig. 13.4) [2,5–7].

Articular cartilage injury and repair

Mechanical injuries to articular cartilage occur when repetitive and prolonged joint overloading or sudden impact produces high compressive stress throughout the tissue and high shear stress at the subchondral bone

junction. These stresses cause injuries that can be separated into three distinct types: microdamage to the cells and matrix without visible disruption of the articular surface, macrodisruption of the articular cartilage alone (chondral fractures) and fracture of the articular cartilage and the subchondral bone (osteochondral fractures).

It is well known that the capacity of articular cartilage for repair is limited. Injuries of the articular cartilage that do not penetrate the subchondral bone do not heal and usually progress to degeneration of the articular surface; a short-lived tissue response has been observed, but it fails to provide sufficient cells and matrix to repair even small defects. Partial-thickness defects in articular cartilage do not heal spontaneously. The reasons for this phenomenon are not well understood. The most frequent hypothesis is that, because there are no blood vessels in mature articular cartilage, cells from perivascular mesenchymal pools cannot enter this area. The observations that are described in the report by Hunziker and Rosenberg [8] indicate that this is not the case. Partial-thickness defects do not need access to cells in marrow to undergo repair. Under appropriate conditions, mesenchymal cells can be induced to migrate from the synovial membrane across the articular surface into the defect, where they proliferate and fill its cavity.

As demonstrated in the report by Wakitani and associates [9], autologous, bone-marrow-derived, osteochondral progenitor cells can be isolated and grown *in vitro* without the loss of their capacity to differentiate into cartilage or bone. Osteochondral progenitor cells were used to repair large, full-thickness defects of the articular cartilage that had been created in the knees of rabbits. The periosteal and the bone-marrow-derived cells showed similar patterns of differentiation into articular cartilage and subchondral bone. Sufficient autologous cells can be generated to initiate the repair of articular cartilage and the reformation of subchondral bone. The repair tissues appear to undergo the same developmental transitions that originally led to the formation of articular tissue in the embryo. This approach to the repair of defects of the articular cartilage may have useful applications in the repair of large, full-thickness defects of joint surfaces.

It seems that foetal articular cartilage has an excellent potential to heal spontaneously. This has been demonstrated by Namba and associates [10] on a foetal lamb model which was developed to investigate the capacity of foetal articular cartilage for repair after the creation of a superficial defect. Superficial defects, 100 μm deep, were made in the articular cartilage of the trochlear groove in the distal aspect of the femur in 18 foetal lambs that were halfway through the 145-day gestational period; the contralateral limb was used as a sham control. The wounds were allowed to heal *in utero* for 3, 7, 14, 21, or 28 days. Seven days after the injury, the defects were filled with a hypocellular matrix, which stained lightly with safranin O. At 28 days, the staining of the matrix was similar to that of the sham controls and the chondrocyte density and the architectural arrangement of the cell layers had been restored. An inflammatory response was not elicited, and no fibrous scar tissue was observed. The clinical relevance of this study is very significant: an orderly sequence of repair of articular cartilage was observed after the creation of partial-thickness defects in the distal aspect of the femur of mid-gestational foetal lambs. The foetal lamb model may be useful for the investigation of interactions between the chondrocyte and extracellular matrices after mechanical stimulation. Fundamental knowledge of the metabolism of foetal articular cartilage may provide an insight into the latent reparative processes of mature cartilage.

Injuries that penetrate the subchondral bone undergo repair through the formation of tissues usually characterised as fibrous, fibrocartilaginous or hyaline-like cartilaginous, depending on the species, the age of the animal, and the location and size of the injury. However, these reparative tissues, even those that resemble hyaline cartilage histologically, differ from normal hyaline cartilage both biochemically and biomechanically, and by 6 months, fibrillation, fissuring and extensive degenerative changes occur in the reparative tissues of approximately half of the full-thickness defects. Similarly, the degenerated cartilage seen in osteoarthrosis does not usually undergo repair but progressively deteriorates.

A clinical role for motion in cartilage repair was described by DePalma and associates [11] who suggested that weight-bearing and motion could improve the healing of cartilage defects. In a major series of studies, Salter and associates [12] studied the influence of continuous passive motion (CPM) on cartilage healing. In studies of the formation of new cartilage from periosteal grafts, CPM was found to aid repair more than either immobilisation or normal cage activity. Numerous laboratory and clinical studies reported in the literature clearly show that immobilisation is detrimental to

cartilage development and repair. However, the major mechanical forces that influence cartilage repair remain unclear, nor is it clear what type and frequency of force provides optimal repair in different areas of the joint.

It seems that full thickness articular cartilage defects continue to progress and deteriorate, although at a slow rate. In a study, reported by Biswal *et al.* [13] at the Radiological Society of North America (RSNA) Annual Meeeting in 1998, 25 patients had undergone repeat magnetic resonance imaging (MRI) of the knee with a time interval between two studies of more than 1 year. Only three patients had completely normal cartilage on both baseline and follow-up studies. In another 22 patients, approximately 50% of focal areas of signal heterogeneity of the articular cartilage progressed to more advanced stage of cartilage pathology, over a 1- to 2-year period.

Chondral damage in ACL deficiency

Continuous multiplane instability and repetitive pivoting in chronic anterior cruciate ligament (ACL) deficient knees result in arthroscopically obvious superficial chondral damage. Additionally, chronic impingement of the tibial eminence on the femoral condyles seems to result in a shearing effect which gradually damages articular cartilage and menisci. There is a possible parallel in the mechanism of chondral injury in the ACL-deficient knee and aetiology of osteochondritis dissecans. Indirect trauma has been discussed extensively as a possible aetiological factor in the development of osteochondritis dissecans lesions of the knee. Fairbank [14] proposed that repetitive impingement of the tibial spine on the lateral aspect of the medial femoral condyle during internal rotation of the tibia is a causative factor in osteochondritis dissecans. This theory was later supported by Smillie [15], who thought that concomitant ligamentous laxity was an associated factor.

However, initial chondral damage is probably much more subtle. It probably starts as a bone bruise (bone marrow oedema) which is very often seen on the MRI in acute ACL injury and affects mainly the lateral femoral and tibial condyles. Spindler *et al.* [16] found an 80% incidence of a bone bruise in knees with acute ACL tears. A bone bruise, assuming that it involves a blunt injury to hyaline articular cartilage and subchondral bone, may be a predictor of future chondral degeneration, even in the absence of a visible articular cartilage injury. Johnson *et al.* [17] confirmed this clinical suspicion: arthroscopic inspection, biopsy and histological examination of articular cartilage and subchondral bone overlying lateral femoral condyle bone bruise, diagnosed previously with MRI, revealed substantial osteochondral damage. All 10 patients had significant cartilage irregularity and other findings including softening, fissuring or overt chondral fracture. Histological examination revealed degeneration of the chondrocytes, loss of proteoglycans, necrosis of osteocytes in the subchondral bone and empty lacunae. Speer *et al.* [18] examined 54 patients with acute complete ACL tears and found an interesting pattern in osseous injuries: the MRI findings revealed that 83% of the knees had an osseous injury (bone bruise) that was located directly over the lateral femoral condyle sulcus terminalis. The lesions varied from a faint increase in signal on T2-weighted images to a frank osteochondral fracture.

In his review of articular cartilage injuries, Mankin [19,20] states that changes consistent with osteoarthritis are likely to result from a single, superphysiological impaction or repeated lesser blows that exceed a critical threshold. Dye and Chew [21,22] reported increased osseous metabolic activity in 85% of patients with a chronically symptomatic tear of the ACL, often in the presence of normal osseous findings on radiographs and MRI scans.

The mechanism of injury involved in the majority of acute tears of the ACL is severe anterior subluxation of the tibia with impaction on the anterior aspect of the femur and the posterior aspect of the tibia. This finding is supported by the statistically significant relationship that exists between anterior lateral femoral condyle and the posterior lateral tibial plateau bone bruising with ACL tears. All of these studies indicate that blunt trauma to articular cartilage, even when clinically quiet and not readily visible on the MRI, may have profound effects on future cartilage metabolism.

Bobic [23] reported a very high incidence of chondral damage to femoral and tibial condyles. In a series of 369 patients who had undergone reconstruction for chronic ACL deficiency, 79% had some form of chondral damage, on Noyes [24] point scaling system for analysis of articular cartilage surfaces. In many chronic ACL-deficient knees, deep and long chondral fissures of medial and lateral tibial condyles were seen, mainly close to tibial eminences, but also close to intact menisci (Fig. 13.5).

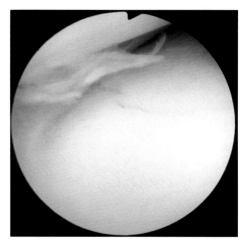

Figure 13.5 – *Arthroscopic view of tibial chondral fissure.*

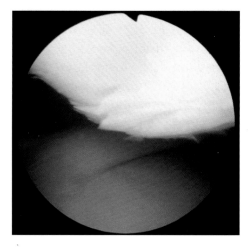

Figure 13.6 – *Arthroscopic view of filleted femoral articular cartilage, in ACL and meniscal deficient knee.*

A high incidence of 'filleted' articular cartilage of both femoral condyles was also seen frequently (Fig. 13.6). Chondral lesions are usually close to the lateral tibial intercondylar tubercle, or close to the junction of the middle and posterior thirds of the lateral meniscus, but usually without major meniscal tears. Fine *et al.* [25] have reported similar asymptomatic lesions immediately adjacent to the inner edge of the lateral meniscus. On arthroscopy, all patients with chronic ACL deficiency had numerous thin slivers and fragments of articular cartilage suspended in the synovial fluid, floating about the joint (Fig. 13.7). However, this has not been observed on arthroscopy of thousands of stable knees. In this cohort of patients with chronic ACL deficiency, 36% of patients had full-thickness femoral chondral defects with subchondral involvement.

In a patient with an injured ACL there is a close relationship between ligament injury (instability) and articular cartilage deterioration. In a study of ACL injuries, researchers have demonstrated a consistent

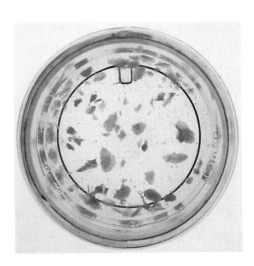

Figure 13.7 –
Chondral flakes (slivers) washed out from chronic ACL-deficient knee.

rapid elevation of the enzyme stromelysin and other cytokines that damage the articular cartilage. It seems that, apart from obvious negative mechanical effects of instability, an unstable joint environment unleashes a destructive biochemical process that may result in a progressive deterioration of its articular cartilage [26].

The reported incidence of articular cartilage injury associated with acute or chronic ACL deficiency varies from 20 to 46% [27–31]. The ACL-deficient knee is obviously exposed to chondral damage of variable severity, ranging from superficial damage and chondral fissures to large full-thickness chondral defects. A full-thickness chondral lesion, however small it may be, requires treatment, but at present we are unable to treat it quickly and appropriately. Fibrocartilage cover is an acceptable short-term solution to this problem; however, one should aim to repair a chondral defect on a more permanent basis. It is fairly obvious that, if neglected, chondral defects are likely to progress, resulting in early degeneration of the joint. Inevitably, this will devalue the long-term outcome of the ACL reconstruction.

The incidence and long-term effect of bone marrow oedema and chondral injury associated with acute ACL injury and chronic ACL deficiency remain unclear. However, one should not forget that sectioning of the ACL is used in animal studies of osteoarthritis to induce rapid joint degeneration, through accelerated articular cartilage wear. On the other hand, several recent studies have shown that a significant percentage of patients with ACL rupture will develop X-ray evidence and clinical symptoms of osteoarthritis, despite having the ligament reconstructed. Often no correlation exists between knee stability and the development of degenerative arthritis. However, the commonly held belief that a knee with a chronic ACL injury automatically develops cartilage wear and degeneration because of instability requires further thought: it seems that a bone bruise, trauma to articular cartilage and subsequent degeneration of both are important variables in the equation for risk of arthritis. Patients with subsequent ACL reconstruction and resulting stability may undergo a slow but inevitable degeneration of menisci and articular cartilage. In patients with persistent instability, this inevitable progression may simply accelerate.

Classification of chondral damage

Several major systems have been used to classify the extent of articular cartilage injury, on the basis of arthroscopic appearance. The Noyes [24] point scaling system for analysis of articular cartilage surfaces is based on four separate and distinct variables: the description of the articular surface, the extent (depth) of involvement, the diameter of the lesion and the location of the lesion. Although somewhat qualitative and subjective, a point scaling system facilitates computerisation and statistical analysis of the data. The Outerbridge classification system was developed for assessing chondromalacia patellae and is often used to classify articular cartilage injury elsewhere in the knee [32]. This system grades the progression of cartilage defects primarily according to their depth. Grade 0 represents normal articular cartilage. Grade I is softening and swelling of the cartilage. Grade II demonstrates early fissuring that does not reach the subchondral bone, nor does its size exceed 0.5 inch. With grade III, fissuring reaches the subchondral bone, which is not exposed, in an area with a diameter over 0.5 inch. In grade IV, the subchondral bone is exposed. In an alternative classification system, Bauer and Jackson classify lesions of the articular surface according to cartilage fracture patterns (type I: linear crack, type II: stellate fracture, type III: flap, type IV: crater, type V: fibrillation, type VI degrading).

However, most classification systems for analysis of articular cartilage surfaces are insufficient for contemporary clinical requirements and qualitative and quantitative evaluation of articular cartilage damage and repair. Giurea *et al.* [33], in a recent review article on classification of articular cartilage lesions, suggest separate systems for communication and research purpose [33].

In October 1997, the International Cartilage Repair Society (ICRS) was founded in Fribourg, Switzerland.

The new Society concluded that it is essential to establish an international cartilage evaluation system, which should be based on accurate anatomical locations, objective arthroscopic measurements and appropriate MRI protocols. The separate task group was set up to complete the Standard Cartilage Evaluation Form [34]. At the meeting, it was proposed to establish a consensus on classification of cartilage injuries and an evaluation system for cartilage repair. The proposed classification and documentation form is already available from the ICRS. Periodic updates will be published in the *ICRS Newsletter* and on the ICRS web site: www.cartilage.org.

The evaluation of damaged articular cartilage remains difficult and unreliable. The visual arthroscopic inspection and probing are currently widely used invasive options. Cartilage stiffness testing with indentation probes has become available as well. However, there is a need for non-invasive diagnosis and monitoring of progression of articular cartilage defects, and for the evaluation of repaired cartilage. This is already possible by using appropriate imaging methods, such as MRI.

Diagnosis of chondral defects

The articular cartilage defect should be diagnosed and treated early, before it becomes a large and deep osteochondral defect. The diagnosis of articular cartilage injury is difficult and unreliable. Clinical examination, standard X-ray and standard clinical MRI generally provide low sensitivity and moderate diagnostic accuracy.

Arthroscopic examination

In most clinical environments, arthroscopy is still the most helpful diagnostic tool in experienced hands. Careful visual arthroscopic inspection and probing of articular surfaces are essential. Large osteochondral defects can be covered with a thick layer of fibrocartilage, which may escape a surgeon's attention. This tissue is usually very soft and semidetached from subchondral bone, and does not have the glossy appearance of normal hyaline cartilage. Delaminated and semidetached chondral flaps also may become visible only when carefully probed. Articular cartilage damage should be described and recorded in an arthroscopic surgery report (fissures, chondral flaps, partial and full-thickness defects, etc.). A classification of chondral injuries should include assessment of the size, the depth, the location and the condition of the opposing articular surface. In

the measurement of the injury size the longest diameter and the longest perpendicular diameter in mm should be recorded. The location of the chondral lesion needs precise anatomical description. It is also important to describe other injuries (menisci, patella, ligaments) and axial angulation. Adequate documentation of arthroscopic findings is essential (videoprints, videorecording, digital images, etc.).

Articular cartilage softening is one of the first signs of the degenerative process. Softening precedes the macroscopic degeneration of the articular surface. The softening is proportional to the degree of superficial loss or redistribution of proteoglycans or collagens in the cartilage. Usually, softening is diagnosed subjectively by palpating the cartilage surface with an arthroscopic probe. A small arthroscopic indentation instrument (Fig. 13.8) has been developed and tested in clinical practice (ArtScan, Helsinki, Finland). The clinical measurements reveal a topographic variation of the stiffness of a normal knee joint (femoral articular cartilage is stiffer than in the tibia or patella). In patients with chondromalacia, patellar cartilage is demonstrably softer (33%) than normal cartilage. It is possible that this clinical instrument could be a valid method for evaluation of the articular cartilage damage and repair outcomes.

Magnetic resonance imaging

Although the MRI of cartilage has been extensively researched and used in clinical practice, there is considerable disagreement with regard to the MRI appearance of normal cartilage, the best technique for imaging cartilage abnormalities, and the accuracy of these techniques in the detection of abnormalities. A study published by Wojtys and associates [35] in 1987

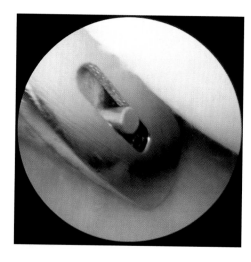

Figure 13.8 – *Articular cartilage stiffness tester (ArtScan).*

and a study published in 1994 by Ochi and associates [36], indicate that although the sensitivity to early changes of chondral lesions was low, confirming the limitation of MRI at that stage, it has been demonstrated that MRI can delineate intracartilaginous changes associated with softening and thickening of cartilage that cannot be detected even with arthroscopy.

Kneeland [37] states that cartilage has proven exceedingly difficult to evaluate accurately with MRI. A standard clinical MRI scan has low sensitivity in diagnosing isolated chondral delamination when compared with arthroscopic findings. Levy *et al.* [38] reported that preoperative MRI scans correctly identified only 21% of the chondral lesions seen at arthroscopic examination (five out of 23 knees in 15 high-calibre soccer players). Bone bruise, or bone marrow oedema, which is a frequent MRI diagnosis following acute knee injuries, is an indicator of severe injury to the articular cartilage. Although the chondral injury is not visible as such, bone bruise represents substantial subchondral changes following traumatic events, especially following ACL injury. Standard clinical MRI is still unable to diagnose superficial and delaminated articular cartilage injury, especially if clinical suspicion is low. However, with advanced MRI techniques, special articular cartilage scanning protocols, and increased awareness of chondral injury, MRI has begun to replace more conventional methods in evaluation of articular cartilage damage and repair [39–42].

Magnetic resonance imaging methods

Chondral injury such as fissures, erosions, fibrillation, and clefts, produce alteration in the morphology of the cartilage, which can be seen on MRI scans as surface irregularities and focal defects filled with joint fluid. Numerous studies have been performed in an attempt to identify the optimum technique for the detection of these cartilage abnormalities. The most commonly advocated MRI technique for showing articular cartilage is a *fat-suppressed three-dimensional T1-weighted gradient echo technique*. Reported sensitivities for the detection of chondral lesions range from 75% to 93%. However, this technique has several limitations: the long imaging time and inadequate visualisation of ligamentous and meniscal pathology, necessitating additional sequences. Gradient echo sequences are prone to magnetic susceptibility artefact, which is accentuated in the presence of orthopaedic instruments (including arthroscopic instruments), limiting evaluation of chondral defects and repaired cartilage following surgical intervention.

The Radiology Department of the University of California San Francisco, Stanford Healthcare, Stanford, California, is at the forefront of development of MRI techniques to minimise the effects of metallic artefacts in cartilage imaging. Two techniques have been developed: view-angle tilting and spectroscopic imaging, which allow imaging of cartilage at short echo times while offering immunity to metallic fragments left in the joint. This is especially important in cases such as multiple osteochondral autograft transplantation, which leaves considerable metallic artefacts.

Spectral-spatial three-dimensional magnetisation transfer was also developed at Stanford and provides high-resolution 3D imaging of the entire joint with excellent cartilage to bone and cartilage to fluid contrast. Use of the spectral-spatial pulse provides superior lipid suppression to other methods.

High-resolution short echo time spectroscopic imaging: short echo times are essential to visualise zonal areas of cartilage and are more sensitive for cartilage pathology. This method provides ultra-short echo time and high resolution images of cartilage over a small area, in addition to spectroscopic data. It is possible that this method can be used to distinguish between hyaline and fibrocartilage. This technique is also unique to Stanford and includes immunity to metallic artefacts and the ability to examine spectra from specific areas within the transplant (Fig. 13.9) [43].

Dynamic studies in the iMRI (MRT): interventional MRI systems with the double doughnut design allow upright imaging during static weight-bearing conditions and during weight-bearing motion studies. General Electric has installed these machines at 14 centres worldwide (Fig. 13.10). The site in the UK is at Imperial College School of Medicine at St Mary's Hospital in London.

Armstrong and Mow [3], in a review of the intrinsic mechanical properties of human articular cartilage, concluded that the visual or histological appearance of a cartilage specimen is a poor indicator of its function to bear weight in the intact joint. They stated that a biomechanical or biochemical analysis is a much more relevant determination. The iMRI may prove useful in a non-invasive biomechanical evaluation of repaired or transplanted articular cartilage.

Many new MRI sequences are currently available and are being developed, for imaging articular cartilage defects and repair. This requires a standardised protocol that provides guidelines for imaging of articular cartilage,

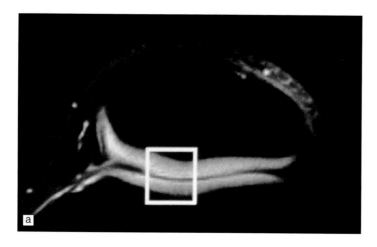

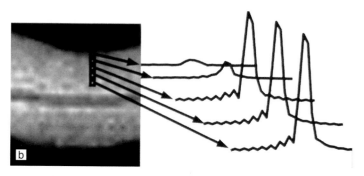

Figure 13.9 – *High-resolution ultra-short echo time spectroscopic imaging, showing fine detail of patellofemoral cartilage (MR image: Stanford University Medical Center, California, US).*

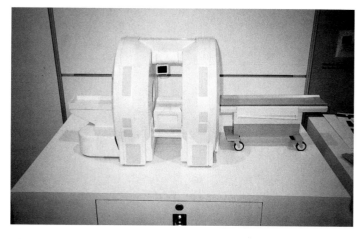

Figure 13.10 – *Interventional 'double-doughnut' MR (iMRI or MRT).*

using hardware and pulse sequence techniques which are available in most centres.

Whatever type of MRI is used, there are certain technical prerequisites for adequate articular cartilage imaging: a high field strength magnet is preferred, because of the superior signal-to-noise ratio (1.5 Tesla magnet is optimal), a circumferential dedicated knee coil is required in order to obtain adequate spatial resolution and signal-to-noise ratio. The recommended sequences for imaging articular cartilage, that are generally available, are a 2D fat-saturated proton density fast spin-echo sequence (FSE), and a 3D fat-suppressed spoiled gradient-echo sequence (SPGR).

In order to detect early pathology in osteoarthritis, new non-invasive methods need to be developed. Gadolinium (Gd-$DTPA^{2-}$) is a charged paramagnetic contrast compound. *In vitro* experiments and recent clinical trials have shown a relationship between Gd-$DTPA^{2-}$ uptake and cartilage proteoglycan content. It seems that articular cartilage changes, consistent with early osteoarthritis, can be non-invasively visualised by Gd-$DTPA^{2-}$ enhanced MRI [44].

Recent advances in MRI technology appear to be very promising. Magnetic resonance is already an effective method to diagnose chondral injury, to aid in the selection of therapeutic intervention and to assess the long-term follow-up of repaired articular cartilage. MRI has unique capabilities to evaluate cartilage non-invasively. It seems that second-look arthroscopy and cartilage biopsy may become obsolete fairly soon.

Key points

- The capacity of articular cartilage for repair is very limited.
- Partial-thickness defects in the articular cartilage do not heal spontaneously.
- Full-thickness defects that involve the subchondral bone undergo repair through the formation of fibrocartilage.
- Growth factors have profound effects on chondrocytes.
- The articular cartilage derives its mechanical properties from its matrix.
- Magnetic resonance imaging is a very useful tool in the evaluation of articular cartilage injury and repair.

CHAPTER 14

Current concepts of treatment of articular cartilage defects in the knee

V. Bobic

Repair versus regeneration

In selecting methods of restoring the damaged articular surface, it is important to distinguish articular cartilage repair from articular cartilage regeneration. *Repair* refers to the healing of injured tissues or replacement of lost tissues by cell proliferation and synthesis of new extracellular matrix. Unfortunately, repaired articular cartilage generally fails to replicate the structure, composition and function of normal articular cartilage. *Regeneration* in this context refers to the formation of an entirely new articulating surface that essentially duplicates the original articular cartilage [1]. Therefore, the best that can be done at present is to repair the chondral defect.

Treatment methods

Historically, there have been a number of attempts to develop clinically useful procedures to repair damaged articular cartilage, but these have not yet proved successful. Treatment options are limited and the long-term outcome is still uncertain. This chapter is an overview of currently available treatment options.

Considerable efforts have been made to address this problem, mainly based on the treatment of chondromalacia patellae and osteochondritis dissecans [2–6]. Table 14.1 shows the range of methods that have been tried.

No treatment

It is generally assumed that untreated focal defects in articular cartilage lead to symptomatic progressive arthrosis. This is probably a correct assumption, but the

Table 14.1 – Range of attempts to repair damaged articular cartilage [7]

- Abrasion arthroplasty
- Allograft and autograft osteochondral transplantation
- Autogenous bone grafting
- Carbon fibre resurfacing
- Debridement and curettage
- Implantation of autologous cultured chondrocytes
- Induction of cartilage repair with growth hormones
- Lavage
- Microfracture
- Perichondrial transplantation
- Periosteal transplantation
- Refixation of chondral fragments
- Subchondral drilling
- Supervised neglect

number of patients who live normal lives with no knee symptoms and without significant functional problems is unknown. Some reports document good outcomes in most patients as long as 14 years after diagnosis of severe chondral damage of the knee.

Chondroprotective agents

Expanding knowledge regarding cartilage biochemistry and the pathogenesis of osteoarthritis (OA) has focused research on slowing the progression of OA and promoting cartilage matrix synthesis. This research has identified substances, termed chondroprotective agents, which counter arthritic degenerative processes and encourage normalisation of the synovial fluid and cartilage matrix. Chondroprotective agents are compounds that stimulate chondrocyte synthesis of collagen and proteoglycans, as well as synoviocyte production of hyaloronan, inhibit cartilage degradation and prevent fibrin formation in the subchondral and synovial vasculature. Examples of compounds that exhibit some of these characteristics are the endogenous molecules of the articular cartilage, including hyaluronic acid, chondroitin sulphate and glucosamine.

Hyaluronic acid

Intra-articular injections of hyaluronic acid (HA) are widely used in the Asian and European orthopaedic communities for controlling the pain and loss of joint function resulting from osteoarthritis. In more than 10 years, it has been used in approximately 1 million patients in 20 countries. The substance is hyaluronate, a naturally occurring viscoelastic agent that supposedly acts as a shock absorber and lubricant in the knee joint. Preliminary results of animal studies demonstrate that intra-articular injection of hyaluronic acid may have protective effects on the articular cartilage. It is indicated for osteoarthritic pain of the knee in patients who have failed to respond adequately to non-operative treatment and other pain medication. Studies of the injectable viscosupplement include a 26-week, double-blind, multi-centre trial carried out in the US of 495 patients with knee pain due to OA. HA is well tolerated with no demonstrable toxicity and few side effects. Because it is injected directly into the joint, the onset of action is rapid. Possible mechanisms by which HA may act therapeutically include: providing additional lubrication of the synovial membrane and controlling permeability of the synovial membrane, thereby controlling effusions and directly blocking inflammation by scavenging free radicals. However, the exact mechanisms of action, articular cartilage changes and short- and long-term results remain unknown [8].

Glucosamine and chondroitin sulphate

In contrast to HA, numerous *in vitro* studies have demonstrated that glucosamine stimulates the synthesis of proteoglycans and collagen by chondrocytes. Since OA results when cartilage breakdown exceeds the synthetic capacity of chrondrocytes, providing exogenous glucosamine increases matrix production and seems likely to alter the natural history of OA. Glucosamine also has a mild anti-inflammatory activity that is unrelated to prostaglandin metabolism. In randomised, double-blind, placebo-controlled clinical trials using oral preparations, glucosamine salts have been verified as efficacious in the management of OA, and have not demonstrated any toxicity, severe side effects, or abnormal clinical, biochemical or haematological changes. Chondroitin sulphate is the most abundant glycosaminoglycan in articular cartilage. It plays an important structural role in articular cartilage, notably for its role in binding with collagen fibrils. As a chondroprotective agent, it also has a metabolic effect: its action is to inhibit competitively many of the degradative enzymes that break down the cartilage matrix and synovial fluid in OA. Because its additional mechanism of action is via the prevention of fibrin thrombi in synovial or subchondral microvasculature, chondroitin sulphate has been investigated for its anti-atherosclerotic effect.

When used together, it seems that glucosamine and chondroitin sulphate combine effects to stimulate the metabolism of chondrocytes and synoviocytes, inhibit degradative enzymes, and reduce fibrin thrombi in peri-articular microvasculature. Numerous clinical studies performed on horses at US veterinary schools have supported this combination and synergistic effect. Randomised, double-blind clinical trials in humans are currently under way [9].

Arthroscopic lavage and debridement

Lavage is one of the most basic of traditional arthroscopic techniques. Dr Robert Jackson, the pioneer of arthroscopy in North America, observed that in the course of performing diagnostic arthroscopies, patients with intra-articular knee problems had significant pain relief following joint lavage. Exactly how arthroscopic lavage and debridement may help the early symptoms of OA is still not entirely clear. Joint lavage removes loose intra-articular tissue debris and inflammatory mediators known to be generated by the synovial lining. In the early stages, removing these degradative enzymes from the joint may allow chondrocytes to increase their biosynthetic activity. Another mechanism by which lavage may relieve the symptoms and increase the resilience and stiffness of articular cartilage is through changing the ionic environment within the synovial fluid. In Jackson's study, lavage resulted in symptomatic improvement at 3.5 years in 45% of the patients. When mechanical debridement is added to lavage, results seem to be somewhat better. In a follow-up study, 88% of the patients experienced improvement, and 68% had continued improvement at 3 years. Lavage may provide pain relief in some patients with advanced degenerative disease of the knee, which may last as long as 3 years. However, lavage provides only short-term symptomatic relief without correction of underlying pathology. If predisposing malalignment is not corrected, the beneficial effects seem to be minimised. The outcome of this simple procedure is generally insufficient for an active young population.

Bone marrow-stimulating techniques

Many clinicians have attempted to repair damaged articular cartilage with the mesenchymal stem cell stimulation techniques: Magnusson in 1946, Smith-Peterson in 1948, Pridie in 1959, Insall in 1974, Ficat in 1979, Sprague in 1981, Ogilvie-Harris and Jackson in 1984, Schonholtz and Ling in 1985, Johnson in 1986, Rae and Noble in 1989 and Rodrigo *et al.* in 1994. These techniques include abrasion arthroplasty, subchondral drilling and microfracture. These treatments involve disruption of subchondral bone in an attempt to induce fibrin clot formation and to initiate primitive stem cell migration from the bone marrow into the cartilage defect site. These techniques utilise primitive stem cells, which are capable of differentiating into bone and cartilage under the influence of various biological and mechanical intra-articular factors. The subchondral bone is penetrated in order to reach a zone of vascularisation, stimulating the formation of a fibrin clot containing pluripotential stem cells. This clot differentiates and remodels, resulting in fibrocartilaginous repair tissue. Although fibrocartilage often appears to offer the patient significant pain relief, this tissue lacks several key structural components to perform the mechanical functions, as a wear-resistant and weight-bearing surface. The fibrocartilage repair tissue does not produce adequate compressive stiffness against the applied mechanical load and thus is subjected to excessive deformation under physiological loading. This is turn causes mechanical failure of the repaired tissue and eventually leads to a recurrence of degeneration of the repaired cartilage. The appropriate histological, biochemical and biomechanical studies are warranted, as the long-term efficacy of these treatments remains unpredictable and controversial.

Subchondral drilling

The concept of drilling through eburnated bone to stimulate reparative cartilage formation was originally described by Pridie in 1959. Arthroscopic drilling with a thin K wire or a drill is aimed at repairing cartilage through formation of fibrocartilaginous tissue. The area of the defect is drilled through the subchondral bone in pinpoint fashion, resulting in fibrin clot formation. The repair tissue filling drill holes has been shown to include fibrocartilage and some hyaline cartilage. However, animal studies have shown that the reparative tissue loses its hyaline appearance after 8 months, and at 1 year resembles dense collagenous tissue with apparent surface fibrillation. In one study, a group of patients who underwent subchondral drilling and high tibial valgus osteotomy showed superior results to those receiving osteotomy alone. This further illustrates the importance of unloading damaged or repaired articular cartilage.

Microfracture

Dr Richard Steadman, from Vail, Colorado, has developed a procedure referred to as the 'microfracture' [10]. Once the full-thickness chondral lesion is identified, the exposed bone is debrided of loose articular cartilage. Steadman believes, on the basis of laboratory research, that the removal of the calcified layer is extremely important. Damage to the subchondral bone should be avoided. An arthroscopic awl is used to make multiple holes (microfracture) in the exposed subchondral bone (Fig. 14.1). The holes should be approximately 3–4 mm apart, and the depth should be about 4 mm. The goal is for a blood clot rich in pluripotential marrow elements (mesenchymal stem cells) to form and to stabilise while covering the lesion. The microfracture technique produces a rough surface in the lesion to which the blood clot can adhere more

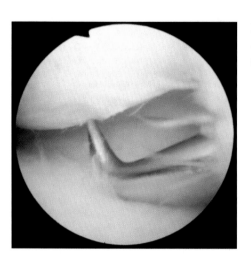

Figure 14.1 – *Microfracture with arthroscopic awl.*

easily, yet the integrity of the subchondral bone is maintained for joint surface shape. The advantage of microfracture over drilling is that the arthroscopic awls produce much less thermal necrosis. Histologically, the microfracture regenerated tissue appears to be a hybrid of hyaline cartilage and fibrocartilage, with viable chondrocytes in lacunae with a uniform matrix. Most rehabilitation protocols call for some form of protective weight-bearing and continuous passive motion. In addition, it is believed that significant predisposing factors such as malalignment or obesity need to be corrected to obtain better results. This allows redistribution of load and protects the fragile fibrocartilage. Follow-up studies of this procedure with postoperative continuous passive motion have reported significant improvement at second-look arthroscopy [10]. However, it appears that initial good results deteriorate over time because of the poor wear characteristics of the repair tissue.

Abrasion arthroplasty

Abrasion arthroplasty of full-thickness articular cartilage defects with motorised instruments was introduced by Johnson in 1981 [11]. This technique is essentially an extension of the Pridie procedure with the exception that a superficial layer of subchondral bone approximately 1–3 mm thick is removed to expose intraosseous vessels. There has been disagreement as to the depth of drilling and whether debridement of the sclerotic lesion should be intracortical or cancellous. This technique also involves debriding the articular defect to a normal tissue edge. The repair tissue formed in the fibrin clot can make a connection with the normal articular cartilage.

Theoretically, the resulting haemorrhage exudate forms a fibrin clot and allows for the formation of fibrous repair tissue over the exposed bone. This immature repair tissue should be protected from excessive loading after the procedure for a minimum of 6–8 weeks. At second-look arthroscopy and biopsy, Johnson *et al.* showed that the cartilage defect was filled with fibrocartilage and that the reparative fibrocartilage maintained its integrity with the host hyaline cartilage up to 6 years [11]. However, some authors believe that abrasion arthroplasty and the Pridie procedure do not appear to offer any benefit in the treatment of degenerative arthritis of the knee [12].

Combined abrasion arthroplasty and high tibial osteotomy

Effective methods of repairing articular cartilage must provide a mechanical and biological environment that promotes synthesis and maintenance of articular cartilage matrix. The value of abrasion arthroplasty combined with high tibial osteotomy (HTO) is minimal. Akizuki *et al.* reported on the results of this combined procedure and concluded that the postoperative improvement, at 2–9 years, was totally unrelated to the abrasion arthroplasty [13]. There was no significant long-term improvement. Although the abrasion arthroplasty promotes limited repair and some improvement of the eburnated surfaces within 1 year, the composition and mechanical quality of this repair tissue is inferior. The clinical outcome depends largely on the redistribution of compartmental load and mechanical improvement. It seems that realignment on its own results in short-term improvement, while abrasion arthroplasty does not contribute at all [13].

Perichondrial transplantation

Animal studies showed that neochondrogenesis of hyaline cartilage is also possible using autologous perichondrial grafts sutured or glued with the cambium layer facing the joint. It has already been demonstrated that perichondrium taken from the cartilaginous covering of a rib could be placed in a joint, where it would develop into hyaline cartilage. Homminga and co-workers performed the first clinical study of perichondrial grafting on 25 patients with symptomatic chondral lesions. One year after surgery, 18 of the 25 patients were completely symptom-free and had resumed previous occupational and athletic activities. However, at 5–7 years postoperatively, 60% of the patients had graft failure (20 of the 30 grafts in this series developed enchondral ossification), with pain and graft degeneration [14].

Periosteal transplantation

This technique involves excavating the pathological tissue from osteochondral defect, leaving only acceptable cartilage and subchondral bone. It is important that this is done right down into the subchondral bone, because the recipient area must be deep for the technique to work. A periosteal graft, harvested from the proximal tibia, is then sutured into the defect in an inverted position, with the cambium layer facing up. The sutures are tied through drill holes in the sides of the femur or into the intercondylar notch. In a follow-up survey of 15 patients, O'Driscoll [15] reported that nine were satisfactory. The six unsatisfactory results were clear-cut failures. In reviewing his 10-year experience O'Driscoll found that his early results may have been better than his later results. Periosteal transplantation is not yet ready for general clinical application for articular cartilage repair [16,17].

Autologous chondrocyte implantation (ACI)

The idea of using autologous chondrocytes as a source of matrix-generating cells is very exciting scientifically. However, this approach has many problems: a source of chondrocytes, maintaining their phenotype, and providing an appropriate three-dimensional matrix. Early attempts using chondrocyte grafts resulted in the formation of fibrocartilage, or cartilage surrounded by fibrous tissue, and the potential of cultured chondrocytes to form repair cartilage was considered to be limited [18–20]. Lindahl *et al.* presented results of an autologous chondrocyte implantation study at the meeting of the Swedish Medical Society in 1986, demonstrating the effectiveness of autologous chondrocytes versus control defects with periosteum alone in rabbits. However, the first published report of successful repair of articular cartilage using a chondrocyte matrix prepared *in vitro* was by Itay *et al.* [21]. Grande *et al.* [22] also reported successful repair in a rabbit model in which cultured chondrocytes were

placed into defects and a periosteal flap was used to retain the gel in the lesion. Based on the successful results obtained from this and other animal studies, Brittberg and co-workers [23] in Sweden decided to attempt the same technique in patients with cartilage defects in the knee. Two years postoperatively, 14 of 16 patients with femoral condylar transplants had good to excellent results. The two patients with poor results suffered severe central wear in their grafts, 11 and 14 months after the procedure. Eleven of the 15 biopsy specimens revealed an intact articular cartilage with a hyaline appearance. Further histological and immunohistochemical findings indicated that near-normal hyaline cartilage had 'regenerated' in the defect. This initial series of 23 patients yielded highly promising results. The technique of autologous chondrocyte implantation (ACI) has received a great deal of attention in the press and in the scientific literature, since its publication [23]. This article generated enormous pressure on the international orthopaedic community and has led the public and the media to believe that it is already possible to reconstruct almost any part of the body. Since the publication of this article, a further 251 patients have been treated with ACI, as reported by Peterson and co-workers in 1996, at the annual meeting of the American Academy of Orthopaedic Surgeons (AAOS). More than 80% of patients have noted improvement after 2 years of follow-up. So far, over 2000 patients have been treated with the ACI.

ACI surgical technique

Cultured chondrocytes that are harvested from the patient are reimplanted after 3–4 weeks of culturing. At implantation, the osteochondral defect is debrided of all fibrous tissue, and a periosteal flap is sewn to the edge of normal articular cartilage. The cultured chondrocytes are then placed underneath the periosteal flap, and the flap is sealed (Fig. 14.2). It is important that the cambium layer of the periosteum is facing the joint, as it may serve as a source of growth factors or cells for the new matrix. The cultured chondrocytes begin to produce an extracellular matrix that closely resembles hyaline cartilage. Histological biopsies, however, reveal that there is still some disorganisation of the chondrocytes and collagen matrix. Therefore, the repaired tissue only can be called hyaline-like articular cartilage [24]. A number of questions need to be answered, for example: (1) Does initial overpopulation

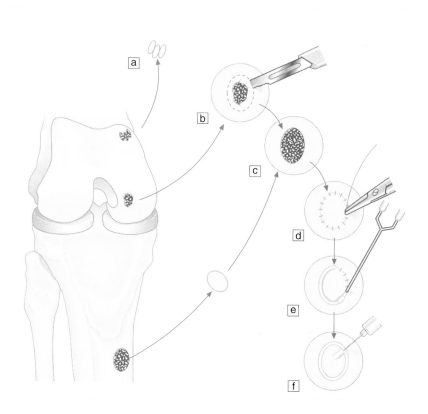

Figure 14.2 – *Autologous chondrocyte implantation. (a) Healthy cartilage previously harvested for tissue culture. (b) Chondral defect debrided to edge of normal articular cartilage. (c) Defect site prepared for patch and cells. (d) Periosteal patch sutured in place. (e) Patch sealed with fibrin glue (optional). (f) Cultured chondrocytes injected underneath periosteal patch. (ACI, Carticel.)*

of 100% chondrocytes cause death of a large number of cells, because chondrocytes are used to a low cellular environment? (2) What is the ratio of chondrocytes to extracellular matrix after 1 or 2 years after implantation (normal ratio is 1:9)? (3) Does 'regenerated' tissue restore congruency of the articulating surface? (4) What are the biomechanical properties of this surface? (5) What happens with the interface of transplanted chondrocyte mass to subchondral bone, in terms of reproduction of the tidemark?

The results of the original experiment in rabbits could not be reproduced in the canine model. The circular femoral trochlear chondral defects were treated with autologous cultured chondrocytes with periosteal flap, periosteal flap only or nothing, and analysed 12 or 18 months after healing. Authors could not detect significant differences among the three groups with regard to any of the parameters used to assess the quality of the repair; the autologous chondrocytes had no effect on the healing of defects in the distal part of the canine femur and suturing a periosteal flap to the defect was detrimental to the adjacent cartilage. The reasons remain unclear and the long-term efficacy of this treatment is unknown at present.

One of the concerns about ACI is the expense. Interestingly, research laboratories in the US, UK and several European countries grow the chondrocytes at a fraction of the charges billed by commercial enterprises. In addition, it has not been shown that the outcome of this technique is any better than that of patients who are treated with other techniques, including the fibrocartilage-generating bone marrow stimulating technique and osteochondral autograft or allograft transplantation.

The main concern with this excellent scientific idea is that the clinical application may be ahead of its time. In 1996 the AAOS issued an advisory statement to orthopaedic surgeons to exercise caution with their patients in the use of cell and tissue engineered products and similar emerging technologies. In 1998 *The Wall Street Journal* published an article on chondrocyte transplantation with a comment that: 'this was marketed before a lot of the science and clinical studies were done'. The editorial published in the *Journal of Bone and Joint Surgery*, in October 1998 [25], reinforces the public concern about this and other recent scientific publications: 'Hasty publications in prominent medical journals appear to provide the data used by doctors to recommend treatment .... Hasty publications can scare the public, generate enormous cost for the health-care system, and produce unwanted repercussions affecting all segments of society.'

Transforming growth factors

The dilemma in the ability to restore articular surfaces appears to lie with the chondrocytes. The chondrocytes are the metabolic power plants that produce the extracellular matrix. Once chondrocytes mature or differentiate, their capacity to reproduce slows down, but they continue with their metabolic activities, embedded in lacunae within the extracellular matrix they are producing. Although isolated, the chondrocytes can respond to growth factors, cytokines and exogenous mechanical stimuli. Changes in those chondrocyte stimulators have been shown to have a profound effect on the degeneration and synthesis of articular cartilage.

Transforming growth factors have been shown to affect chondrocyte metabolism and chondrogenesis. The bone matrix contains a variety of these molecules, including transforming growth factor-beta (TGF-β), insulin-like growth factors, bone morphogenetic proteins and platelet-derived growth factors. In addition, mesenchymal cells, endothelial cells and platelets produce many of these factors. Thus, osteochondral injuries and exposure of bone due to loss of articular cartilage may release these agents that affect the formation of cartilage repair tissue, and they probably have an important role in the formation of new articular surfaces after currently used operative procedures, including abrasion arthroplasty, microfracture, periosteal grafting and possibly osteotomy. Local treatment of chondral or osteochondral defects with growth factors has the potential to stimulate the restoration of an articular surface that is superior to that formed after the penetration of subchondral bone alone, especially in joints with normal alignment and a normal range of motion and with limited regions of cartilage damage. A recent experimental study of the treatment of partial-thickness cartilage defects with enzymatic digestion of proteoglycans that inhibit adhesion of cells to articular cartilage, followed by implantation of a fibrin matrix and timed release of TGF-β, showed that this growth factor can stimulate cartilage repair. The cells that filled the chondral defects migrated into the defects from the synovial tissue and formed a fibrous matrix [26]. Despite the promise of this approach, the wide variety of growth factors, their multiple effects, their interactions, the possibility that the responsiveness of cells to growth factors may decline with age and the limited understanding of their effects in osteoarthritic joints make it difficult to develop a simple strategy for the use of these agents to manage patients who have osteoarthrosis. However, the development of growth-factor-based treatment for younger patients who have an isolated chondral or osteochondral defect and early degenerative changes of cartilage appears promising.

Growth factors are likely to revolutionise the treatment of articular cartilage defects. These substances will take the field of orthopaedics into the 21st century, going beyond reactive treatment to the replacement and regeneration of osteochondral defects and pre-emptive treatment of small chondral defects. There is no doubt that this is the future of orthopaedic surgery; it has already started.

Artificial matrices

The treatment of chondral defects with growth factors or cell transplants requires a method of delivering and stabilising the growth factors or cells in the defect. In addition, an artificial matrix may allow and, in some instances, stimulate ingrowth of host cells, matrix formation and binding of new cells and matrix to host tissue. Researchers have found that implants formed from a variety of biological and non-biological materials, including treated cartilage and bone matrices, collagens, collagens and hyaluronan, fibrin, carbon fibre, hydroxyapatite, porous polylactic acid, polytetra-fluoroethylene, polyester and other synthetic polymers, facilitate the restoration of an articular surface. A lack of data makes it difficult to compare the relative merits of different types of artificial matrices and to evaluate the possibility that some implanted materials may cause synovitis; however, the available evidence indicates that at least some types of artificial matrices can carry out the function of an articular surface. In animal experiments, fibrous polyglycolic acid, collagen gels and fibrin have proved to be effective matrices for the implantation of cells, and fibrin has been used to implant and allow timed release of a growth factor. The treatment of osteochondral defects with use of carbon-fibre pads in rats and rabbits resulted in the restoration of a smooth articular surface consisting of firm fibrous tissue that filled the pads. Muckle and Minns [27] used the same approach to treat osteochondral defects of the knee in humans. Satisfactory results were obtained in 77% of 47 patients who were evaluated clinically and arthro-scopically 3 years after the operation. Minns recently reported that the matrix support material is safe, with no evidence of mutagenicity, toxicity or carcinogenicity in over 5000 implants up to 17 years of use. Overall pain relief and functional clinical scores suggest 70–80% excellent or good results after at least 5 years of implantation from 10 studies of implantation in over 1500 joints. Carbon fibre pads and rods appear to work best on the femoral condyle and the femoral trochlea. Brittberg and associates [28] also studied the use of carbon-fibre pads for the treatment of articular surface defects: they noted a good or excellent result in 83% of 36 patients at an average of 4 years.

New developments in this field include multiple hexagonal absorbable carriers which develop into a firm articulating surface when invaded by pluripotent cells and chondrocytes. It may also be possible to use a combination of inert permanent or resorbable carriers and TGF enhanced autologous chondrocytes.

Coblation in articular cartilage repair

This technique is based on a process of energy-mediated, low-temperature tissue removal and it is known as *coblation*, because of its cool ablative properties. A recently published preliminary report on the use of coblation in articular cartilage surgery demonstrates that this technique is suitable for partial-thickness chondral defects with unstable borders where the primary goal is stabilisation, and for types II and III chondromalacia for cleanly removing loose articular fragments. This approach could also be useful in chondral grafting procedures to stabilise the articular cartilage in the area around the chondral plug, and to prevent synovial penetration. The University of Miami Medical Center now has a series of 130 patients who have undergone coblation-based articular surgery for whom long-term follow-up is available. Initial clinical and magnetic resonance imaging (MRI) observations, with articular cartilage scanning protocol, seem to be encouraging [29]. However, more research is needed to define optimal parameters for the use of this technology. It remains unclear whether this method causes transient or long-term superficial and deep thermal chondral damage.

Allograft transplantation

In 1908, Lexer reported the first series of fresh osteochondral transplants into human joints, and he stated that the function of the joint was good in each patient after incorporation of the allograft. However, Burkle-de la Camp, who studied the histological

characteristics of two of Lexer's osteochondral grafts 14 and 16 years after transplantation, found that the articular cartilage had been completely replaced by fibrous tissue.

However, contemporary rationale for fresh osteochondral allografts is clinical and experimental evidence of maintenance of viability and function of chondrocytes after fresh transplantation (95% at 5 years, 77% at 10 years and 66% at 20 years). There is also histological evidence that the bony part of these grafts can be replaced by host bone in a uniform fashion in 2–3 years. The survivorship is very encouraging, as shown by Allan Gross in numerous articles. Garrett [30] produced excellent results for patients treated for traumatic defects and osteochondritis dissecans, which may be the best indication for allograft transplantation.

Fresh osteochondral shell allografting for localised defects in articular cartilage is a relatively new procedure. It is indicated in young patients in whom previous more conservative procedures have failed and for whom arthroplasty and arthrodesis are not indicated. A success rate of approximately 75% at 2–5 years postoperatively and survival for as long as 14 years have been reported.

According to the criteria of the American Association of Tissue Banks, all grafts must be procured within 24 hours of the donor's death. It seems that the storage time (the time between procurement and surgery) can be extended to a maximum of 7 days at 4°C. Also, donors should be under 30 years of age to ensure that the grafts have healthy cartilage and strong bone [31].

Paste grafting: combined autologous chondral and cancellous bone grafting

Dr Kevin Stone, from San Francisco, California, has developed a technique to harvest a mixture of articular cartilage and cancellous bone. The idea is that the pluripotent cells found in cancellous bone, combined with the presence of the extracellular matrix found in the articular cartilage, and the growth factors found in the associated blood clot, would be significant to stimulate the regeneration of hyaline-like cartilage if treated with continuous passive motion and non-weight-bearing. Additionally, the author had noted that the intercondylar notch regenerated hyaline-like cartilage, after notchplasty was performed during anterior cruciate ligament (ACL) reconstruction. Since 1992 this technique has been used on 60 patients. Gross healing occurred in all but two lesions examined by second-look arthroscopy. The surgical appearance of the lesions has been generally smooth with colour varying from greyish translucent to normal white. Immature, hyaline-like cartilage was seen in four of 10 biopsies available for review. The mixture of hyaline and fibrocartilage was seen in five biopsies. Collagen typing showed a mixture of type I and II collagen. The tissue formed has durable characteristics over 6.5 years follow-up [32]. Because the biopsy data are limited, and because biomechanical analysis is not available, one can only speculate about the quality and durability of the repair tissue in the long term. However, it seems that this procedure offers pain relief and the possibility of limited articular cartilage repair in patients with painful osteochondral lesions.

Osteochondral autograft transplantation (OAT)

The recorded history of autologous osteochondral grafting for the repair of osteochondral defects dates back to early 1990. Several groups have published clinically significant work: Wilson and Jacobs [33] in 1952, Müller [34] in 1978, and Yamashita *et al.* [35] in 1985, published results of the transplantation of autogenic osteochondral grafts, with the successful outcome and survivorship of the hyaline cartilage, from

6 months to over 10 years [36,37]. A similar clinical study, on treating osteochondritis dissecans lesions with osteochondral autografts, was reported at the annual AOSSM (American Orthopaedic Society for Sports Medicine) conference, by Fabbriciani and associates [38] in 1991. In 1993, Matsusue and associates [39] published the first case report and the technique of arthroscopic osteochondral autograft transplantation in an ACL deficient knee.

In 1995 Outerbridge *et al.* [40] published long-term outcome of treating osteochondral defects of the femoral condyle with patellar block osteochondral grafts in 10 patients and found that the function of the knee improved and symptoms were alleviated in all patients at an average of 6.5 years after transplantation. Hyaline cartilage survived up to 9 years.

Open and arthroscopic MosaicPlasty technique, using small multiple autologous osteochondral grafts (Fig. 14.3) was reported by Hangody *et al.* [41–43] in 1996 and 1997. The extensive clinical experience on over 600 procedures and the longest follow-up of 6 years clearly demonstrate survival of transplanted hyaline cartilage. The biopsy at 4.5 years showed that retrieved specimens were composed of 70–80% hyaline cartilage. Biopsies also demonstrated normal appearing chondrocytes, high glucosamine glycan (GAG) content, normal orientation of chondrocytes and matrix elements, and matrix integration between the hyaline and the fibrocartilage

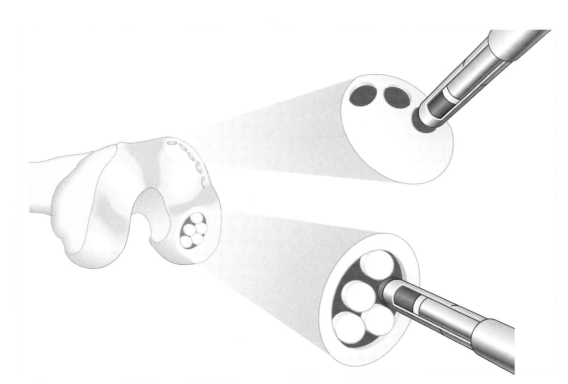

Figure 14.3 – *MosaicPlasty (Smith & Nephew, Acufex).*

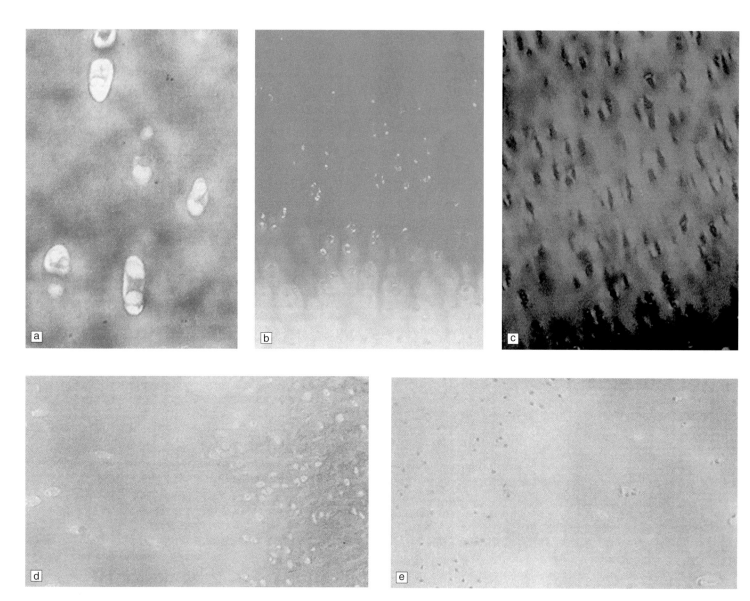

Figure 14.4 – *Histological analysis of MosaicPlasty (osteochondral autologous graft over 4 years after transplantation). (Courtesy of Dr L. Hangody.)*

(Fig. 14.4). The MosaicPlasty technique has been used for the repair of focal osteochondral lesions of the talar dome. All donor grafts were harvested from the ipsilateral knee.

In 1996 Bobic [44] published the first series of 12 patients undergoing ACL reconstruction with patellar tendon graft, using arthroscopic technique, modified tubular instruments and multiple osteochondral cylinders harvested from the notchplasty area. Second-look arthroscopy at 2 years clearly demonstrated a normal shiny appearance and colour of the grafted area, and a thin shallow halo at the interface of the recipient and grafted articular hyaline cartilage in each case. On close inspection all grafted areas appear slightly more prominent than the surrounding area, which is due to the different curve radius of the donor site. Transplanted grafts appeared satisfactory in 10 patients. In two cases multiple concentric grafts were either too prominent or sunk-in, due to inadequate surgical technique and instruments. Two randomly selected cases were biopsied 2 years postoperatively. A 2 mm core specimen, obtained from the transplanted area, showed no signs of histological degeneration and was composed of hyaline cartilage. The border between the transplanted and recipient articular cartilage was made of fibrocartilage. The donor site on the anterolateral aspect of distal femur was difficult to identify arthroscopically, being covered with fibrous tissue.

Indications for osteochondral autograft transplantation (OAT)

The concept that small lesions are insignificant is not supported in the study of 23 isolated chondral defects in 15 high-calibre soccer players: 33% of the lesions were less than 10 mm in diameter, but all players had knee pain. Pain probably occurs because of the stimulation of nerve endings of the subchondral bone, which is caused by the compromised load-transmitting and energy-absorbing capabilities [45].

The 'ideal' chondral lesion is a relatively small, 10–20 mm in diameter, full-thickness chondral defect. Quite frequently this type of the lesion will be present in the weight-bearing area of medial femoral condyle, in an ACL-deficient knee. Although it may be easier to microfracture or drill this lesion, this will produce fibrocartilage or hyaline-like cartilage cover (Fig. 14.5).

Osteochondral autograft transplantation can repair the defect with autologous hyaline cartilage, which will survive and restore the height and the shape of the defect. The main reason for the long-term survival of transplanted hyaline cartilage seems to be the preservation of an intact tidemark and cancellous bone carrier. The bone base of the transplant acts as an anchor, within its own environment, and enables secure fixation and integration with surrounding bone. It seems that this procedure does not disturb the main nutritional pattern of the articular cartilage.

Deep and large osteochondral defects are not suitable for osteochondral autograft transplantation, mainly because of the limited availability of autologous osteochondral grafts. Also, it is difficult to reconstruct subchondral bone and restore the contour of the defect

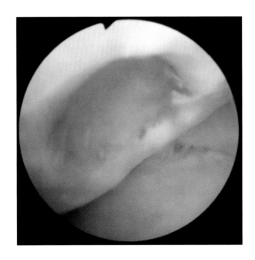

Figure 14.6 – *Large, crater-like osteochondral defect (Dr V. Bobic).*

area, and to cover the entire defect area with hyaline articular cartilage (Fig. 14.6).

Osteochondral autograft transfer system (OATS)

A set of purpose-designed tubular osteochondral harvesters was released commercially in February 1996 (OATS, Arthrex Inc., US). The instruments were developed by Vladimir Bobic, MD, Liverpool, UK, and Reinhold Schmieding, CEO Arthrex, and improved through clinical use by Craig Morgan, MD, Wilmington, Delaware, and Steven Burkhard, MD, San Antonio, Texas. The following paragraphs will describe the OAT System (OATS) surgical technique and clinical experience in detail. This arthroscopic technique is still evolving, as there is a considerable learning curve.

OATS surgical technique: step-by-step guide

Step 1: selection of donor site

The potential donor sites lie in an area along the outer edge of the lateral femoral condyle, above the *sulcus terminalis*. This area is exposed to significantly less contact pressure than other areas commonly recommended by various authors [46]. This area has a convex articular surface similar to that of the central weight-bearing areas of both femoral condyles. When inspected during a large number of total knee replacement procedures, this area is seldom worn out, even in advanced osteoarthrosis where the rest of femoral condyles are eburnated. Access to this donor area is made through a standard lateral portal with the knee flexed only about 30°. The decision to transplant

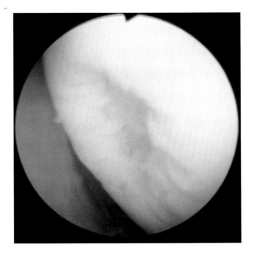

Figure 14.5 – *Small chondral defect (Dr V. Bobic).*

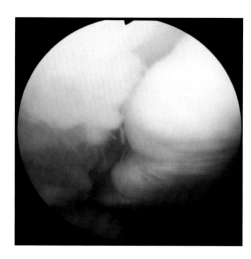

Figure 14.8 – *Femoral chondro-osteophyte.*

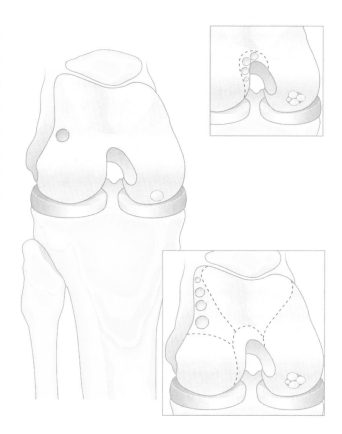

Figure 14.7 – *OAT donor sites.*

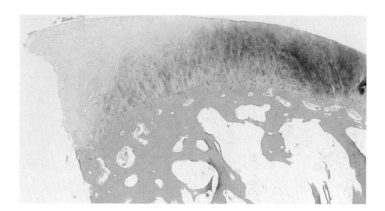

Figure 14.9 – *Chondro-osteophyte histology.*

single or multiple osteochondral grafts should be based on the size and location of the lesion, harvest site accessibility and the convex to concave relationships of donor and recipient sites. An alternative donor site for multiple small grafts is directly adjacent to the superolateral margin of the intercondylar notch, in the notchplasty and roofplasty area in ACL reconstruction (Fig. 14.7).

Chondro-osteophyte in chronic ACL deficiency

This site is a usable alternative to regular donor sites, for multiple small grafts. Histological analysis demonstrates normal architecture and composition of hyaline articular cartilage that covers lateral and proximal aspect of the medial femoral notch osteophyte in ACL deficiency. However, in chronic ACL deficiency the peripheral area of the chondro-osteophyte may contain a high percentage of fibrocartilage (Figs 14.8, 14.9).

Step 2: chondral defect size determination and surgical planning

The chondral defect is inspected arthroscopically and the size of the lesion is measured using a range of appropriate

colour-coded sizers. These instruments are also used to evaluate potential donor sites. The appropriately sized donor graft harvester is introduced into the joint and placed over the selected hyaline cartilage harvest site. It is essential that the harvester is perpendicular to the donor articular cartilage area. The T mark and the depth markings on the barrel of the harvester should be clearly visible, and should be carefully observed during impaction. Using a mallet, the tubular harvester is driven into the subchondral bone to a depth of approximately 15 mm. Care should be taken not to change the angle or to rotate the tube harvester during impaction. It is very important to insert the harvester at an appropriate angle (90°) in order to obtain a circular graft. If this is not done properly, the graft may not fit the recipient area and transplanted cartilage may not be flush with the recipient cartilage (Fig. 14.10).

Step 3: donor core harvesting

Once the selected depth has been attained, remove the tubular harvester containing the graft, by rotating the

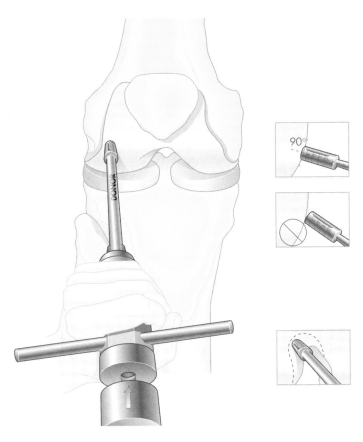

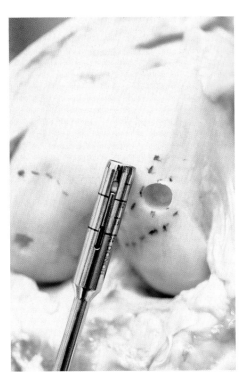

Figure 14.11 – *OATS, tubular harvester with osteochondral autograft.*

Figure 14.10 – *OATS, perpendicular orientation of the graft harvester.*

driver/extractor 90° clockwise and counter-clockwise. The handle of the driver/extractor should be rocked gently up and down, to fracture the cancellous base of the bone core for removal. Once removed, the donor core length and hyaline cartilage thickness can be seen through the slots in the harvester, and measured for overall length with a calibrated alignment stick (Fig. 14.11).

Tubular harvester versus drilling
Laboratory, cadaver and clinical trials clearly demonstrate that drilling of the recipient area, even at slow speeds, causes thermal damage and circular necrosis. Drilling of the recipient site does not provide press-fit graft fixation, and produces tissue debris (Fig. 14.12). Harvesting of osteochondral grafts using a power trephine or a drill, as opposed to a manual punch technique, causes significantly greater chondrocyte death. Improved tubular harvesters with a specially designed 'atraumatic' cutting edge uniformly provide precise recipient site and cut sharp recipient cartilage edges, with minimal peripheral trauma (Fig. 14.13). Extensive cadaver trials in the US and UK demonstrated

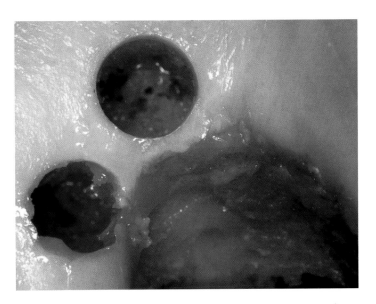

Figure 14.12 – *Drilling produces irregular recipient site and tissue debris.*

uniform quality of the osteochondral grafts and the recipient area (Fig. 14.14).

Step 4: recipient socket creation
If a single core transfer has been selected to repair the defect, the recipient tube harvester is positioned to cover the entire defect and is driven into the subchondral bone to depth of approximately 13 mm. During socket creation, attention to maintaining the

175

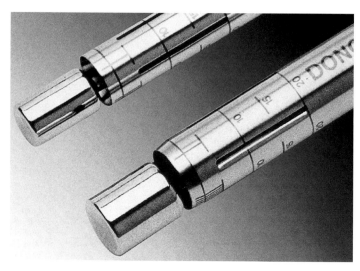

Figure 14.13 – *A set of OATS tubular harvesters (new design).*

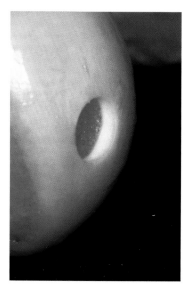

Figure 14.14 – *OATS recipient site (cadaver trials).*

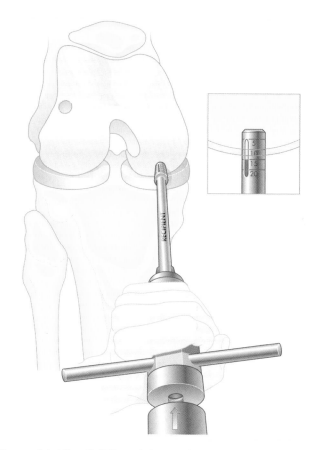

Figure 14.15 – *OATS, recipient socket creation.*

harvester at a 90° angle to the articular cartilage in both the sagittal and coronal planes is very important to achieve a flush transfer. Prior to harvesting, rotate the barrel of the tube harvester, until the depth markings can be clearly seen. Care must be taken to adjust the insertion and knee flexion angle to ensure that the end of the tube harvester is flush with the chondral surface prior to impaction. Using a sturdy mallet, the tube harvester is then driven into subchondral bone. Care should be taken not to change the angle of insertion or to rotate the tube harvester during impaction. Once the selected depth has been attained, the tube harvester containing the captured bone should be rotated 90° clockwise and counter-clockwise, and pulled out (Fig. 14.15).

Step 5: use of alignment sticks

A calibrated alignment stick of the appropriate diameter may be used to measure the recipient socket depth and to align correctly the angle of the recipient socket in relation to the position of the insertion portal when using an arthroscopic approach. The alignment stick may be used as an impactor to 'fine-tune' recipient socket length, to match the length of the donor core (Fig. 14.16).

Step 6: donor core insertion

The donor tube harvester containing the collared pin and autograft core to be transferred are reinserted into the driver/extractor, the impaction cap is unscrewed and the T-handled mid-section removed. This exposes the end of the collared pin which is used to advance the graft into the recipient socket. A flat pin calibrator is inserted over the guide pin and pressed onto the open back end of the driver/extractor (Fig. 14.17).

Step 7: final donor core seating

The donor tube harvester's bevelled edge is inserted fully into the recipient socket. This stabilises the harvester during autograft impaction and correctly seats the

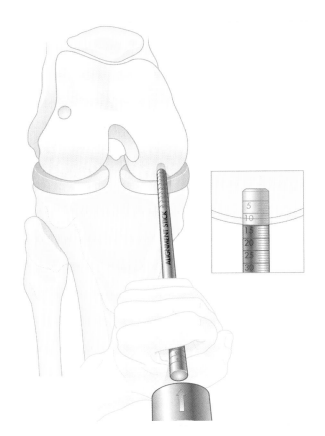

Figure 14.16 – *OATS alignment stick (donor socket fine-tuning).*

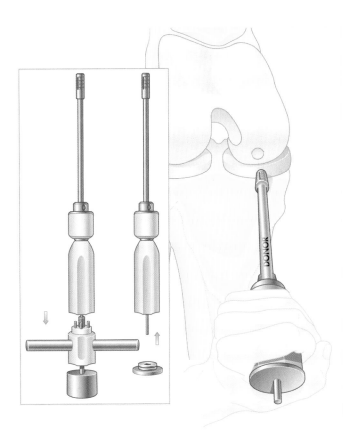

Figure 14.17 – *OATS donor core insertion.*

harvester for proper insertion depth control. A mallet is used to lightly tap the end of the collared pin and drive the graft into the recipient socket. The collared pin should be gently advanced until the end of the pin is flush with the pin calibrator. This provides exact mechanical control to ensure proper graft insertion. The pre-determined length of the collared pin is designed to advance the graft so that 1 mm of the graft will be exposed. A sizer, measuring at least 1 mm in diameter larger than the diameter of the graft, is positioned over the graft core. Final seating of the graft is achieved by tapping the tamp lightly, until the articular cartilage is flush with the recipient cartilage (Fig. 14.18).

Multiple osteochondral transfers

When multiple cores of various diameters are elected to be harvested and transferred into specific areas of the defect, each core transfer should be completed prior to creation of the further recipient socket. This prevents potential recipient tunnel wall fracture and allows subsequent cores to be placed directly adjacent to previously inserted bone cores. The fibrocartilage layer between osteochondral grafts will form and provide additional support to multiple osteochondral grafts (Fig. 14.19).

Donor sockets are routinely left open after harvesting and have been shown to fill in with cancellous bone and fibrocartilage within 12 weeks (Fig. 14.20). At 1 year the defect is typically filled with soft fibrous tissue which is level with the surrounding articular cartilage (Fig. 14.21). Re-arthroscopy at 3 years demonstrates level surface filled with cartilage-like tissue which is hard on probing and visually indistinguishable from surrounding cartilage. Cancellous bone removed from the recipient area may be inserted into donor sites and should be impacted firmly into the donor site with an alignment stick to compress and widen the cancellous bone. Alternatively, porous hydroxyapatite rods (5–10 mm in diameter) can be used for this purpose.

Complications include haemarthrosis, effusion, pain, donor site pain, graft fracture, potential for condylar fracture and avascular necrosis if a large number of small grafts is harvested from the same area, and loose bodies.

Rehabilitation

If the surgical technique is correct there is no need for restrictions or immobilisation: early movement and weight-bearing are essential for normal joint function. This is not a fracture situation, as the graft is press-fitted

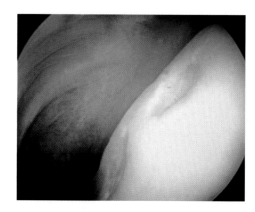

Figure 14.20 – *OATS donor sites at 3 months.*

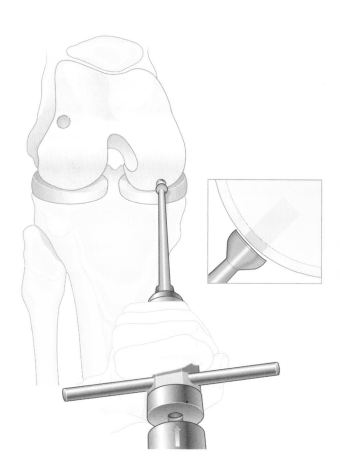

Figure 14.18 – *OATS final donor core seating.*

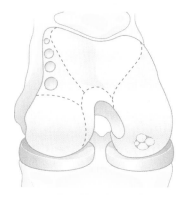

Figure 14.19 – *OATS multiple osteochondral transfers.*

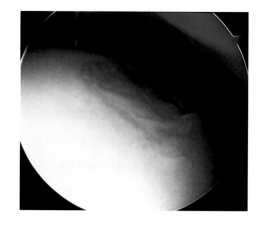

Figure 14.21 – *OATS donor sites at 12 months (arthroscopic photograph: Craig Morgan, 1998).*

into a compacted half-tunnel (similar to patella tendon bone block in ACL reconstruction) of the same size. In trochlear grafting, the knee is kept at 30° of flexion, to keep patella pressure on the graft, which tends to be shorter because of the hard subchondral bone in this area. Haemarthrosis, effusion and pain tend to slow rehabilitation down during the initial 2–4 weeks. Adequate pain management and swelling control are essential.

The evaluation of osteochondral grafting

The second-look arthroscopy
Figures 14.22 and 14.23 show examples of second-look arthroscopy.

Magnetic resonance imaging
Magnetic resonance imaging (MRI) can be used instead of second-look arthroscopy and biopsy [47–50]. MRI evaluation of the osteochondral autograft transplantation, with the OATS technique and instrumentation (Arthrex, Inc.) has been used in Liverpool, UK, since late 1996 in 18 patients, at 3–12 months after transplantation. Appropriate high-resolution sequences and the scanning protocol for articular cartilage imaging has been used for both clinical and research MRI. The development of optimal scanning protocols for imaging articular cartilage and research evaluation of the OAT is a part of an ongoing project, with the Radiology Department of the Liverpool University Hospitals, UK [51–53].

MRI of the single 10 mm osteochondral autograft transplant to isolated medial femoral condylar cartilage

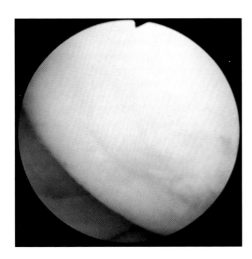

Figure 14.22 – *Single 10 mm OATS graft after 3 years (Dr V. Bobic, PEOH Exeter, 1996).*

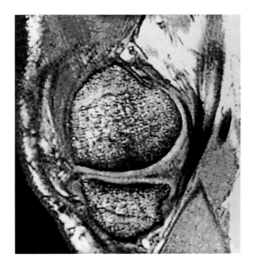

Figure 14.24 – *MRI of single 10 mm OATS graft after 6 months (University of Liverpool MARIARC MRI).*

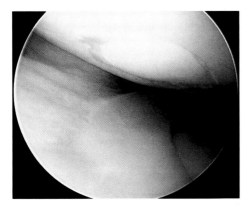

Figure 14.23 – *Single 10 mm OATS graft after 1 year (Craig Morgan, 1998).*

defect is done simultaneously with the BPTB ACL reconstruction. MRI scan after 6 months shows satisfactory bone-to-bone integration, excellent cartilage cover, matching cartilage curvature and thickness and congruent articular surface (Fig. 14.24).

Metallic artefacts

Metallic particles are minute, generally not visible on the standard radiographs and MRI sequences. They are the residual metallic debris, following the use of surgical instruments. Metallic artefacts are visible as a cluster of black speckles within soft tissues.

Technical problems

The picture and serial MRI images clearly demonstrate that the wrong angle during harvesting and inserting the graft will result in incongruent transplant that is too proud on one side and sunken on the opposite side (Fig. 14.25).

OAT transplant MRI analysis

The orange pixels correspond to normal T2 values for bone. The blue and purple pixels are anomalous: the T2

relaxation times are elevated because the tissue is 'wetter' than normal. This shows the fluid interface between recipient and donor bone (Fig. 14.26).

OAT comparative analysis of normal and transplanted bone core

The mean T2 value of normal bone is 84.0 ms. In the region of the implant the T2 value is elevated to 116.3 ms. The synovial fluid has T2 values greater than 200 ms. The incorporation of the implant in the surrounding bone can be objectively followed and compared between patients, either pixel by pixel, or using histogram and profile analysis of T2 relaxation time maps. The variation in T2 values at the margin of the implant provides an objective measure of the magnitude of the discontinuity between the implant and surrounding bone (Fig. 14.27).

OAT new developments

Indications for osteochondral grafting have been extended to treatment of the patellar and trochlear chondral defects, osteochondritis dissecans, allograft transplantation, bone grafting and focused bone core biopsy, including joints other than the knee (chondral defects of the talus, femoral head, humeral head, etc.). Large harvesters (10–35 mm) can be used for fresh osteochondral 'shell' or block allografts (Fig. 14.28). Porous hydroxyapatite rods have been used for grafting donor sites, to obliterate deep dead spaces between osteochondral autografts, and to provide scaffolding in the reconstruction of subchondral bone. A blood clot has been inserted into the recipient site to enhance early bone-to-bone healing and full integration of cancellous bone. Locally produced autologous chondrocytes are applied to mechanical carrier (cancellous bone or

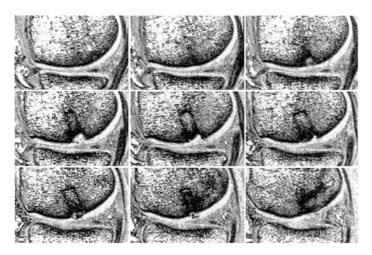

Figure 14.25 – *Serial MRI of single OATS graft, harvested and inserted under the wrong angle. This is the most common cause of OATS graft failure (University of Liverpool MARIARC MRI).*

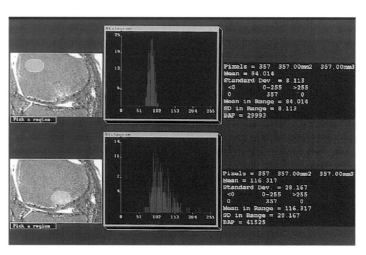

Figure 14.27 – *OAT comparative MRI analysis (University of Liverpool, MARIARC MRI).*

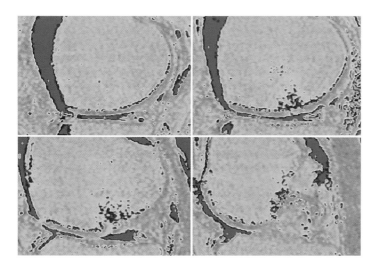

Figure 14.26 – *OAT transplant MRI analysis (University of Liverpool, MARIARC).*

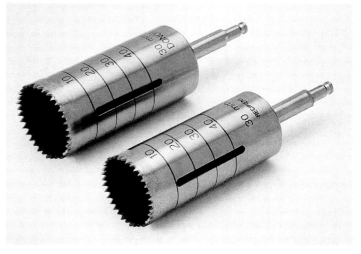

Figure 14.28 – *Arthrex 30 mm allograft harvesters (developed with Dr J. Garrett).*

hydroxyapatite) to obliterate dead spaces between circular osteochondral autografts. Growth factors (TGF-β) could be used to stimulate cell production and integration of hyaline cartilage (recipient–donor interface), with biological glues to seal cartilage–cartilage interface.

OAT problems

Like many orthopaedic procedures that require the use of autologous tissues, this is the 'rob Peter to pay Paul' situation. The main problem and limitation is availability of grafts. The size and depth of defects are also significant limiting factors. The dead spaces between circular grafts, integration of donor and recipient hyaline cartilage, different position, thickness and mechanical properties of donor and recipient hyaline cartilage are further sources of clinical concern.

OAT summary

This technique does not offer a long-term solution to all chondral problems. The quantity and quality of osteochondral grafts is very limited and, therefore, large, deep, osteochondral lesions are beyond the limits of this procedure. Although it seems that hyaline cartilage remains viable on macroscopic and microscopic examination for at least 5–7 years, little is known about the mechanical properties and the long-term survival of transplanted hyaline cartilage.

Buckwalter and Mankin, in their comprehensive review of articular cartilage repair techniques, state: '. . . Because of the small number of possible donor sites from which osteochondral autologous grafts may be obtained, use of these grafts has been limited to selected localised regions of damaged articular cartilage. In a small number of patients, surgeons have replaced damaged or lost articular surfaces with autologous grafts of articular cartilage . . ., and the results have shown that this technique can restore an articular surface. The long-term follow-up of small series of patients has shown that the transplantation of osteochondral autologous grafts . . . can be effective for the treatment of focal defects of articular cartilage in selected patients. . .' [1].

At present, osteochondral autograft transplantation seems to be the only surgical technique that can replace and retain hyaline articular cartilage, connected to and supported by firm cancellous bone carrier and with tidemark. Osteochondral autograft transplants have been associated with a good rate of success; however, the experience with this procedure is limited and further long-term follow-up is essential.

The clinical algorithm

It is important to understand that the outcome of articular cartilage repair depends on many complex issues: chronic or acute condition, previous repair, location of the defect, defect thickness, size of the lesion, degree of containment of the lesion, ligament and meniscal integrity and alignment. The planned treatment should be safe and effective. The anticipated outcome of the treatment should be clear and realistic. Goals should be set before the surgery so that the patient understands the problem, treatment plan, and what to expect. Although most treatment options will produce fibrocartilage or hyaline-like cartilage, which are unable to restore the original mechanical properties of the damaged articulating surface, the elimination of pain, swelling, stiffness, grinding and locking may be satisfactory enough to enable people to return to work and sports.

It is worth remembering that partial-thickness lesions (fissures) do not heal. They seem to remain static, at least for a while. We do not know for how long, and what happens with this lesion in the long run. Full-thickness lesions heal with fibrocartilage that lacks structure to withstand cyclic compression and articulation and to maintain integrity in the long run.

For practical purposes, chondral defects can be divided into groups of lesions less than 2 cm^2 and over 2 cm^2. The lesions that have the best prognosis are femoral condylar defects less than 2 cm^2. If the lesion is stable and contained, it is appropriate to consider one of the bone marrow (mesenchymal) stimulating techniques: debridement and microfracture or drilling. If there is no major associated ligament, meniscal or alignment pathology, one may expect such treatment results to be reasonably successful in the short term, 3–5 years, probably without progression to arthritis. Alternatively, such a lesion can be treated with OAT or with ACI, if this option is deemed cost-effective. The probability of progressing into arthritis is higher in knees with femoral lesions greater than 2 cm^2, since the repair tissue (fibrocartilage) will be unable to contain the defect. In the low-demand patient the bone marrow stimulation may be acceptable as a primary approach. In the higher-demand group OAT or ACI should be considered the primary approach. The OAT provides firm and congruent repair almost immediately, but it is limited by the number of autologous grafts required to cover the entire lesion. Failure of both techniques may be revised by using the osteochondral autograft. Tertiary failure of OAT or ACI transplantation may require realignment and block allograft or arthroplasty.

For femoral osteochondritis dissecans lesions the initial approach should include fixation with absorbable pins. This probably works only on relatively fresh osteochondral rather than chondral fragments. If this fails, OAT and ACI should be considered, especially in large and deep osteochondral lesions. It the lesion is particularly deep, it may require a large cylindrical osteochondral allograft or a staged procedure with an initial bone graft followed by ACI.

The treatment of patellar chondral defects is very difficult and results are generally poor in the long run. The main problem with patellar articular cartilage repair is its thickness and shape, as well as the enormous compression and shearing forces in the patellofemoral joint. It is essential to correct the patellofemoral alignment. It seems that trochlear defects can be treated successfully with a couple of a large osteochondral autografts. However, the experience is limited and the follow-up of a small number of cases is fairly short.

Treating tibial chondral lesions has been challenging, to say the least. The results have been generally unsatisfactory with ACI and OAT. Neither technique is recommended in patients with this type of lesion [54].

Clinical assessment of articular cartilage repair

The evaluation of repaired articular cartilage remains difficult and unreliable. The visual arthroscopic inspection, probing, and stiffness testing with indentation probes are currently widely used invasive options. However, the repaired area should be monitored periodically by non-invasive imaging methods, such as MRI.

The International Cartilage Repair Society (ICRS) provides the Standard Cartilage Evaluation Form which should be used for standardised evaluation purposes, available from the ICRS (www.cartilage.org).

The problem with all current articular cartilage repair techniques and derived studies to date has been the lack of standardised outcome assessment. It is imperative to use a clinical outcome tool to measure the patient's subjective symptoms.

The modified Cincinnati rating scale is an excellent tool for clinical assessment because it allows both the patient and the clinician to rate symptoms quantitatively in relation to severity and functional level. The functional level ranges from sedentary life to full return to sport (from 2 for poor overall condition: significant limitations that affect activities of daily living, up to 10 for excellent overall condition: able to do any sport with no problems).

It is also important to record treatment outcomes in terms of short and long-term improvement in mobility, joint line pain, crepitus, swelling and giving way.

A quality of life survey, such as the SF36 health survey (Health Assessment Lab, www.SF36.com), which is part of the International Quality of Life (IQOLA) Project, helps to define optimally the impact of the problem and interventions on the patient.

Summary

At the present time, debridement to bleeding bone and stimulation of the fibrocartilage growth remains the most common surgical treatment for a chondral lesion in a young adult. However, we must not forget that the fibrocartilage primarily functions as a resistor to tension, whereas the hyaline cartilage is mainly subject to and resists compressive forces. Therefore, the end product is inadequate biomechanically, and is bound to fail in the long run.

The choice of surgical techniques that can restore and maintain hyaline cartilage is very limited. At this moment, the osteochondral autograft transplantation seems to be the only surgical technique that can restore the height and the shape of articulating surface in osteochondral defects, with composite autologous material that contains all necessary ingredients: hyaline articular cartilage, intact tidemark and a firm carrier in the form of its own subchondral bone.

Tissue engineering has recently emerged as a new interdisciplinary science to repair injured body parts. It seems that techniques like ACI and TGF have significant treatment potential at the cellular level. Cellular engineering and implantation may be able to replace large and deep hyaline cartilage defects in the not too distant future. However, none of the experimental methods for facilitating the repair of cartilage, when applied to osteoarthritic joints, has been shown to stimulate formation of a surface durable enough to function as articular cartilage for a long period of time. One should be careful in recommending these treatments to young patients as a means of repairing chondral defects and preventing arthritis in the future.

The challenge to restore a damaged articular surface is a multidisciplinary challenge which has generated tremendous interest amongst research scientists, clinicians and patients. Many new articular cartilage repair techniques have emerged in the past 4–6 years, most of which appear to be very promising. The current state of the art of articular cartilage repair is the result of the increased awareness of the significance of articular cartilage damage, the explosive interest, the intense research and rapid development of clinical applications. The final product is still in its infancy and far from being finished, but it is this systematic, and rapid sequential progression that will lead to future developments. At this rapid pace, further advances in articular cartilage research, leading to clinical application with the reliable long-term outcome, are not far away.

However, we must not forget Dr Mankin's thoughts: '. . . it should be clear that cartilage does not yield its secrets easily and that inducing cartilage to heal is not simple. The tissue is difficult to work with, injuries to joint surface – whether traumatic or degenerative – are unforgiving, and the progression to osteoarthritis is sometimes so slow that we delude ourselves into thinking we are doing better than we are. It is important, however, to keep trying' [12].

Key points

■ Treatment options are limited and the long-term outcome is still uncertain.

■ The choice of surgical techniques that can restore and maintain hyaline cartilage is very limited.

■ The best that can be achieved at present is to repair the chondral defect.

References

Chapter 1

1. Fergusson CM. The aetiology of osteoarthritis. A review. *Postgrad Med J* 1987; **63**: 439–45.
2. Meyers MH, Akeson W, Convery FR. Resurfacing of the knee with fresh osteochondral allograft. *J Bone Jt Surg (Am)* 1989; **71**: 705–13.
3. Brittberg M, Faxen E, Peterson L. Carbon fiber scaffolds in the treatment of early knee osteoarthritis. a prospective 4-year follow-up of 37 patients. *Clin Orthop* 1994; **307**: 155–64.
4. Brittberg M, Lindahl A, Nilsson A *et al.* Treatment of deep cartilage defects in the knee with autologous chondocyte transplantation. *N Engl J Med* 1994; **331**: 889–95.
5. Breinan HA, Minas T, Hsu H *et al.* Effect of cultured autologous chondrocytes on repair of chondral defects in a curine model. *J Bone Jt Surg (Am)* 1997; **79**: 1439–51.
6. Bobic V. Arthroscopic osteochondral autograft transplantation in anterior cruciate ligament reconstruction: a preliminary clinical study. *Knee Surg Sports Traumatol Arthrosc* 1996; **3**: 262–4.
7. Roos H, Adalbert T, Dahlberg L, Lohmander LS. Osteo-arthritis of the knee after injury to the anterior cruciate ligament or meniscus: the influence of time and age. *Osteoarthritis Cartilage* 1995; **3**: 261–7.
8. Cooper C, McAlindon T, Snow S *et al.* Mechanical and constitutional risk factors for symptomatic knee osteo-arthritis: differences between medial tibiofemoral and patello-femoral disease. *J Rheumatol* 1994; **21**: 307–13.
9. Doherty M, Watt I, Dieppe P. Influence of primary generalised osteoarthritis on development of secondary osteoarthritis. *Lancet* 1983; **2**: 8–11.
10. Odenbring S, Lindstrand A, Egund N *et al.* Prognosis for patients with medial gonarthrosis: a 16-year follow-up study of 189 knees. *Clin Orthop* 1991; **266**: 152.
11. Bert JM, Maschka K. The arthroscopic treatment of unicompartmental gonarthrosis: a five-year follow-up study of abrasion arthroplasty plus arthroscopic debridement and arthroscopic debridement alone. *Arthroscopy* 1989; **5**: 25–32.
12. Burks RT. Arthroscopy and degenerative arthritis of the knee: a review of the literature. *Arthroscopy* 1990; **6**: 43–7.
13. Ogilvie-Harris DJ, Fitsialos DP. Arthroscopic management of the degenerative knee. *Arthroscopy* 1991; **7**: 151–7.
14. Schonholtz GJ. Arthroscopic debridement of the knee joint. *Orthop Clin North Am* 1989; **20**: 257–63.
15. Sprague NF III. Arthroscopic debridement for degenerative joint disease. *Clin Orthop* 1974; **101**: 61.
16. Timoney JM, Kneisl JS, Barrack RL *et al.* Arthroscopy in the osteo-arthritic knee. *Orthop Rev* 1990; **19**: 371–9.
17. Jackson RW. The role of arthroscopy in the management of the arthritic knee. *Clin Orthop* 1974; **101**: 28–35.
18. Edelson R, Burks RT, Bloebaum RD. Short-term effects of knee washout for osteoarthritis. *Am J Sports Med* 1995; **23**: 345–9.
19. Jackson RW, Rousse DW. The results of partial arthroscopic meniscectomy in patients over 40 years of age. *J Bone Jt Surg (Br)* 1982; **64**: 481.
20. Pridie KH. A method of resurfacing osteoarthritic knee joints. *J Bone Jt Surg (Br)* 1959; **41**: 618.
21. Magnuson PB. Technique of debridement of the knee joint for arthritis. *Surg Clin North Am* 1946; **24**: 249.
22. McEldowney AJ, Weiker GG. Open knee Magnuson debridement as conservative treatment for degenerative osteo-arthritis of the knee. *J Arthroplasty* 1995; **10**: 805–9.
23. Coventry MB. Current concepts review. Upper tibial osteotomy for osteoarthritis. *J Bone Jt Surg (Am)* 1985; **67**: 1136–40.
24. Maquet P. The treatment of choice in osteoarthritis of the knee. *Clin Orthop* 1985; **192**: 108.
25. Hernigou P. [A 20-year follow-up study of internal gonarthrosis after tibial valgus osteotomy: single versus repeated osteotomy]. *Rev Chir Orthop Reparatrice Appar Mot* 1996; **82**: 241–50.
26. Insall JN, Joseph DM, Msika C. High tibial osteotomy for varus gonarthrosis: a long-term follow-up study. *J Bone Jt Surg (Am)* 1984; **66**: 1040–8.
27. Prodromos CC, Andriacchi TP, Galante JO. A relationship between gait and clinical changes following high tibial osteotomy. *J Bone Jt Surg (Am)* 1985; **67**: 1188–94.
28. Wang J-W, Kuo KN, Andriacchi TP, Galante JO. The influence of walking mechanics and time on the results of proximal tibial osteotomy. *J Bone Jt Surg (Am)* 1990; **72**: 905–9.

29. Learmonth ID. A simple technique for varus supracondylar osteotomy in genu valgum. *J Bone Jt Surg (Br)* 1990; **72**: 235–7.

30. McDermott AGP, Finklestein JA, Farine I *et al*. Distal femoral varus osteotomy for valgus deformity of the knee. *J Bone Jt Surg (Am)* 1988; **70**: 110–16.

31. Holden DL, James SL, Larson RL, Slocum DB. Proximal tibial osteotomy in patients who are fifty years old or less. A long-term follow-up study. *J Bone Jt Surg (Am)* 1988; **70**: 977–82.

32. Ivarsson I, Myrnerts R, Gillquist J. High tibial osteotomy for medial osteoarthritis of the knee: a 5 to 7 and an 11 to 13 year follow-up. *J Bone Jt Surg (Br)* 1990; **72**: 238–44.

33. Murphy SB. Tibial osteotomy for genu varum. Indications, preoperative planning and technique. *Orthop Clin North Am* 1994; **25**: 477–82.

34. Windsor RE, Insall JN, Vince KG. Technical considerations of total knee arthroplasty after proximal tibial osteotomy. *J Bone Jt Surg (Am)* 1988; **70**: 547–55.

35. Lattermann C, Jakob RP. High tibial osteotomy alone or combined with ligament reconstruction in anterior cruciate ligament-deficient knees. *Knee Surg Sports Traumatol Arthrosc* 1996; **4**: 32–8.

36. Dalury DF, Ewald FC, Christie MJ, Scott, RD. Total knee arthroplasty in a group of patients less than 45 years of age. *J Arthroplasty* 1995; **10**: 598–602.

37. Diduch DR, Insall JI, Scott WN *et al*. Total knee replacement in young active patients. Longterm follow-up and functional outcome. *J Bone Jt Surg (Am)* 1997; **79**: 575–82.

38. Stuart MJ, Rand JA. Total knee arthroplasty in the young adult. *Orthop Trans* 1987; **11**: 441–2.

39. Ewald F, Christie MJ. Results of cemented total knee replacement in young patients. *Orthop Trans* 1987; **11**: 442.

40. Rand JA, Ilstrup DM. Survivorship analysis of total knee arthroplasty. Cumulative rates of survival of 9200 total knee arthroplasties. *J Bone Jt Surg (Am)* 1991; **73**: 397–409.

41. Stern SH, Becker MW, Insall JN. Unicondylar knee arthroplasty. An evaluation of selection criteria. *Clin Orthop* 1993; **286**: 143–8.

Chapter 2

1. Rand JA, Bryan RS. Reimplantation for the salvage of an infected total knee arthroplasty. *J Bone Jt Surg (Am)* 1983; **65**: 1081–8.

2. Rand JA, Bryan RS, Morrey BF *et al*. Management of infected total knee arthroplasty. *Clin Orthop* 1986; **205**: 75–9.

3. Bengston S, Knutson K, Lidgren L. Treatment of infected knee arthroplasty. *Clin Orthop* 1989; **245**: 173–8.

4. Bengston S, Blomgren G, Knutson K *et al*. Haematogenous infection after knee arthroplasty. *Acta Orthop Scand* 1987; **58**: 529–32.

5. Wilson MG, Kelley K, Thornhill TS. Infection as a complication of total knee arthroplasty. *J Bone Jt Surg (Am)* 1990; **72**: 878–83.

6. Garner RW, Mowat AC, Hazelman BL. Wound healing after operations on patients with rheumatoid arthritis. *J Bone Jt Surg (Br)* 1973; **55**: 134–7.

7. Insall JN, Hass SB. Complications of total knee arthroplasty. In: Insall J N, Windsor R E, Scott W N *et al.*, eds. *Surgery of the Knee*. New York: Churchill Livingstone 1993.

8. Schoifet SD, Morrey BF. Treatment of infection after total knee arthroplasty by debridement with retention of the components. *J Bone Jt Surg (Am)* 1990; **72**: 1383–8.

9. Henderson JJ, Bamford DJ, Noble J, Brown JF. The value of skeletal scintigraphy in predicting the need for revision surgery in total knee replacement. *Orthopaedics* 1996; **19**: 295–9.

10. Oishi CS, Elliott ML, Colwell CW. Recurrent hemarthrosis following a total knee arthroplasty. *J Arthroplasty* 1995; **10 (Suppl)**: 56–8.

11. Dennis DA, Channer M. Retained distal femoral osteophyte. An infrequent cause of postoperative pain following total knee arthroplasty. *J Arthroplasty* 1992; **7**: 193–5.

12. Larson JE, Becker DA. Fabellar impingement in total knee arthroplasty. A case report. *J Arthroplasty* 1993; **8**: 95–7.

13. Scher DM, Paumier JC, Di-Cesare PE. Pseudomeniscus following total knee arthroplasty as a cause of persistent knee pain. *J Arthroplasty* 1997; **12**: 114–18.

14. Ritter MA, Faris PM, Keating EM. Anterior femoral notching and ipsilateral supracondylar femur fracture in total knee arthroplasty. *J Arthroplasty* 1988; **3**: 185–9.

15. Austin KS, Siliski JM. Symptomatic heterotopic ossification following total knee arthroplasty. *J Arthroplasty* 1995; **10**: 695–8.

16. Lewonowski K, Dorr LD, McPherson EJ *et al*. Medialisation of the patella in total knee arthroplasty. *J Arthroplasty* 1997; **12**: 161–7.

17. Doerr TE, Eckhoff DG. Lateral patellar burnishing in total knee arthroplasty following medialisation of the patellar button. *J Arthroplasty* 1995; **10**: 540–2.

18. Braakman M, Verburg AD, Bronsema G *et al*. The outcome of three methods of patellar resurfacing in total knee arthroplasty. *Int Orthop* 1995; **19**: 7–11.

19. Campbell DG, Mintz AD, Stevenson TM. Early patellofemoral revision following total knee arthroplasty. *J Arthroplasty* 1995; **10**: 287–91.

20. Bocell JR, Thorpe CC, Tullos JH. Arthroscopic treatment of symptomatic total knee arthroplasty. *Clin Orthop* 1991; **271**: 125–34.

21. Beight JL, Yao B, Hozack WJ *et al*. The patella 'clunk' syndrome after posterior stabilised total knee arthroplasty. *Clin Orthop* 1994; **299**: 139–42.

22. Vernace JV, Rothman RH, Booth RE, Balderston RA. Arthroscopic management of the patellar clunk syndrome following posterior stabilised total knee arthroplasty. *J Arthroplasty* 1989; **4**: 179–84.

23. Diduch DR, Scuderi GR, Scott WN *et al*. The efficacy of arthroscopy following total knee replacement. *Arthroscopy* 1997; **13**: 166–71.

24. Krackow KA, Weiss PC. Recurvatum deformity complicating performance of total knee arthroplasty: a brief note. *J Bone Jt Surg (Am)* 1990; **72**: 268–9.

25. Emerson RH, Head WC, Malinin TI. Reconstruction of patellar tendon rupture after total knee arthroplasty with an extensor mechanism allograft. *Clin Orthop* 1990; **260**: 154–6.

26. Murena PF, Pasqualini M. Should total prosthetization of the patella be used in knee surgery? A review of the literature and personal experience. *Chir Organi Mov* 1995; **80**: 323–8.

27. Bourne RB, Rorabeck CH, Vaz M *et al.* Resurfacing versus not resurfacing the patella during total knee replacement. *Clin Orthop* 1995; **321**: 156–61.

28. Keblish PA, Varma AK, Greenwald AS. Patellar resurfacing or retention in total knee arthroplasty. A prospective study of patients with bilateral replacements. *J Bone Jt Surg (Br)* 1994; **76**: 930–7.

29. Enis JE, Gardner R, Robledo MA *et al.* Comparison of patellar resurfacing versus nonresurfacing in bilateral total knee arthroplasty. *Clin Orthop* 1990; **260**: 38–42.

30. Smith SR, Stuart P, Pinder IM. Nonresurfaced patella in total knee arthroplasty. *J Arthroplasty* 1989; **4**: S81–6.

31. Barrack RL, Wolfe MW, Waldman DA *et al.* Resurfacing of the patella in total knee arthroplasty. A prospective, randomised, double-blind study. *J Bone Jt Surg (Am)* 1997; **79**: 1121–31.

32. Kajino A, Yoshino S, Kameyama S *et al.* Comparison of the results of bilateral total knee arthroplasty with and without patellar replacement for rheumatoid arthritis. *J Bone Jt Surg (Br)* 1997; **79**: 570–4.

33. Nicholls DW, Dorr LD. Revision surgery for stiff total knee arthroplasty. *J Arthroplasty* 1990; **5(Suppl)**: 73–7.

34. Katz MM, Hungerford DS, Krackow KA, Lennox DW. Reflex sympathetic dystrophy as a cause of poor results after total knee arthroplasty. *J Arthroplasty* 1986; **1**: 117–23.

35. Yashar AA, Adler RS, Grady-Benson JC *et al.* An ultrasound method to evaluate polyethylene component wear in total knee replacement arthroplasty. *Am J Arthroplasty* 1996; **25**: 702–4.

36. Yoshii I, Whiteside LA, Anouchi YS. The effect of patella button placement and femoral component design on patellar tracking in total knee arthroplasty. *Clin Orthop* 1992; **275**: 211–19.

37. Markel DC, Luessenhop CP, Windsor RE *et al.* Arthroscopic treatment of peripatellar fibrosis after total knee arthroplasty. *J Arthroplasty* 1996; **11**: 293–7.

38. Johanson DR, Friedman RJ, McGinty JB *et al.* The role of arthroscopy in the problem total knee replacement. *Arthroscopy* 1990; **6**: 30–2.

39. Wilde AH. Management of infected knee and hip prostheses. *Curr Opin Rheumatol* 1993; **5**: 317–21.

40. Isiklar ZU, Landon GC, Tullos HS. Amputation after failed total knee arthroplasty. *Clin Orthop* 1994; **299**: 173–8.

41. Dellon AL, Mont MA, Mullick T *et al.* Partial denervation for persistent neuroma pain around the knee. *Clin Orthop* 1996; **329**: 216–22.

42. Insall JN, Hass SB. Complications of total knee arthroplasty. In: Insall JN, Windsor RE, Scott WN *et al.*, eds., *Surgery of the Knee*. New York: Churchill Livingstone, 1993: 891–934.

Chapter 3

1. Commission on the Provision of Surgical Services. *Report of the Working Party on the Management of Patients with Major Injury*. Royal College of Surgeons of England, November 1988.

2. Noyes FR, Butler DL, Grood ES *et al.* Clinical paradoxes of anterior cruciate instability and a new test to detect its instability. *Orthop Trans* 1978; **2**: 36.

3. Bollen SR, Scott BW. Rupture of the anterior cruciate ligament – a quiet epidemic? *Injury* 1996; **27**: 407–9.

4. Nicholl JP, Coleman P, Williams BT. Injuries in Sport and Exercise. Main report. *A National Study of the Epidemiology of Exercise-Related Injury and Illness*. A Report to the Sports Council, 1991.

5. Kujala UM, Taimela S, Antti-Poika I *et al.* Acute injuries in soccer, ice-hockey, volleyball, basketball, judo and karate: analysis of National Registry data. *Br Med J* 1995; **311**: 1465–8.

6. Miyasaka KC, Daniel DM, Shore ML, Hirsham P. The incidence of knee ligament injuries in the general population. *Am J Knee Surg* 1991; **4**: 3–8.

7. Nielsen AB, Yde J. Epidemiology of acute knee injuries: a prospective hospital investigation. *J Trauma* 1991; **31**: 1644–8.

8. Matthewson MH, Dandy DJ. Osteochondral fractures of the lateral femoral condyle. A result of indirect violence to the knee. *J Bone Joint Surg (Br)* 1978; **60**: 199–202.

9. Meyers MH, McKeever FM. Fracture of the intercondylar eminence of the tibia. *J Bone Jt Surg (Am)* 1959; **41**: 209–22.

10. Galway RD, Beaupré A, MacIntosh DL. Pivot shift: a clinical sign of symptomatic anterior cruciate insufficiency. *J Bone Jt Surg (Br)* 1972; **54**: 763–4.

11. Irvine GB, Dias JJ, Finlay DBL. Segond fractures of the lateral tibial condyle: brief report. *J Bone Jt Surg (Br)* 1987; **69**: 613–4.

12. Segond P. Recherches cliniques et experimentales sur les epanchements sanguins du genou par entorse. *Prog Med* 1879; **7**: 297–9, 319–21, 340–1. Symptomes - Marche - Diagnostic: 379–81, 400–1. Traitement: 419–21.

13. Allum RL, Jones JR. The locked knee. *Injury* 1986; **17**: 256–8.

14. Gilquist J, Hagberg G, Oretorp N. Arthroscopy in acute injuries of the knee joint. *Acta Orthop Scand* 1977; **48**: 190–6.

15. Noyes FR, Bassett RW, Grood ES, Butler DL. Arthroscopy in acute traumatic hemarthrosis of the knee. Incidence of anterior cruciate tears and other injuries. *J Bone Jt Surg (Am)* 1980; **62**: 687–95.

16. De Haven KE. Diagnosis of acute knee injuries with hemarthrosis. *Am J Sports Med* 1980; **8**: 9–14.

17. Jones JR, Allum RL. Acute traumatic haemarthrosis of the knee: expectant treatment or arthroscopy? *Ann R Coll Surg Engl* 1989; **71**: 40–3.

18. Casteleyn PP, Handelberg F, Opdecam P. Traumatic haemarthrosis of the knee. *J Bone Jt Surg (Br)* 1988; **70**: 404–6.

19. Maffuli N, Binfield PM, King JB, Good CJ. Acute haemarthrosis of the knee in athletes. A prospective study of 106 cases. *J Bone Jt Surg (Br)* 1993; **75**: 945–9.

20. Chissell HR, Allum RL, Keightley A. MRI of the knee: its cost-effective use in a district general hospital. *Ann R Coll Surg Engl* 1994; **76**: 26–9.

21. Goodfellow J. He who hesitates is saved. *J Bone Jt Surg (Br)* 1980; **62**: 1–2.

22. Goodfellow J. Closed meniscectomy. *J Bone Jt Surg (Br)* 1983; **65**: 373–4.

23. Indelicato PA. Non-operative treatment of complete tears of the medial collateral ligament of the knee. *J Bone Jt Surg (Am)* 1983; **65**: 323–9.

24. Sandberg R, Balkfors B, Nilsson B, Westlin N. Operative versus non-operative treatment of recent injuries to the

ligaments of the knee. A prospective randomised study. *J Bone Jt Surg (Am)* 1987; **69**: 1120–6.

25. Reider B, Sathy MR, Talkington J *et al*. Treatment of isolated medial collateral ligament injuries in athletes with early functional rehabilitation. A five-year follow-up study. *Am J Sports Med* 1994; **22**: 470–7.

26. Shelbourne KD, Porter DA. Anterior cruciate ligament - medial collateral ligament injury. Nonoperative management of medial collateral ligament tears with anterior cruciate ligament reconstruction: a preliminary report. *Am J Sports Med* 1992; **20**: 283–6.

27. Hughston JC, Jacobsen KE. Chronic posterolateral rotatory instability of the knee. *J Bone Jt Surg (Am)* 1985; **67**: 351–9.

28. Clancy WG Jr, Meister K, Craythorne CB. Posterolateral corner collateral ligament reconstruction. In: Jackson DW, ed. *Reconstructive Knee Surgery. Master Techniques in Knee Surgery*. New York, NY: Raven Press, 1995; 143–59.

29. Veltri DM, Warren RF. Instructional course lectures, the American Academy of Orthopaedic Surgeons. Posterolateral instability of the knee. *J Bone Jt Surg (Am)* 1994; **76**: 460–72.

30. Mohtadi NGH, Webster-Bogaert S, Fowler PJ. Limitation of motion following anterior cruciate ligament reconstruction: a case–control study. *Am J Sports Med* 1991; **19**: 620–5.

31. Shelbourne KD, Wilckens JH, Mollabashy A, DeCarlo M. Arthrofibrosis in acute anterior cruciate ligament reconstruction. The effect of timing of reconstruction and rehabilitation. *Am J Sports Med* 1991; **19**: 331–6.

32. Harner CD, Irrgang JJ, Paul J *et al*. Loss of motion following anterior cruciate ligament reconstruction. *Am J Sports Med* 1992; **20**: 499–506.

33. Marcacci M, Zaffagnini S, Iacono F *et al*. Early versus late reconstruction for anterior cruciate ligament rupture. Results after five years of followup. *Am J Sports Med* 1995; **23**: 690–3.

34. Majors RA, Woodfin B. Achieving full range of motion after anterior cruciate ligament reconstruction. *Am J Sports Med* 1996; **24**: 350–5.

35. O'Neill DB. Arthroscopically assisted reconstruction of the anterior cruciate ligament. A prospective randomised analysis of three techniques. *J Bone Jt Surg (Am)* 1996; **78**: 803–13.

Chapter 4

1. Wojtys EM. The ACL deficient knee. *Am Acad Orthop Surg Monogr* 1994: 93.

2. Graf B, Uhr F. Complications of intra-articular anterior cruciate reconstruction. *Clin Sports Med* 1988; **7**: 835–48.

3. Sachs RA, Daniel DM, Stone ML, Garfein RF. Patellofemoral problems after anterior cruciate ligament reconstruction. *Am J Sports Med* 1989; **17**: 760–5.

4. Fu FH, Irrgang JJ, Harner CD. Loss of motion following anterior cruciate ligament reconstruction. In: Jackson DW, ed. *The Anterior Cruciate Ligament, Current and Future Concepts*. New York, NY: Raven Press, 1993: 373–80.

5. Harner CD, Irrgang JJ, Paul J *et al*. Loss of motion after anterior cruciate ligament reconstruction. *Am J Sports Med* 1992; **20**: 499–506.

6. Shelbourne KD, Patel DV, Martini DJ. Classification and management of arthrofibrosis of the knee after anterior cruciate ligament reconstruction. *Am J Sports Med* 1996; **24**: 857–62.

7. Mohtadi NGH, Webster-Bogaert S, Fowler PJ. Limitation of motion following anterior cruciate ligament reconstruction. A case–control study. *Am J Sports Med* 1991; **19**: 620–5.

8. Shelbourne KD, Wilckens JH, Mollabashy A, DeCarlo M. Arthrofibrosis in acute anterior cruciate ligament reconstruction. The effect of timing of reconstruction and rehabilitation. *Am J Sports Med* 1991; **19**: 331–6.

9. Majors RA, Woodfin B. Achieving full range of motion after anterior cruciate ligament reconstruction. *Am J Sports Med* 1996; **24**: 350–5.

10. Marcacci M, Zaffagnini S, Iacono F *et al*. Early versus late reconstruction for anterior cruciate ligament rupture. Results after five years of followup. *Am J Sports Med* 1995; **23**: 690–3.

11. O'Neill DB. Arthroscopically assisted reconstruction of the anterior cruciate ligament. A prospective randomised analysis of three techniques. *J Bone Jt Surg (Am)* 1996; **78**: 803–13.

12. Howell SM, Clark JA, Farley TE. A rationale for predicting anterior cruciate graft impingement by the intercondylar roof. A magnetic resonance imaging study. *Am J Sports Med* 1991; **19**: 276–82.

13. Howell SM, Barad SJ. Knee extension and its relationship to the slope of the intercondylar roof. Implications for positioning the tibial tunnel in anterior cruciate ligament reconstructions. *Am J Sports Med* 1995; **23**: 288–94.

14. Jackson DW, Schaefer RK. Cyclops syndrome: loss of extension following intra-articular anterior cruciate ligament reconstruction. *Arthroscopy* 1990: **6**: 171–8.

15. Shelbourne KD, Nitz P. Accelerated rehabilitation after anterior cruciate ligament reconstruction. *Am J Sports Med* 1990; **18**: 292–9.

16. Paulos LE, Rosenberg TD, Drawbert J *et al*. Infrapatellar contracture syndrome. An unrecognised cause of knee stiffness with patellar entrapment and patella infera. *Am J Sports Med* 1987; **15**: 331–41.

17. Paulos LE, Wnorowski DC, Greenwald AE. Infrapatellar contracture syndrome. Diagnosis, treatment, and long term followup. *Am J Sports Med* 1994; **22**: 440–9.

18. O'Brien SJ, Warren RF, Pavlov H *et al*. Reconstruction of the chronically insufficient anterior cruciate ligament with the central third of the patellar ligament. *J Bone Jt Surg (Am)* 1991; **73**: 278–86.

19. Dandy DJ, Desai SS. Patellar tendon length after anterior cruciate ligament reconstruction. *J Bone Jt Surg (Br)* 1994; **76**: 198–9.

20. Shelbourne KD, Foulk DA. Timing of surgery in acute anterior cruciate ligament tears on the return of quadriceps muscle strength after reconstruction using an autogenous patellar tendon graft. *Am J Sports Med* 1995; **23**: 686–9.

21. Fitzgibbons RE, Shelbourne KD. 'Aggressive' nontreatment of lateral meniscal tears seen during anterior cruciate ligament reconstruction. *Am J Sports Med* 1995; **23**: 156–9.

22. Shelbourne KD, Johnson GE. Locked bucket-handle meniscal tears in knees with chronic anterior cruciate ligament deficiency. *Am J Sports Med* 1993; **21**: 779–82.

23. Hillard-Sembell D, Daniel DM, Stone ML *et al*. Combined injuries of the anterior cruciate and medial collateral ligaments of the knee. Effect of treatment on stability and function of the joint. *J Bone Jt Surg (Am)* 1996; **78**: 169–76.

24. Shelbourne KD, Porter DA. Anterior cruciate ligament – medial collateral ligament injury. Nonoperative management of medial collateral ligament tears with anterior cruciate ligament reconstruction: a preliminary report. *Am J Sports Med* 1992; **20**: 283–6.

25. Brown HR, Indelicato PA. Complications of anterior cruciate ligament reconstruction. *Oper Tech Orthop* 1992; **2**: 125–35.

26. Watanabe BM, Howell SM. Arthroscopic findings associated with roof impingement of an anterior cruciate ligament graft. *Am J Sports Med* 1995; **23**: 616–25.

Chapter 5

1. Gillquist J. Repair and reconstruction of the ACL. Is it good enough? *Arthroscopy* 1993; **9**: 68–71.

2. Jaureguito JW, Paulos LE. Why grafts fail. *Clin Orthop* 1996; **325**: 25–41.

3. Ritchie JR, Parker RD. Graft selection in anterior cruciate ligament revision surgery. *Clin Orthop* 1996; **325**: 65–78.

4. O'Brien WR, Friederich NF. Isometric placement of cruciate ligament substitutes. In: Fagin JA, ed. *The Crucial Ligaments* 2nd edn. New York: Churchill Livingstone 1994: 595-604.

5. Howell SM, Taylor MA. Failure of reconstruction of the anterior cruciate ligament due to impingement by the intercondylar roof. *J Bone Jt Surg (Am)* 1993; **75**: 1044–55.

6. Kurosaka M, Yoshya S, Andrish JT. A biomechanical comparison of different surgical techniques of graft fixation in anterior cruciate reconstruction. *Am J Sports Med* 1987; **15**: 225–9.

7. Shelbourne KD, Nitz P. Accelerated rehabilitation after anterior cruciate ligament reconstruction. *Am J Sports Med* 1990; **18**: 292–9.

8. Harner C (ed). Failed anterior cruciate ligament surgery a symposium. *Clin Orthop* 1996; **325**: 2–130.

9. Frank CB, Jackson DW. The science of reconstruction of the anterior cruciate ligament. *J Bone Jt Surg (Am)* 1997; **79**: 1156–76.

10. Casteleyn PP. Handelberg F. Nonoperative management of anterior cruciate ligament injuries in the general population. *J Bone Jt Surg (Br)* 1996; **78**: 446–51.

11. Andersson C, Odensten M, Good L, Gillquist J. Surgical or non-surgical treatment of acute rupture of the anterior cruciate ligament: a randomised study with long term follow-up. *J Bone Jt Surg (Am)* 1989; **71**: 965–74.

12. Ciccotti MG, Lombardo SJ, Nonweiler B, Pink M. Non-operative treatment of ruptures of the anterior cruciate ligament in middle-aged patients: results after long term follow-up. *J Bone Jt Surg (Am)* 1994; **76**: 1315–26.

13. Daniel DM, Stone ML, Dobson BE *et al.* Fate of the ACL-injured patient: a prospective outcome study. *Am J Sports Med* 1994; **22**: 632–44.

14. Pattee GA, Fox JM, Del Pizzo W, Friedman MJ. Four to ten year follow-up of unreconstructed anterior cruciate ligament tears. *Am J Sports Med* 1989; **17**: 430–5.

15. Shirakura K, Teranchi M, Kizuki S *et al.* The natural history of untreated anterior cruciate ligament tears in recreational athletes. *Clin Orthop* 1995; **317**: 227–36.

16. Noyes FR, Matthews DS *et al.* The symptomatic anterior cruciate deficient knee. Part II: the results of rehabilitation activity modification and counseling on functional disability. *J Bone Jt Surg (Am)* 1983; **65**: 63–74.

17. Rosenberg TD, Paulos LE, Parker RD *et al.* The forty-five degree postero-anterior flexion weight-bearing radiograph of the knee. *J Bone Jt Surg (Am)* 1988; **70**: 1479–83.

18. Outerbridge RE. The aetiology of chrondromalacia patellae. *J Bone Jt Surg (Br)* 1961; **43**: 752–7.

19. Rodeo SA, Arnoczky SP, Torzilli PA *et al.* Tendon healing in a bone tunnel – a biomechanical and histological study in the dog. *J Bone Jt Surg (Am)* 1993; **75**: 1795–1803.

20. Brown CH, Hecker AT, Hipp JA *et al.* The biomechanics of interference screw fixation of patellar tendon anterior cruciate ligament grafts. *Am J Sports Med* 1993; **21**: 880–6.

21. Kohn D, Rose C. Primary stability of interference screw fixation: influence of screw diameter and insertion torque. *Am J Sports Med* 1994; **22**: 334–8.

22. Jonha NM, Raso V, Leung P. Effect of varying angles on the pullout strength of interference screw fixation. *Arthroscopy* 1993; **9**: 580–3.

23. Fink C, Benedetto KP, Hackl W *et al.* Bioabsorbable polyglyconate interference screw fixation in ACL reconstruction: a prospective, CT controlled study presented at 8th Congress of the European Society of Sports Traumatology, Knee Surgery and Arthroscopy April 29 – May 2 1998: Nice, France.

24. Martinek V, Schwanborn T, Thomas M. Bioabsorbable interference screws in ACL reconstruction: a prospective clinical and MRI study. Presented at 8th Congress of the European Society of Sports Traumatology, Knee Surgery and Arthroscopy April 29 – May 2 1998: Nice, France.

25. Steiner ME, Hecker A, Brown CH *et al.* Anterior cruciate ligament graft fixation: comparison of hamstring and patellar tendon grafts. *Am J Sports Med* 1992; **22**: 240–6.

26. Höhes J, Vogrin TM, Withrow JD *et al.* Hamstring graft constructs stretch out under cyclic loading – a biomechanical study. *Arthroscopy* 1993; **9**: 580–3.

27. Giurea M, Amis AA, Aichroth PM, Duri L. Cyclic load testing of anchors used for hamstring tendon ACL reconstructions. Presented at 8th Congress of the European Society of Sports Traumatology, Knee Surgery and Arthroscopy April 29 – May 2 1998: Nice, France.

28. Dye SF. The knee as a biologic transmission with an envelope of function: a theory. *Clin Orthop* 1996; **325**: 10–19.

29. Jenny J-Y, Christel Pascal D, Jian P and French Society for Arthroscopy. Revision arthroscopic anterior cruciate ligament replacement. Presented at 8th Congress of the European Society of Sports Traumatology, Knee Surgery and Arthroscopy April 29 – May 2 1998: Nice, France

30. Safran MR, Harner CD. Technical considerations of revision anterior cruciate ligament surgery. *Clin Orthop* 1996; **325**: 50–64.

31. Johnson DL. Revision anterior cruciate ligament surgery. In: Fu FH, Harner CD, Vince KG, eds. *Knee Surgery Vol 1.* Baltimore: Williams & Wilkins, 1994; 877–95.

32. Frank CB. Future directions of anterior cruciate ligament research. In: Jackson D W, Arnoczky S P (ed). *The Anterior Cruciate Ligament: Current and Future Concepts.* New York: Raven Press; 1993: 4449–50.

33. Dye SF. The future of anterior cruciate ligament restoration. *Clin Orthop* 1996; **325**: 130–9.

Chapter 6

1. Bergfeld JA. Diagnosis and non-operative treatment of acute posterior cruciate ligament injuries. *Instr Course Lect AAOS* 1990; 208.
2. Fanelli GC. Posterior cruciate ligament injuries in trauma patients. *Arthroscopy* 1993; **9**: 291–4.
3. Miller MD, Johnson DL, Harner CD, Fu FH. Posterior cruciate ligament injuries. *Orthop Res* 1993; **22**: 1201–10.
4. Girgis FG, Marshall JL, Monajem ARS. The cruciate ligaments of the knee joint. *Clin Orthop* 1976, **106**: 216–31.
5. De Lee, JC, Riley MB, Rockwood CA. Acute postero-lateral rotatory instability of the knee. *Am J Sports Med* 1983; **11**: 199–207.
6. Nielsen S, Helmig P. The static stabilizing function of the popliteus tendon in the knee. *Arch Orthop Trauma Surg* 1986; **104**: 357–62.
7. Gollehon DL, Torzilla P, Warren RF. The role of the postero-lateral and cruciate ligaments in the stability of the human knee. A biomechanical study. *J Bone Jt Surg (Am)* 1987; **69**: 233–42.
8. Cross MJ, Powell JF. Long-term follow-up of posterior cruciate rupture: a study of 116 cases. *Am J Sports Med* 1984; **12**: 292–7.
9. Torg JS, Barton TM, Pavlov H, Stine R. Natural history of the posterior cruciate deficient knee. *Clin Orthop* 1989; **246**: 208–16.
10. Dandy D, Pusey R. The long term results of unrepaired tears of the posterior cruciate ligament. *J Bone Jt Surg (Br)* 1982; **64**: 92–4.
11. Fowler PJ, Messieh SS. Isolated posterior cruciate injuries in athletes. *Am J Sports Med* 1987; **15**: 553–7.
12. Insall JN, Hood RM. Bone-block transfer of the medial head of the gastrocnemius for posterior cruciate insufficiency. *J Bone Jt Surg (Am)* 1982; **64**: 691–9.
13. Dejour H, Walch G, Peyrot J, Eberhard P. The natural history of the rupture of the posterior cruciate ligament. *Orthop Trans* 1987; **11**: 146.
14. Keller PM, Shelbourne D, McCaroll JR, Rettig AC. Non operatively treated isolated posterior cruciate ligament injuries. *Am J Sports Med* 1993; **21**: 132–6.
15. Rubinstein RA, Shelbourne KD. Diagnosis of posterior cruciate ligament injuries and indications for non-operative and operative treatment. *Operative Tech Sports Med* 1993; **1**: 99–103.
16. Clancy WG, Shelbourne KD, Zoellner GB. Treatment of knee joint instability secondary to the rupture of the posterior cruciate ligament. *J Bone Jt Surg (Am)* 1983; **65**: 310–22.
17. Shelbourne KD, Rubinstein RA. Methodist Sports Centre's experience with acute and chronic isolated posterior cruciate ligament injuries. *Clin Sports Med* 1994; **13**: 531–43.
18. Jakob RP, Hassler H, Staübli H-U. Observations on rotatory instability of the lateral compartment of the knee – experimental studies on the functional anatomy and pathomechanism of the true and reverse pivot shift sign. *Acta Orthop Scand* 1981; **191(Suppl)**: 6–27.
19. Hughston JC, Norwood LA. The posterolateral drawer test and external rotational recurvation test for postero-lateral rotatory instability of the knee. *Clin Orthop Rel Res* **147**: 82–7.
20. Sonin AM, Fitzgerald SM, Hoff FL *et al*. Imaging of the posterior cruciate ligament. Normal, abnormal and associated injury patterns. *Radiographics* 1995; **15**: 55–61.
21. Spindler KP, Benson EM. Natural history of posterior cruciate ligament injury. *Sports Med Arthrosc Rev* 1994; **2**: 73–80.
22. Parolie JM, Bergfeld JA. Long term results of non-operative treatment of isolated posterior cruciate ligament injuries in the athlete. *Am J Sports Med* 1986; **14**: 35–8.
23. Trickey EL. Injuries to the posterior cruciate ligament: diagnosis and treatment of early injuries and reconstruction of late instability. *Clin Orthop Rel Res* 1980; **147**: 76–81.
24. Bousquet G, Charmion L, Passot JP *et al*. Stabilization du condyle externe du genou dans les laxites anterieurs chronique. Importance du muscle poplitie. *Rev Chir Orthop* 1986; **72**: 427–34.
25. Hughston JC, Jacobson KE. Chronic postero-lateral rotatory instability of the knee. *J Bone Jt Surg (Am)* 1985; **67**: 351–9.
26. Sidles JA, Larson RV, Garbini J. Ligament length relationships in the moving knee. *J Orthop Res* 1988; **6**: 593–610.
27. Clancy WG. Repair and reconstruction of the posterior cruciate ligament. In: Chapman M, ed. *Operative Orthopaedics*. Philadelphia: Lippincott, 1988: 1651–66.
28. Staübli H-U, Birrer S. The popliteus tendon and its fascicles at the popliteus hiatus: gross anatomy and functional arthroscopic evaluation with or without anterior cruciate ligament deficiency. *Arthroscopy* 1990; **6**: 209–20.

Chapter 7

1. O'Brien SJ, Warren RF, Paulou H *et al*. Reconstruction of the chronically insufficient anterior cruciate ligament with the central third of the patellar ligament. *J Bone Jt Surg (Am)* 1991; **73**: 278–85.
2. Butler DL, Noyes FR, Grood ES. Ligamentous restraints to anterior–posterior drawer in the human knee. *J Bone Jt Surg (Am)* 1980; **62**: 259–70.
3. Allen AA, Harner CD, Fu FH. Anatomy and biomechanics of the posterior cruciate ligament. *Sports Med Arthrosc Rev* 1994; **2**: 81–7.
4. Slocum DB, Larson RL, James SL. Late reconstruction of the injuries of the medial compartment of the knee. *Clin Orthop* 1974; **100**: 23–55.
5. Kaplan EB. The fabello-fibular and short lateral ligaments of the knee joint. *J Bone Jt Surg (Am)* 1961; **43**: 169–71.
6. Seebacher JR, Inglis AE, Marshall JL, Warren RF. The structure of the postero-lateral aspect of the knee. *J Bone Jt Surg (Am)* 1982; **64**: 536–41.
7. Grana WA, Janssen T. Lateral ligament injury of the knee. *Orthopaedics* 1987; **10**: 1039–44.
8. Johnson LL. Lateral capsular ligament complex. Anatomical and surgical considerations. *Am J Sports Med* 1979; **7**: 156–60.
9. Gollehon DC, Torzilli PA, Warren RF. The role of the postero-lateral and cruciate ligaments in stability of the human knee. A biomechanical study. *J Bone Jt Surg (Am)* 1987; **69**: 233–42.
10. Grood ES, Stowers SF, Noyes FR. Limits of movement in the human knee. Effects of sectioning the posterior cruciate ligament and postero-lateral structures. *J Bone Jt Surg (Am)* 1988; **70**: 88–97.

11. Wroble RR, Grood ES, Cummings JS. The role of the lateral extra-articular restraints in the anterior cruciate deficient knee. *Am J Sports Med* 1993; **21**: 257–63

12. Shields L, Mital M, Cave EF. Complex dislocation of the knee: experience at the Massachusetts General Hospital. *J Trauma* 1969; **9**: 192–215.

13. Meyers MH, Moore TM, Harvey JP Jr. Traumatic dislocation of the knee joint. *J Bone Jt Surg (Am)* 1975; **57**: 430–3.

14. Sisto DJ, Warren RF. Complete knee dislocations. A follow-up study of operative treatment. *Clin Orthop* 1985; **198**: 94–101.

15. Noyes FR, Dunworth LA, Andriacchi TP *et al.* Knee hyperextension gait abnormality in unstable knees. Recognition and preoperative gait retraining. *Am J Sports Med* 1996; **4**: 35–45.

16. Hughston JC, Norwood LA. The postero-lateral drawer test and external rotation recurvation test for postero-lateral rotatory instability of the knee. *Clin Orthop* 1980; **147**: 82–7.

17. Jakob P, Staübli H-U. The reversed pivot shift sign – a new diagnostic aid for postero-lateral rotatory instability of the knee: its distinction from the true pivot shift sign. *Orthop Trans* 1981; **5**: 587.

18. Warren LF, Marshall JJ. The supporting structures and layers on the medial side of the knee. *J Bone Jt Surg (Am)* 1979; **61**: 56–62.

19. Watanabe Y, Morriya H, Takahasi K *et al.* Functional anatomy of the postero-lateral structures of the knee. *Arthroscopy* 1993; **9**: 57.

20. Tria AJ, Klein KS. *An Illustrated Guide to the Knee.* New York: Churchill Livingstone, 1992: 84.

21. Hughston JC, Jacobson KE. Chronic postero-lateral rotatory instability of the knee. *J Bone Jt Surg (Am)* 1985; **67**: 351–9.

22. Muller W. *The Knee: Form, Function and Ligament Reconstruction.* Berlin: Springer-Verlag, 1983.

23. Noyes FR, Barber-Westin SD. Surgical restoration to treat chronic deficiency of the postero-lateral complex and cruciate ligaments of the knee joint. *Am J Sports Med* 1996; **24**; 415–26.

24. Noyes FR, Roberts CS. High tibial osteotomy in knees with associated chronic ligament deficiencies. In: Jackson DW, ed. *Master Techniques in Orthopaedic Surgery. Reconstructive Knee Surgery.* New York: Raven Press, 1995: 185–210.

25. Jakob RP. Posterior, postero-lateral and postero-medial instability of the knee. Diagnosis and treatment. In: *European Institute Course Lecture.* London: British Editorial Society of Bone and Joint Surgery, 1995(2): 27–40.

26. Dandy DJ, Pusey RJ. The long term results of unrepaired tears of the posterior cruciate ligament. *J Bone Jt Surg (Br)* 1982; **6**: 92–4.

27. Torg JS, Barton TM, Pavlov H, Stine R. Natural history of the posterior cruciate ligament deficient knee. *Clin Orthop* 1989; **246**; 208–16.

28. Keller PM, Shelbourne KD, McCarroll JR, Rettig AC. Non-operatively treated isolated posterior cruciate ligament injuries. *Am J Sports Med* 1993; **21**: 132–6.

29. Green NE, Allen BL. Vascular injuries associated with dislocations of the knee. *J Bone Jt Surg (Am)* 1977; **59**: 236–9.

30. Taylor AR, Arden GP, Rainey HA. Traumatic dislocations of the knee. A report of 43 cases with special reference to conservative treatment. *J Bone Jt Surg (Br)* 1972; **54**: 96–102.

31. Frassica FJ, Sim FH, Staeheli JW, Pairolero PC. Dislocation of the knee. *Clin Orthop* 1991; **263**; 200–5.

32. Insall JN, Windsor RE, Scott WN *et al.*, eds. *Surgery of the knee* (2nd edn). New York: Churchill Livingstone, 1993.

Chapter 8

1. Arrol B, Ellis-Pegler E, Edwards A, Sutcliffe G. Patello-femoral pain syndrome. A critical review of the clinical trials on non-operative therapy. *Am J Sports Med* 1997; **25**: 207–12.

2. Merchant AC. Classification of patello-femoral disorders. *Arthroscopy* 1988; **4**: 235.

3. Powers CM, Maffucci R, Hampton S. Rearfoot posture in subjects with patello-femoral pain. *J Orthop Sports Phys Ther* 1995; **22**: 155–60.

4. Ficat P, Ficat C, Bailleux A. Syndrome d'hyperpression externe de la rotule (SHPE): son interet pour la connaissance de l'arthrose. *Rev Chir Orthop* 1975; **61**: 39–59.

5. Winslow J, Yoder E, Patello-femoral pain in female ballet dancers: correlation with iliotibial band tightness and tibial external rotation. *J Orthop Sports Phys Ther* 1995; **22**: 18–21.

6. Cicuttini FM, Baker J, Hart DJ, Spector TD. Choosing the best method for radiological assessment of patello-femoral osteo-arthritis. *Ann Rheum Dis* 1996; **55(2)**: 134–6.

7. Beaconsfield T, Pintore E, Maffulli N, Petri GJ. Radiological measurements in patello-femoral disorders. A review. *Clin Orthop* 1994; **308**: 18–28.

8. Popp JE, Yu JS, Kaeding CC. Recalcitrant patellar tendinitis. Magnetic resonance imaging, histologic evaluation and surgical treatment. *Am J Sports Med* 1997; **25**: 218–22.

9. Dye SF, Boss DA. Radionuclide imaging of the patello-femoral joint in young adults with anterior knee pain. *Orthop Clin North Am* 1986; **17**: 249.

10. Jones RB, Barlett EC, Vainright JR, Carroll RG. CT determination of tibial tubercle lateralization in patients presenting with anterior knee pain. *Skeletal Radiol* 1995; **24**: 505–9.

11. Kannus P, Niittywaki S. Which factors predict outcome in the non-operative treatment of patello-femoral pain syndrome? A prospective follow-up study. *Med Sci Sports Exerc* 1994; **26**: 289–96.

12. Callaghan MJ, Oldham JA. The role of quadriceps exercise in the treatment of patello-femoral pain syndrome. *Sports Med* 1996; **21**: 384–91.

13. Harrison E, Magee D, Quinney H. Development of a clinical tool and patient questionnaire for evaluation of patello-femoral pain syndrome patients. *Clin J Sport Med* 1996; **6**: 163–70.

14. McConnell J. The management of chondromalacia patellae: a long-term solution. *Aust J Physiother* 1986; **32**: 215.

15. Witvrouw E, Sneyers C, Lysens R *et al.* Reflex response times of vastus medialis oblique and vastus lateralis in normal subjects and in subjects with patello-femoral pain syndrome. *J Orthop Sports Phys Ther* 1996; **24**: 160–5.

16. Stiene HA, Brosky T, Reinking MF *et al.* A comparison of closed kinetic chain and isokinetic joint isolation exercise in patients with patello-femoral dysfunction. *J Orthop Sports Phys Ther* 1996; **24**: 136–41.

17. Cushnaghan J, McCarthy C, Dieppe P. Taping the patella medially: a new treatment for osteo-arthritis of the knee joint? *Br Med J* 1994; **308**: 753–5.

18. Kowall MG, Kolk G, Nuber GW *et al*. Patellar taping in the treatment of patello-femoral pain. A prospective randomized study. *Am J Sports Med* 1996; **24**: 61–6.
19. Greenwald AE, Bagley AM, France EP *et al*. A biomechanical and clinical evaluation of a patello-femoral knee brace. *Clin Orthop* 1996; **324**: 187–95.
20. Bentley G. Anterior knee pain: diagnosis and management. *J R Coll Surg Edinb* 1989; **2**: S2-3.
21. Fulkerson JP, Shea KP. Disorders of patello-femoral alignment. *J Bone Jt Surg (Am)* 1990; **72**: 1424.
22. Kinnard P, Levesque RY. The plica syndrome: a syndrome of controversy. *Clin Orthop* 1984; **183**: 141.
23. Matsusue Y, Yamamuro T, Hama H *et al*. Symptomatic type D (separated) medial plica: clinical features and surgical results. *Arthroscopy* 1994; **10**: 281–5.
24. Fulkerson JP, Hungerford DS. Patellar subluxation. In: Fulkerson JP, Buuck DA, Post WR, eds. *Disorders of the Patellofemoral Joint*, 3rd edn. Baltimore: Lippincott, Williams & Wilkins 1996: 175–97.
25. Henry JE, Pflum FA Jr. Arthroscopic proximal patella realignment and stabilization. *Arthroscopy* 1995; **11**: 424–5.
26. Shelbourne KD, Porter DA, Rozzi W. Use of a modified Elsmslie–Traillat procedure to improve abnormal patellar congruence angle. *Am J Sports Med* 1994; **22**: 318–23.
27. Mori Y, Okumo H, Iketani H, Kuroki Y. Efficacy of lateral retinacular release for painful bipartite patella. *Am J Sports Med* 1995; **23**: 13–18.
28. Macquet P. Advancement of the tibial tuberosity. *Clin Orthop* 1976; **115**: 225.
29. Jenny J-Y, Sader Z, Henry A *et al*. Elevation of the tibial tubercle for patello-femoral pain syndrome. An 8–15 year follow-up. *Knee Surg Sports Traumatol Arthrosc* 1996; **4**: 92–6.
30. Miller JB, Larochelle PJ. The treatment of patello-femoral pain by combined rotation and elevation of the tibial tubercle. *J Bone Jt Surg (Am)* 1986; **68**: 419.
31. Fulkerson JP. Anteromedialization of the tibial tuberosity for patellofemoral malalignment. *Clin Orthop* 1983; **177**: 176–81.
32. Fulkerson JP, Becker GJ, Meaney JA *et al*. Anteromedial tibial tubercle transfer without bone graft. *Am J Sports Med* 1990; **18**: 490.
33. Morshuis WJ, Pavlov PW, De Rooy KP. Anteromedialization of the tibial tuberosity in the treatment of patello-femoral pain and malalignment. *Clin Orthop* 1990; **255**: 242.
34. Morsher E. Osteotomy of patella in chondromalacia patellae. *Arch Orthop Trauma Surg* 1978; **92**: 139.
35. Hejgaard N, Arnoldi CC. Osteotomy of the patella in the patello-femoral pain syndrome. The significance of increased intra-osseous pressure during sustained knee flexion. *Int Orthop* 1984; **8**: 189–94.
36. Kelly MA, Insall JN. Patellectomy. *Orthop Clin North Am* 1986; **17**: 289.
37. Lennox IA, Cobb AG, Knowles J, Bentley G. Knee function after patellectomy. A 12–48 year follow-up. *J Bone Jt Surg (Br)* 1994; **76**: 485–7.
38. Watkins MP, Harris BA, Wender S *et al*. Effect of patellectomy on the function of the quadriceps and hamstrings. *J Bone Jt Surg (Am)* 1983; **65**: 390.
39. Feller JA, Bartlett RJ. Patellectomy and osteo-arthritis: arthroscopic findings following previous patellectomy. *Knee Surg Sports Traumatol Arthrosc* 1993; **1**: 159–61.

Chapter 9

1. Brattstrom H. Shape of the intercondylar groove normally and in recurrent dislocation of the patella. *Acta Orthop Scand* 1964; **68(Suppl)**.
2. Lloyd-Roberts GC, Thomas TG. The etiology of quadriceps contracture in children. *J Bone Jt Surg (Br)* 1964; **46**: 498–502.
3. Goutallier D, Bernageau J, Lecudonnec B. Mesure de l'écart tuberosité tibiale antérieure – gorge de la trochlée (TA–GT): technique, résultats, intérêt. *Rev Chir Orthop* 1978; **64**: 423–8.
4. Coleman HM. Recurrent osteochondral fracture of the patella. *J Bone Jt Surg (Br)* 1948; **30**: 153–7.
5. Insall JN, Salvati E. Patella position in the normal knee joint. *Radiology* 1971; **101**: 101–4.
6. Blackburne JS, Peel TE. A new method of measuring patellar height. *J Bone Jt Surg (Br)* 1977; **59**: 241–2.
7. Caton J, Mironneau A, Walch C *et al*. Adolescent idiopathic patella alta: a review of 61 cases treated surgically. *French J Orthop Surg* 1990; **4**: 196–203.
8. Dejour H, Walch G, Nove-Josserand L, Guier C. Factors of patellar instability: an anatomic radiologic study. *Knee Surg Sports Traumatol Arthrosc* 1994; **2**: 19–26.
9. Blumensaat C. Die Lageabuweichungen und Verrenkurigan der Kniescheibe. *Ergebnisse Chir Orthop* 1938; **31**: 149–223.
10. Merchant AC, Mercer RL, Jacobsen RH, Cool CR. Roentgenographic analysis of patellofemoral congruence. *J Bone Jt Surg (Am)* 1974; **56**: 1391–6.
11. Dandy DJ. *Arthroscopy of the Knee: A Diagnostic Atlas.* London: Gower-Butterworth, 1984.
12. Dandy DJ, Griffiths D. Lateral release for recurrent dislocation of the patella. *J Bone Jt Surg (Br)* 1989; **71**: 121–5.
13. Hauser EDW. Total tendon transplant for slipping patella. *Surg Gynecol Obstet* 1938; **66**: 199–214.
14. Maquet P. Advancement of the tibial tuberosity. *Clin Orthop* 1974; **115**: 225–7.
15. Dandy DJ, Desai SS. The results of arthroscopic lateral release of the extensor mechanism for recurrent dislocation of the patella after 8 years. *Arthroscopy* 1994; **10**: 540–5.
16. Albee FH. *Orthopaedic and Reconstructive Surgery.* Philadelphia: W B Saunders, 1919: 627.
17. Goldthwait JE. Slipping or recurrent dislocation of the patella with a report of eleven cases. *Boston Med Surg J* 1904; **150**: 169–74.
18. Nakamura N, Ellis M, Seedhom BB. Advancement of the tibial tuberosity: a biomechanical study. *J Bone Jt Surg (Br)* 1985; **67**: 255–60.
19. Fulkerson JP. Anteromedial tibial tubercle transfer without bone graft. *Am J Sports Med* 1982; **10**: 47.
20. Dandy DJ. *Arthroscopic Management of the Knee*, 2nd edn. Edinburgh: Churchill Livingstone, 1987.
21. Metcalf RW. An arthroscopic method for lateral release of the subluxating and dislocating patella. *Clin Orthop* 1982; **167**: 11–18.
22. Conn HR. A new method for operative reduction of congenital luxation of the patella. *J Bone Jt Surg* 1925; **7**: 370–3.
23. Green JP, Waugh W. Congenital lateral dislocation of the patella. *J Bone Jt Surg (Br)* 1968; **50**: 285–9.
24. Fielding JW, Liebler WA, Tambakis A. The effect of a tibial tubercle transplant in children on the growth of the upper tibial epiphysis. *J Bone Jt Surg (Am)* 1960; **42**: 1426–34.

25. Pappas AM, Anas P, Toczylowski HM. Asymmetrical arrest of the proximal tibial epiphysis and genu recurvatum deformity. *J Bone Jt Surg (Am)* 1984; **66**: 575–81.
26. Baker RH, Carrol N, Dewar P, Hall JE. Semitendinosus tenodesis for recurrent dislocation of the patella. *J Bone Jt Surg (Br)* 1972; **54**: 103–9.
27. Carter C, Sweetnam R. Familial joint laxity and recurrent dislocation of the patella. *J Bone Jt Surg (Br)* 1958; **40**: 664–7.
28. Dandy DJ. Recurrent subluxation of the patella on extension of the knee. *J Bone Jt Surg (Br)* 1971; **53**: 483–7.
29. Jackson AM. Recurrent dislocation of the patella. *J Bone Jt Surg (Br)* 1994; **74**: 2–4.
30. Crosby EB, Insall JN. Recurrent dislocation of the patella. *J Bone Jt Surg (Am)* 1976; **58**: 9–13.

Chapter 10

1. St-Pierre DM. Rehabilitation following arthroscopic meniscectomy. *Sports Med* 1995; **20**: 338–47.
2. Thompson WO, Fu FH. *Clin Sport Med* 1993; **12**: 771–96.
3. Annandale T. An operation for displaced semilunar cartilage. *Br Med J* 1885; **1**: 779.
4. Quigley TB. Knee injuries incurred in sports. *J Am Med Surg* 1959; **171**: 1666.
5. Smillie JS. *Injuries of the Knee Joint*. 4th edn. Edinburgh: Churchill Livingstone, 1971; 68.
6. Jackson JP. Degenerative changes in the knee after meniscectomy. *Br Med J* 1968; **2**: 525–7.
7. Fairbank TJ. Knee joint changes after meniscectomy. *J Bone Jt Surg (Br)* 1948; **30**: 664–70.
8. Tapper EM, Hover NW. Late results after meniscectomy. *J Bone Jt Surg (Am)* 1969; **51**: 517–26.
9. Medlar RC, Manidberg JJ, Lyne ED. Meniscectomies in children – a report of long term results. *Am J Sports Med* 1980; **8**: 87–92.
10. Clark CR, Ogden JA. Development of the menisci of the human knee joint. *J Bone Jt Surg (Am)* 1983; **65**: 538–47.
11. Aspen RM, Yarker YE, Hukins DWL. Collagen orientations in the meniscus of the knee joint. *J Anat* 1985; **140**: 371–380.
12. Shim SS, Leung G. Blood supply of the knee joint. A microangiographic study in children and adults. *Clin Orthop* 1986; **208**: 119–25.
13. Arnoczky SP, Warren RF. Microvasculature of the human meniscus. *Am J Sports Med* 1982; **10**: 90–5.
14. Danzig L, Resnick D, Gonsalves M, Akeson WH. Blood supply to the normal and abnormal menisci of the human knee. *Clin Orthop* 1983; **172**: 271.
15. Cipolla M, Cerullo G, Puddu G. Microvasculature of the human medial meniscus: operative findings. *Arthroscopy* 1992; **8**: 522–5.
16. Cabaud H, Rodkey W, Fitzwater J. Medial meniscal repairs: an experimental and morphologic study. *Am J Sports Med* 1981; **19**: 129.
17. Johnson RJ, Kettelkamp DB, Clark W, Leaverton P. Factors affecting late results after meniscectomy. *J Bone Jt Surg (Am)* 1974; **56**: 719–29.
18. McDevitt C, Webber R. The ultrastructure and biochemistry of the meniscal cartilage. *Clin Orthop* 1990; **252**: 8–18.
19. Renstrom P, Johnson R. Anatomy and biomechanics of the menisci. *Clin Sports Med* 1990; **9**: 523–38.
20. Bullough PG, Munueral L, Murphy J, Weinstein AM. The strength of the menisci of the knee as it relates to their fine structure. *J Bone Jt Surg (Br)* 1970; **52**: 564–70.
21. Brady O, Hurson B. Acute injuries of the meniscus. In: *Oxford Textbook of Sports Medicine*. Oxford: Oxford Medical Publishing, 1998, 342–62.
22. Verdonk R. Alternative treatments for meniscal injuries. *J Bone Jt Surg (Br)* 1997; **79**: 866–73.
23. Swenson T, Harner C. Knee ligament and meniscal injuries, current concepts. *Orthop Clin North Am* 1995; **26**: 529–46.
24. Walker P, Erkman MJ. The role of the menisci in force transmission across the knee. *Clin Orthop* 1975; **252**: 8–18.
25. Simpson DA, Thomas NP, Aichroth PM. Open and closed meniscectomy. A comparative analysis. *J Bone Jt Surg* 1986; **68**: 301–4.
26. Levy I, Torzolli P, Warren R. The effect of medial meniscectomy on the anterior-posterior motion of the knee joint. *J Bone Jt Surg (Am)* 1989; **71**: 401.
27. Baker BE, Peckham AC, Pupparo F, Sanborn JC. Review of meniscal injury and associated sports. *Am J Sports Med* 1985; **13**: 1.
28. Ciccotti M, Shields C, El Attache N. Meniscectomy. In: Fu F, Harner C, Vance K, eds. *Knee Surgery*. Baltimore: Williams & Wilkins, 1994: 602.
29. Noyes FR, Bassett RW, Grood ES, Butler DL. Arthroscopy in acute traumatic haemarthrosis of the knee: incidence of anterior cruciate tears and other injuries. *J Bone Jt Surg (Am)* 1980; **62**: 687–95.
30. Rappeport ED, Wieslander SB, Stephensen S, Lausten GS, Thomsen HS. MRI preferable to diagnostic arthroscopy in knee joint injuries. *Acta Orthop Scand* 1997; **68**: 277–81.
31. Mackenzie R, Palmer CR, Lomas DJ, Dixon AK. Magnetic resonance imaging of the knee: diagnostic performance studies. *Clin Radiol* 1996; **51**: 251–7.
32. Andrade A, Thomas NP. Correlation of MRI and operative finding in injuries to the MPFL. Poster ESSKA, Nice, 1998.
33. DeHaven KE. Decision making factors in the treatment of meniscal lesions. *Clin Orthop* 1990; **252**: 49–54.
34. Weiss CB, Lundberg M, Hamberg P *et al*. Non-operative treatment of meniscal tears. *J Bone Jt Surg (Am)* 1989; **71**: 811.
35. Metcalf R. Operative arthroscopy of the knee. *Am Acad Orthop Surg Instruct Course Lectures* 1981; **30**: 357.
36. Cox JS, Nye CE, Schafer WW *et al*. The degenerative effects of partial and total resection of the medial meniscus in dogs' knees. *Clin Orthop* 1975; **109**: 178–83.
37. Baratz ME, Fu FH, Mengato R. Meniscal tears: the effect of meniscectomy and of repair on the intra-articular contact areas and stresses in the human knee. *Am J Sports Med* 1988; **16**: 1.
38. Seedholm BB. Transmission of the load in the knee joint with special reference to the role of the menisci: I. Anatomy, analysis, and apparatus. *Eng Med* 1979; **8**: 207–19.
39. Seedholm BB, Hargreaves DJ. Transmission of the load in the knee joint with special reference to the role of the menisci: II. Experimental results, discussion, and conclusion. *Eng Med* 1979; **8**: 220.
40. Jackson RW, Dandy DJ. Partial meniscectomy. *J Bone Jt Surg (Am)* 1976; **58**: 87.
41. McGinty JB, Guess LF, Marvin RA. Partial or total meniscectomy. *J Bone Jt Surg (Am)* 1977; **59**: 763.

42. Northmore-Ball MD, Dandy DJ, Jackson RW. Arthroscopic, open partial and total meniscectomy: a comparative study. *J Bone Jt Surg (Br)* 1983; **65**: 400.

43. Dandy DJ, Jackson RW. The diagnosis of problems after meniscectomy. *J Bone Jt Surg (Br)* 1975; **57**: 349.

44. Schimmer RC, Brulhart KB, Duff C, Glinz W. Arthroscopic partial meniscectomy: a 12-year follow-up and two-step valuation of the long-term course. *Arthroscopy* 1998; **14**: 136–42.

45. King D. The healing of semilunar cartilages. *J Bone Jt Surg (Am)* 1936; **18**: 333.

46. Henning CE, Lynch MA, Clark JR. Vascularity for healing of meniscal repairs. *Arthroscopy* 1987; **3**: 13–18.

47. Miller M, Warner J, Harner C. Meniscal repair. In: Fu F, Harner C, Vince K, eds. *Knee Surgery*. Baltimore: Williams & Wilkins, 1994: 616.

48. DeHaven KE, Loher WA, Lovelock JE. Long-term results of open meniscal tear. *Am J Sports Med* 1995; **23**: 524–30.

49. Henning C. Arthroscopic repair of meniscal tears. *Orthopaedics* 1983; **6**: 1130.

50. Barrett GR, Richardson K, Ruff CG, Jones A. The effect of suture type on meniscus repair. A clinical analysis. *Am J Knee Surg* 1997; **10**: 2–9.

51. Asik M, Sener N, Akpinar S *et al.* Strength of different meniscus suturing techniques. *Knee Surg Sport Traumatol Arthrosc* 1997; **5**: 80–3.

52. Post WR, Akers SR, Kish V. Load to failure of common meniscal repair techniques: effects of suture technique and suture material. *Arthroscopy* 1997; **13**: 731–6.

53. Morgan C. The 'all-inside' meniscus repair: technical note. *Arthroscopy* 1991; **7**: 120.

54. Escalas F, Quadras J, Caceres E, Benaddi J. T-fix anchor sutures for arthroscopic meniscal repair. *Knee Surg Sport Traumatol Arthrosc* 1997; **5**: 72–6.

55. Koukoubis TD, Glisson RR, Feagin JA Jr *et al.* Meniscal fixation with an absorbable staple. An experimental study in dogs. *Knee Surg Sport Traumatol Arthrosc* 1997; **5**: 22–30.

56. Albrecht-Olsen P, Lind T, Kristensen G, Falkenberg B. Failure strength of a new meniscus arrow technique: biomechanical comparison with horizontal suture. *Arthroscopy* 1997; **13**: 183–7.

57. Kristensen G *et al.* Biofix-meniscus tacks versus inside-out suturing technique in the treatment of bucket-handle lesions: a random study. *Acta Orthop Scand* 1994; **65(Suppl 260)**.

58. Dervin GF, Downing KJ, Keene GC, McBride DG. Failure strengths of suture versus biodegradable arrow for meniscal repair: an in-vitro study. *Arthroscopy* 1997; **13**: 296–300.

59. Arnoczky S, Warren R, Spivak J. Meniscal repair using an exogenous fibrin clot: an experimental study in dogs. *J Bone Jt Surg (Am)* 1988; **70**: 1209.

60. Henning C, Lynch M, Yearout K *et al.* Arthroscopic meniscal repair using exogenous fibrin clot. *Clin Orthop* 1990; **252**: 64.

61. Rubman MH, Noyes FR, Barber-Westin SD. Arthroscopic repair of meniscal tears that extend into the avascular zone. A review of 198 single and complex tears. *Am J Sports Med* 1998; **26**: 87–95.

62. DeHaven KE. Diagnosis of acute knee injuries with haemarthrosis. *Am J Sport Med* 1980; **8**: 9.

63. Warren RF. Meniscectomy and repair in the anterior cruciate ligament deficient patient. *Clin Orthop* 1990; **252**: 55–63.

64. Rosenberg T, Scott S, Coward D. Arthroscopic meniscal repair evaluated by second look arthroscopy. *Arthroscopy* 1986; **2**: 20.

65. Cannon W, Vittori J. The incidence of healing in arthroscopic meniscal repairs in anterior cruciate ligament reconstructed knees. *Am J Sport Med* 1992; **20**: 176.

66. Ochi M, Kanda T, Sumne Y, Ikuta Y. Changes in the permeability and histologic findings of the rabbit menisci after immobilization. *Clin Orthop* 1997; **334**: 305–15.

67. Dowdy PA, Miniaci A, Arnoczky SP *et al.* The effect of cast immobilisation on meniscal healing. An experimental study in the dog. *Am J Sports Med* 1995; **23**: 721–8.

68. Barber FA, Click SD. Meniscus repair rehabilitation with concurrent anterior cruciate reconstruction. *Arthroscopy* 1997; **13**: 433–7.

69. Harner C. Personal communication.

70. Paletta GA Jr, Manning T, Snell E *et al.* The effect of allograft meniscal replacement on intraarticular contact area and pressures in the human knee. A biomechanical study. *Am J Sports Med* 1997; **25**: 692–8.

71. Gao J, Messner K. Natural healing of anterior and posterior attachments of the rabbit meniscus. *Clin Orthop* 1996; **328**: 276–84.

72. Hamlet W, Lui SH, Yang R. Destruction of a cryopreserved meniscal allograft: a case for acute rejection. *Arthroscopy* 1997; **13**: 517–21.

73. Arnoczky SP, DiCarlo EF, O'Brien SJ, Warren RF. Cellular repopulation of deep-frozen meniscal allografts: an experimental study in the dog. *Arthroscopy* 1992; **8**: 428–36.

74. Arnoczky SP, Warren RF, McDevitt CA. Meniscal replacement using a cryopreserved allograft: an experimental study in the dog. *Clin Orthop* 1990; **252**: 121–8.

75. Stone KR, Steadman JR, Rodkey WG, Li ST. Regeneration of meniscal cartilage with use of a collagen scaffold. Analysis of preliminary data. *J Bone Jt Surg (Am)* 1997; **79**: 1770–7.

76. Stone KR, Rodkey WG, Webber RJ *et al.* Future directions: collagen-based prostheses for meniscal regeneration. *Clin Orthop* 1990; **252**: 129–35.

77. Mooney MF, Rosenberg TD. Meniscus repair, the inside-out technique. In: Jackson DW, ed. Reconstructive Knee Surgery. Philadelphia: Raven Press, 1995: 81.

Chapter 11

1. Paget J. On the production of some of the loose bodies in joints. *St Bartholomew's Hosp Reports* 1870; **6**: 1–4.

2. König F. Euber freie Körper in den Gelenken. *Deutsche Zeitchr Chir Leipz* 1887–1888; **27**: 90–109.

3. Fairbank HAT. Osteochondritis dissecans. *Br J Surg* 1933; **21**: 67–82.

4. Smillie IS. *Osteochondritis Dissecans: Loose Bodies in Joints: Aetiology, Pathology, Treatment.* Edinburgh: E & S Livingstone, 1960.

5. Aichroth PM. Osteochondritis dissecans of the knee: a clinical survey. *J Bone Jt Surg (Br)* 1971; **53**: 440–7.

6. Wilson JN. A diagnostic sign in osteochondritis dissecans of the knee. *J Bone Jt Surg (Am)* 1967; **49**: 447–80.

7. Bradley J, Dandy DJ. Osteochondritis dissecans and other lesions of the femoral condyles. *J Bone Jt Surg (Br)* 1989; **71**: 518–22.

8. Kennedy JC, Grainger RW, McGraw RW. Osteochondritis dissecans fractures of the femoral condyles. *J Bone Jt Surg (Br)* 1966; **48**: 436–40.

9. Landells JW. The reactions of injured human articular cartilage. *J Bone Jt Surg (Br)* 1957; **39**: 548–62.
10. Aichroth PM. Osteochondral fractures and their relationship to osteochondritis dissecans of the knee: an experimental study in animals. *J Bone Jt Surg (Br)* 1971; **53**: 448–54.
11. Bradley J, Dandy DJ. Results of drilling osteochondritis dissecans before skeletal maturity. *J Bone Jt Surg (Br)* 1989; **71**: 642–4.
12. Patel JV, Murphy JP, Aichroth PM. Results of Orthosorb pin fixation of osteochondritis dissecans in the knee: a preliminary report. *The Knee* 1996; **3**: 41–4.
13. Homminga GN, Bulstra SK, Bouwmeester PSM. Perichondrial grafting for cartilage lesions of the knee. *J Bone Jt Surg (Br)* 1990.
14. Stone KR, Walgenbach A. Surgical technique for articular cartilage transplantation to full thickness cartilage defects in the knee joint. *Oper Tech Orthop* 1997; **7**: 305–11.
15. Hangody L, Karpati Z, Szigati I, Sukosk L. Clinical experience with the Mosaic technique. *Rev Osteol* 1996; **4**: 32–6.
16. Bobic V. Arthroscopic osteochondral autograft transplantation in anterior cruciate ligament reconstruction: a preliminary study. *Knee Surg Sports Traumatol Arthrosc* 1996; **3**: 262–4.
17. Aston J, Bentley G. Repair of articular surfaces by allografts of articular and growth-plate cartilage. *J Bone Jt Surg (Br)* 1986; **68**: 29–35.
18. Brittberg M, Lindahl A, Nilsson A *et al.* Treatment of deep cartilaginous defects of the knee with autologous chondrocyte transplantation. *N Engl J Med* 1994; **33**: 889–95.
19. Beaver RJ, Gross AE. Fresh small-fragment osteoarticular allografts in the joint. In: Aichroth PM, Cannon WD, eds. *Knee Surgery Current Practice.* London: M Dunitz 1992; 464–71.
20. Totoritis M. Cartilage Allografts. In: *Recent Advances in Management of Chondral and Osteochondral Defects at the Knee. The Wellington Knee Surgery Unit Proceedings.* 1997.

Chapter 12

1. Merskey H, Bogduk N, eds. *Classification of Chronic Pain: Descriptions of Chronic Pain Syndromes and Definition of Pain Terms.* Seattle: IASP Press, 1994.
2. Stanton-Hicks M, Baron R, Gordh T *et al.* Complex regional pain syndromes: guidelines for therapy. *Clin J Pain* 1998; 14: 155–66.
3. Shumacker HB Jr. A personal view of causalgia and other reflex dystrophies. *Arm Surgery* 1985; **201**: 278–89.
4. Rosen PS, Graham W. The shoulder hand syndrome: historical review with observations on seventy three patients. *Can Med Assoc J* 1957; **77**: 86–91.
5. Katz MM, Hungerford DS. Reflex sympathetic dystrophy affecting the knee. *J Bone Jt Surg (Br)* 1987; **69**: 797–803.
6. Ogilvie-Harris DJ, Roscoe M. Reflex sympathetic dystrophy of the knee. *J Bone Jt Surg (Br)* 1987; **69**: 804–6.
7. Poehling GG, Pollock F, Koman LA, Pollock FE. Reflex sympathetic dystrophy of the knee after sensory nerve injury. *Arthroscopy* 1988; **4**: 31–5.
8. Cooper DE, De Lee JC, Ramamurthy S. Reflex sympathetic dystrophy of the knee. Treatment using epidural anaesthesia. *J Bone Jt Surg (Am)* 1989; **71**: 365–9.

9. Fulkerson JP, Hungerford DS, eds. *Disorders of the Patello-Femoral Joint,* 2nd edn. Baltimore: Williams & Wilkins 1990; 247–64.
10. O'Brien SJ, Ngeow J, Gibney MA *et al.* Reflex sympathetic dystrophy of the knee. Causes, diagnosis and treatment. *Am J Sports Med* 1995; **23**: 655–9.
11. Lindenfield TN, Bach BR, Wojtys EM. Reflex sympathetic dystrophy and pain dysfunction in the lower extremity. An Instructional Course Lecture. The American Academy of Orthopaedic Surgeons. *J Bone Jt Surg (Am)* 1996; **78**: 1936–44.
12. Barasi S, Lynn B. Effects of sympathetic stimulation on mechanoreceptor and nociceptor afferent units with small myelinated and unmyelinated axons innervating the rabbit pinna. *J Physiol* 1983; **341**: 51.
13. Scadding JW. Development of ongoing activity, mechanosensitivity and adrenaline sensitivity in severed peripheral nerve axons. *Exper Neurol* 1981; **75**: 345–64.
14. Devor M, Janig W. Activation of myelinated afferents ending in a neuroma by stimulation of the sympathetic supply in the rat. *Neurosci Lett* 1981; **24**: 43–7.
15. Janig W. Causalgia and reflex sympathetic dystrophy: in what way is the sympathetic nervous system involved? *Trends Neurosci* 1985; **8**: 471–7.
16. Sunderland S. *Nerves and Nerve Injuries,* 2nd edn. New York: Churchill Livingstone, 1978: 377–472.
17. Wall PD, Devor M. The effect of peripheral nerve injury on dorsal root potentials and on transmission of afferent impulses into the spinal cord. *Brain Res* 1981; **209**: 95–111.
18. Atkins RM. Post-traumatic reflex sympathetic dystrophy. *Baillière's Clin Orthop* 1996; **1**: 223–40.
19. Arlet J. The history of reflex sympathetic dystrophy. *Baillière's Clin Orthop* 1996; **1**: 209–21.
20. Melzak R, Wall TD. *Textbook of Pain.* Churchill Livingstone, 1984: 683.
21. Arner S, Meyerson BA. Lack of analgesic effect of opioids on neuropathic and idiopathic forms of pain. *Pain* 1988; **33**: 11–23.
22. Portenoy RK, Foley KM, Inturrisi CE. The nature of opioid responsiveness and its implications for neuropathic pain: a new hypothesis derived from studies of opioid infusions. *Pain* 1990; **43**: 273–86.
23. Rowbotham MC, Resiner Keller LA, Fields HL. Both intravenous lidocaine and morphine reduce the pain of postherpetic neuralgia. *Neurology* 1991; **41**: 1024–8.
24. Mellick GA, Mellicy LB, Mellick LB. Gabapentin in the management of reflex sympathetic dystrophy. *J Pain Symptom Management* 1995; **10**: 265–6.
25. Davis KD, Treede RD, Raja SN *et al.* Topical application of clonidine relieves hyperalgesia in patients with sympathetically mediated pain. *Pain* 1991; **47**: 309–17.
26. Raj PP, Denson DD. Prolonged analgesia technique with local anaesthetics in practical management of pain. In: Raj P, ed. *Practical Management of Pain.* Chicago: Year Book Medical Publishers 1986: 687–700.
27. Rauck RI, Eisnach JC, Jackson K *et al.* Epidural clonidine treatment for refractory reflex sympathetic dystrophy. *Anaesthesiology* 1993; **79**: 1163–9.
28. Barolet G, Schwartsman R, Woo R. Epidural spinal cord stimulation in the management of reflex sympathetic dystrophy. *Stereotact Funct Neurolsurg (Switzerland)* 1989; **53**: 29–39.

29. Hannington Kiff JG. Intravenous block with guanethidine. *Lancet* 1974; **1**: 1010–20.

30. Jadad AR, Carroll D, Glynn CJ, McQuay HJ. Intravenous regional sympathetic blockade for pain relief in reflex sympathetic dystrophy. A systematic review and a randomised, double blind crossover study. *J Pain Symptom Management* 1995; **10**: 13–20.

31. Darzi A, Fell RH. Current research.

Chapter 13

1. Hunter W. On the structure and diseases of articular cartilages. *Philos Trans R Soc London Biol* 1743; **42**: 514–21.

2. Buckwalter JA, Mankin HJ. Articular cartilage. *J Bone Jt Surg (Am)* 1997; **79**: 600–32.

3. Armstrong CG, Mow VC. Variations in the intrinsic mechanical properties of human articular cartilage with age, degeneration, and water count. *J Bone Jt Surg (Am)* 1982; **64**: 88–94.

4. Yao JQ, Seedhom BB. Functional adaptation of the thickness of human articular cartilage. *J Bone Jt Surg (Br)* 1998; **80**: 209–10.

5. Soames RW, (Section ed.) Structure of cartilage, In: Williams PL, ed. *Gray's Anatomy*, 38th edn, London: Churchill Livingstone, 1995: 443–52.

6. Ratcliffe A, Mow VC. The structure, function and biologic repair of articular cartilage. In: Friedlander GE, Goldberg VM, eds. *Bone and cartilage allografts*, AAOS Symposium, AAOS, Park Ridge 1989: 123–54.

7. Jeffery AK. Articular cartilage and the orthopaedic surgeon: structure and function. *Curr Orthop* 1994; **8**: 38–44.

8. Hunziker EB, Rosenberg LC. Repair of partial-thickness defects in articular cartilage: cell recruitment from the synovial membrane. *J Bone Jt Surg (Am)* 1997; **78**: 721–33.

9. Wakitani S, Goto T, Pineda SJ *et al.* Mesenchymal cell-based repair of large, full-thickness defects of articular cartilage. *J Bone Jt Surg (Am)* 1994; **76**: 579–92.

10. Namba RS, Meuli M, Sullivan KM *et al.* Spontaneous repair of superficial defects in articular cartilage in a fetal lamb model. *J Bone Jt Surg (Am)* 1998; **80**: 410.

11. DePalma AF, McKeever CD, Subin DK. Process of repair of articular cartilage demonstrated by histology and autoradiography with tritiated thymidine. *Clin Orthop* 1996; **48**: 229–42.

12. Salter RB, Simmonds DF, Malcolm BW *et al.* The biological effect of continuous passive motion on the healing of full-thickness defects in articular cartilage: an experimental investigation in the rabbit. *J Bone Jt Surg (Am)* 1980; **62**: 1232–51.

13. Biswal S, Dovichi E, Vandeveene J *et al.* Prognostic significance of focal MR signal abnormalities of the knee cartilage: assessment in a longitudinal MR imaging study. RSNA 84th Scientific Assembly and Annual Meeting. *Book of Abstracts*, 1998.

14. Fairbank HA. Osteo-chondritis dissecans. *Br J Surg* 1933; **21**: 67–82.

15. Smillie IS. *Osteochondritis Dissecans*. Edinburgh, Churchill Livingstone, 1960.

16. Spindler KP, Schils JP, Bergfeld JA *et al.* Prospective study of osseous, articular, and meniscal lesions in recent anterior cruciate ligament tears by magnetic resonance imaging and arthroscopy. *Am J Sports Med* 1993; **21**: 551–6.

17. Johnson DL, Urban WP Jr, Caborn DNM *et al.* Articular cartilage changes seen with magnetic resonance imaging-detected bone bruise associated with anterior cruciate ligament rupture. *Am J Sports Med* 1998; **26**: 409–14.

18. Speer KP, Spritzer CE, Bassett FH III. Osseous injury associated with acute tears of the anterior cruciate ligament. *Am J Sports Med* 1992; **20**: 382–9.

19. Mankin HJ. Current concepts review: the response of articular cartilage to mechanical injury. *J Bone Jt Surg (Am)* 1982; **64**: 460–6.

20. Mankin HJ, Buckwalter JA. Restoration of the osteoarthritic joint. Editorial. *J Bone Jt Surg (Am)* 1996; **78**: 1–2.

21. Dye SF, Chew MH. The use of scintigraphy to detect increased osseous metabolic activity about the knee. *J Bone Jt Surg (Am)* 1993; **75**: 1388–406.

22. Dye SF, Chew MH. Restoration of osseous homeostasis after anterior cruciate ligament reconstruction. *Am J Sports Med* 1993; **21**: 748–50.

23. Bobic V. *The Outcome of Accelerated Rehabilitation of ACL Reconstructed Knees*. Proceedings of the 2nd World Congress on Sports Trauma and 22nd AOSSM Annual Meeting, Orlando, Florida 1996.

24. Noyes FR, Stabler CL. A system for grading articular cartilage lesions at arthroscopy. *Am J Sports Med* 1989; **17**: 505–13.

25. Fine KM, Glasgow SG, Torg JS. Tibial chondral fissures associated with the lateral meniscus. *Arthroscopy* 1995; **11**: 292–5.

26. Mandelbaum BR, Browne JE, Fu FH *et al.* Articular cartilage lesions of the knee. *Am J Sports Med* 1998; **26**: 853–61.

27. Noyes FR, Mooar PA, Matthews DS, Butler DL. The symptomatic anterior cruciate-deficient knee. Part I: the long term functional disability in athletically active individuals. *J Bone Jt Surg (Am)* 1983; **65**: 154–62.

28. Pattee GA, Fox JM, Del Pizzo W, Friedman MJ. Four- to ten-year follow-up of unreconstructed anterior cruciate ligament tears. *Am J Sports Med* 1989; **17**: 430–5.

29. Ciccotti MG, Lombardo SJ, Nonweiler B, Pink M. Non-operative treatment of ruptures of the anterior cruciate ligament in middle-aged patients. Results after long term follow-up. *J Bone Jt Surg (Am)* 1994; **76**: 1315–21.

30. Shelbourne KD, Wilckens JH. Intraarticular anterior cruciate ligament reconstruction in the symptomatic arthritic knee. *Am J Sports Med* 1993; **21**: 685–9.

31. Jacobsen K. Osteoarthrosis following insufficiency of the cruciate ligaments in man. *Acta Orthop Scand* 1977; **48**: 520–6.

32. Outerbridge RE. The aetiology of chondromalacea patellae. *J Bone Jt Surg (Br)* 1961; **43**: 752–767.

33. Giurea M, Aichroth PM, Duri Z. Classification of articular cartilage lesion at the knee at arthroscopy. *The Knee* 1998; **5**: 159–64.

34. International Cartilage Repair Society. Introduction to an articular cartilage classification: the knee cartilage standard evaluation form. *ICRS Newsletter*, 1998; **1**: 5–8.

35. Wojtys E, Wilson M, Buckwalter K *et al.* Magnetic resonance imaging of knee hyaline cartilage and intraarticular pathology. *Am J Sports Med* 1987; **15**: 455–63.

36. Ochi M, Sumen Y, Kanda T *et al.* The diagnostic value and limitation of magnetic resonance imaging on chondral lesions in the knee joint. *Arthroscopy* 1994; **10**: 176–83.

37. Kneeland JB. MR imaging of articular cartilage and of cartilage degeneration. In: Stoller DW, ed. *Magnetic Resonance Imaging in Orthopaedics and Sports Medicine*, 2nd edn, CD-ROM. Philadelphia: Lippincott-Raven, 1997.

38. Levy AS, Lohnes J, Sculley S et al. Chondral delamination of the knee in soccer players. *Am J Sports Med* 1996: **24**: 634–9.

39. Linklater JM, Potter HG. Imaging of chondral defects. In: Miller M, ed. *Operative Techniques in Orthopaedics. Treatment of Chondral Injuries*. Philadelphia: Saunders, 1997; 279–88.

40. Potter HG, Linklater JM, Allen AA et al. Magnetic resonance imaging of articular cartilage in the knee. *J Bone Jt Surg (Am)* 1998; **80**: 1276–84.

41. Bobic V. Magnetic resonance imaging of chondral defects. *International Cartilage Repair Society (ICRS) Newsletter*, 1998; **2**: 16–18.

42. Cohen ZA, McCarthy DM, Athesian GA et al. In vivo and in vitro knee joint cartilage topography, thickness, and contact areas from MRI. 43rd Annual Meeting, Orthopaedic Research Society, San Francisco. *Book of Abstracts*, 1997; 625.

43. Lang P, Bergman G. Articular cartilage MR imaging. Personal communication (unpublished clinical data), Stanford University Medical Center, Radiology Department, Stanford, California, 1998.

44. Bashir A, Gray ML, Burstein D. Gd-DTPA^{2-} as a measure of cartilage degradation. *Magn Reson Med* 1996; **36**: 665–73.

Chapter 14

1. Buckwalter JA, Mankin HJ. Articular cartilage. *J Bone Jt Surg (Am)* 1997; **79**: 600–32.

2. Müller W. Osteochondrosis dissecans. In: Hastings DE, ed. *Progress in Orthopaedic Surgery*. New York: Springer, 1978; **3**: 135.

3. Bradley J, Dandy DJ. Osteochondritis dissecans and other lesions of the femoral condyles. *J Bone Jt Surg (Br)* 1989; **71**: 518–22.

4. Dandy DJ, Jackson RW. The impact of arthroscopy on the management of disorders of the knee. *J Bone Jt Surg (Br)* 1975; **57**: 346–8.

5. Mariani PP, Adriani E, Maresca G. Osteochondritis dissecans of the knee: aetiological factors and treatment. An overview. *J Sports Traumatol Rel Res* 1993; **15**: 105–25.

6. Schenck RC, Goodnight JM. Osteochondritis dissecans. Current concepts review. *J Bone Jt Surg (Am)* 1996; **78**: 439–56.

7. Wirth CJ, Rudert M. Techniques of cartilage growth enhancement: a review of the literature. *Arthroscopy* 1996; **12**: 300–8.

8. Beadling L. Hyaluronic acid may prevent cartilage damage. *Orthopaedics Today International* 1998; **1**: 9.

9. Hungerford DS. Treating osteoarthritis with chondro-protective agents. *Orthopedic Spec Ed* 1998; **4**: 1.

10. Steadman JR, Rodkey WG, Singleton SB, Briggs KK. Microfracture technique for full-thickness chondral defects: technique and clinical results. In: Fu FH, ed. *Operative Techniques in Orthopaedics. Treatment of Chondral Injuries*, Guest Ed. Miller MD. 1997; **7**: 300–4.

11. Johnson LL. Arthroscopic abrasion arthroplasty. In: McGinty JB, ed. *Operative Arthroscopy*. New York: Raven Press, 1991: 341–60.

12. Bert JM. Abrasion arthroplasty. In: Fu FH, ed. (Miller MD, guest ed.) *Operative Techniques in Orthopaedics. Treatment of Chondral Injuries*. 1997; **7**: 294–9.

13. Akizuki S, Yasukawa Y, Takizawa T. Does arthroscopic abrasion arthroplasty promote cartilage regeneration in osteoarthrotic knees with eburnation? A prospective study of high tibial osteotomy with abrasion arthroplasty versus high tibial osteotomy alone. *Arthroscopy* 1997; **13**: 9–17.

14. Homminga GN, Bulstra SK, Bouwmeester PSM, Van den Linden AJ. Perichondral grafting for cartilage lesions of the knee. *J Bone Jt Surg (Br)* 1990; **72**: 1003–7.

15. O'Driscoll SW. The healing and regeneration of articular cartilage. *J Bone Jt Surg (Am)* 1998; **80**: 1795–812.

16. Angermann P, Riegels-Nielsen P. Osteochondritis dissecans of the femoral condyle treated with periosteal trans-plantation: a preliminary clinical study of 14 cases. *Orthopaedics International Edition* 1994; **2**: 425–8.

17. Beadling L. Periosteal transplantation not ready for clinical application for cartilage repair. *Orthopaedics Today* 1997; **17**: 18.

18. Aichroth PM, Ellis H. Transplantation of joint surfaces by cartilage grafts. *Br J Surg* 1970; **57**: 855

19. Bentley G, Greer RB III. Homotransplantation of isolated epiphyseal and articular cartilage chondrocytes into joint surfaces of rabbits. *Nature* 1971; **230**: 385–8.

20. Lane JM, Brighton CT, Ottens HR, Lipton M. Joint resurfacing in the rabbit using an autologous osteochondral graft. A biochemical and metabolic study of cartilage viability. *J Bone Jt Surg (Am)* 1977; **59**: 218–22.

21. Itay S, Abramovici A, Yosipovitch Z et al. Correction of defects in articular cartilage by implants of cultured embryogenic chondrocytes. *Trans Orthop Res Soc* 1988; **13**: 112.

22. Grande DA, Pitman MI, Peterson L et al. The repair of experimentally produced defects in rabbit articular cartilage by autologous chondrocyte transplantation. *J Orthop Res* 1989; **7**: 208–18.

23. Brittberg M, Lindahl A, Nilsson A et al. Treatment of deep cartilage defects in the knee with autologous chondrocyte transplantation. *N Engl J Med* 1994; **331**: 889–95.

24. Mankin HJ. Chondrocyte transplantation – one answer to an old question. *N Engl J Med* 1994; **331**: 940–1.

25. Rangaswamy L. Conversations with a cab driver. Editorial. *J Bone Jt Surg (Am)* 1998; **80**: 1407–9.

26. Hunziker EB, Rosenberg L. Induction of repair in partial thickness articular cartilage lesions by timed release of TGF-β. *Trans Orthop Res Soc* 1994; **19**: 236.

27. Muckle DS, Minns RJ. Biological response to woven carbon fibre pads in the knee. A clinical and experimental study. *J Bone Jt Surg (Br)* 1990; **72**: 60–2.

28. Brittberg M, Faxén E, Peterson L. Carbon fiber scaffolds in the treatment of early knee osteoarthritis. A prospective 4-year followup of 37 patients. *Clin Orthop* 1994; **307**: 155–64.

29. Uribe JW, Markarian G, Kaplan L, Tjin-A-Tsoi E. Use of coblation in articular cartilage surgery. *Res Outcomes Arthrosc Surg* 1998; **3**: 1.

30. Garrett JC. Treatment of osteochondral defects of the distal femur with fresh osteochondral allografts: a preliminary report. *Arthroscopy* 1986; **2**: 222–6.

31. Sammarco, VJ, Gorab R, Miller R et al. Human articular cartilage storage in cell culture medium; guidelines for storage of fresh osteochondral allografts (editorial discussion). *Orthopaedics* 1997; **20**: 500.

32. Stone KR, Walgenbach A. Surgical technique for articular cartilage transplantation to full-thickness cartilage defects in the knee joint. In: Fu FH, ed. *Operative Techniques in Orthopaedics. Treatment of Chondral Injuries*, Guest Ed. Miller MD. 1997; **7**: 305–11.

33. Wilson WJ, Jacobs JE. Patellar graft for severely depressed comminuted fractures of the lateral tibial condyle. *J Bone Jt Surg (Am)* 1952; **34**: 436–42.

34. Müller W. Osteochondrosis dissecans. In: Hastings DE, ed. *Progress in Orthopaedic Surgery*. New York: Springer, 1978; **3**: 135.

35. Yamashita F, Sakakida K, Suzu F, Takai S. The transplantation of an autogenic osteochondral fragment for osteochondritis dissecans of the knee. *Clin Orthop* 1985; **201**: 43–50.

36. Dew TL, Martin RA. Functional, radiographic and histological assessment of healing of autogenous osteochondral grafts and full-thickness cartilage defects in the talus of dogs. *Am J Vet Res* 1992; **53**: 2141–52.

37. Roffman M. Autogenous grafting for an osteochondral fracture of the femoral condyle: a case report. *Acta Orthop Scand* 1995; **66**: 571–2.

38. Fabbriciani C, Schiavone Panni A, Delcogliano A, Sagarriga Visconti C. Osteochondral autograft in the treatment of osteochondritis dissecans of the knee. The 17th AOSSM Annual Meeting, Orlando, Florida, *Book of Abstracts* 1991; 67–8.

39. Matsusue Y, Yamamuro T, Hama H. Case report: arthroscopic multiple osteochondral transplantation to the chondral defect in the knee associated with anterior cruciate ligament disruption. *Arthroscopy* 1993; **9**: 318–21.

40. Outerbridge HK, Outerbridge AR, Outerbridge RE. The use of a lateral patellar autologous graft for the repair of a large osteochondral defect in the knee. *J Bone Jt Surg (Am)* 1995; **77**: 65–72.

41. Hangody L, Szigeti I, Kárpáti Z *et al.* Autogenous osteochondral graft technique for replacing knee cartilage defects in dogs. *Orthopaed Int* 1997; **3**: 175–81.

42. Hangody L, Kish G, Kárpáti Z *et al.* Arthroscopic autogenous osteochondral mosaicplasty for the treatment of femoral condylar articular defects. *Knee Surg Sports Traumatol Arthrosc* 1997; **5**: 262–7.

43. Beadling L, Trace R. World of opportunity for osteochondral transplantation. *Orthopaedics Today* 1996; **16**: 17–19.

44. Bobic V. Arthroscopic osteochondral autograft transplantation in anterior cruciate ligament reconstruction: a preliminary clinical study. *Knee Surg Sports Traumatol Arthrosc* 1996; **3**: 262–4.

45. Levy AS, Lohnes J, Sculley S *et al.* Chondral delamination of the knee in soccer players. *Am J Sports Med* 1996; **24**: 634–9.

46. Simonian PT, Sussmann PS, Wickiewicz TL *et al.* Contact pressures at osteochondral donor sites in the knee. *Am J Sports Med* 1998; **26**: 491–4.

47. Cohen ZA, McCarthy DM, Athesian GA *et al.* In vivo and in vitro knee joint cartilage topography, thickness, and contact areas from MRI. 43 Annual Meeting, Orthopaedic Research Society, San Francisco. *Book of Abstracts*, 1997: 625.

48. Linklater JM, Potter HG. Imaging of chondral defects. In: Fu F, ed. *Treatment of Chondral Injuries. Operative Techniques in Orthopaedics.* Guest ed. Miller MD. 1997; **7**: 279–88.

49. Potter HG, Linklater JM, Allen AA *et al.* Magnetic resonance imaging of articular cartilage in the knee. *J Bone Jt Surg (Am)* 1998; **80**: 1276–84.

50. Bobic V. Magnetic resonance imaging of chondral defects. *International Cartilage Repair Society (ICRS) Newsletter*, Summer 1998; **2**: 16–18.

51. Lang P, Bergman G. Articular cartilage MR imaging. Personal communication, unpublished clinical data. Stanford University Medical Center, Radiology Department, Stanford, California 1998.

52. Ritchie D. Articular cartilage MR imaging. Personal communication, unpublished clinical data. Radiology Department, The Royal Liverpool University Hospitals, Liverpool, UK, 1998.

53. Whitehouse GH, Roberts N. Articular cartilage MR imaging. Personal communication, unpublished clinical data. The University of Liverpool, Magnetic Resonance and Image Analysis Research Centre (MARIARC), Liverpool 1998.

54. Mandelbaum BR, Browne JE, Fu FH *et al.* Articular cartilage lesions of the knee. *Am J Sports Med* 1998; **26**: 853–61.

Index